HEALING
MASSAGE

HEALING MASSAGE

An A–Z Guide for More than Forty Medical Conditions

For Professional and Home Use

Maureen Abson

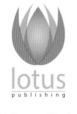

lotus
publishing

Chichester, England

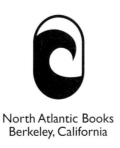

North Atlantic Books
Berkeley, California

First published in 2016 by
Lotus Publishing
Apple Tree Cottage, Inlands Road, Nutbourne, Chichester, PO18 8RJ, and
North Atlantic Books
Berkeley, California

All Drawings Amanda Williams
Photographs Simon Caughey-Rogers
Text Design Mary-Anne Trant
Cover Design Jasmine Hromjak
Printed and Bound in the UK by Bell & Bain Limited

Healing Massage: An A–Z Guide for More than Forty Medical Conditions: For Professional and Home Use is sponsored and published by the Society for the Study of Native Arts and Sciences (dba North Atlantic Books), an educational nonprofit based in Berkeley, California, that collaborates with partners to develop cross-cultural perspectives, nurture holistic views of art, science, the humanities, and healing, and seed personal and global transformation by publishing work on the relationship of body, spirit, and nature.

North Atlantic Books' publications are available through most bookstores. For further information, visit our website at www.northatlanticbooks.com or call 800-733-3000.

British Library Cataloguing-in-Publication Data
A CIP record for this book is available from the British Library
ISBN 978 1 905367 63 4 (Lotus Publishing)
ISBN 978 1 62317 059 2 (North Atlantic Books)

Library of Congress Cataloguing-in-Publication Data
Abson, Maureen, author.
 Healing massage: an A-Z guide for more than forty medical conditions for professional and home use / Maureen Abson.
 p. ; cm.
 Includes bibliographical references and index.
 ISBN 978-1-62317-059-2 (pbk.) — ISBN 978-1-62317-060-8 (ebook)
 I. Title.
 [DNLM: 1. Massage—methods. WB 537]
 RM721
 615.8'22—dc23
2015036296

Contents

Acknowledgements 6

PART I
Massage Techniques 7
Chapter 1 Introduction.....................8
Chapter 2 Hand Massage 14
Chapter 3 Foot Massage 21
Chapter 4 Head Massage.................... 27
Chapter 5 Back Massage 31

PART II
An A–Z of Medical Conditions..41
Ankylosing Spondylitis 42
Anxiety Disorders 49
Asthma.. 56
Cancer 62
Cerebral Palsy 75
Cervical and Thoracic Spondylosis............. 80
Chronic Fatigue Syndrome
   / Myalgic Encephalopathy 86
Constipation 89
Cramp... 92
Down Syndrome 97
Dupuytren's Contracture 101
Eating Disorders.. 104
Emotional Issues and Post-Traumatic
   Stress Disorder 108
Fibromyalgia 116
Foot Drop... 120
Frozen Shoulder 124

Gynecological Issues.. 130
Irritable Bowel Syndrome............................ 135
Lumbar Spondylosis 137
Menopause.. 144
Multiple Sclerosis.. 149
Muscular Dystrophy 154
Parkinson's Disease 159
Peripheral Neuropathy.................................. 163
Plantar Fasciitis 166
Pregnancy... 171
Raynaud's Syndrome....................................... 177
Repetitive Strain Injuries............................. 180
Restless Legs Syndrome................................. 184
Rotator Cuff Injury... 191
Scar Tissue 195
Sciatica.. 198
Scoliosis... 203
Shin Splint Syndrome..................................... 210
Sinusitis 218
Temporomandibular Joint Disorders 222
Tendonitis and Tenosynovitis.................... 227
Tennis Elbow.. 231
Tension Headaches... 234
Trigeminal Neuralgia................................... 238
Whiplash.. 242
Winged Scapula 249
Wrist-Drop 253

Index.. 257

Acknowledgements

There are many people who have made this book possible and to whom I owe a debt of gratitude.

All models in the book are clients who have not only entrusted me with their wellbeing but who also gave up their time to come and take part in the photo shoot. Thank you to photographer Simon Caughey-Rogers and models (in the order that we took the photographs) Dr Michelle Caughey-Rogers, Beverley and Daniel Fong, Sadaf Aleem and Kasam Ganchi, Margaret Walton, Kaarina McCooey, Chris James, Gareth Proud, Sarah Abson, Peter Abson, and Amos Popplewell.

I am indebted to Jon Hutchings from Lotus Publishing who had the faith to commission the book. I came to massage after working in mainstream education for many years and am grateful to those who influenced this new journey. My studies in massage have taken in many modalities but my starting point was to study with, and then work alongside, Brandon Raynor, and I am grateful for this inspiration. My anatomy and physiology were brought to life via death in my explorations with Gil Hedley in his Integral Anatomy dissection class.

My thanks also go to Michael McElroy, acupuncturist and friend, for his technical proofing of the TCM input into this book and to Jeff Shurr for his technical checking of certain chapters and the wisdom he imparted while I worked with him at Chiropractic Associates. I am indebted to Terry Wills and Janet Walmsley who spent many hours correcting my spelling and punctuation in their proofreading.

Finally, but most importantly, my thanks go to my family. To Peter, my husband, without whose unfailing love, support, and encouragement this book would still be in my head. To my daughters Sarah and Caroline and son-in-law-to-be Gareth Proud who delivered numerous cups of tea and coffee to my side while I wrote. To Mollie our dog who made sure I took breaks to go "walkies." This book is only made possible by their support.

Dedication

This book is dedicated to my parents, Joan and Gil Sloan, who instilled in me the belief that I could "do it," no matter what "it" was. For that, and their love, I will always be grateful.

PART I
MASSAGE TECHNIQUES

1 Introduction

This book has been written from years of experience in working with and teaching massage and seeks to provide practical information on using massage to treat a range of medical conditions. Massage has been used for thousands of years to treat a whole array of conditions and was traditionally passed down through families as part of everyday life. With the increase in modern medicine two things have happened: firstly the power of massage has been largely forgotten, and secondly, with the increase of a litigious culture, it has been politicized and people have become scared to touch for fear of litigation.

This book seeks to both educate and empower two groups of people: the qualified massage practitioner wanting a ready reference book for unfamiliar conditions, and everyday people wanting to help a friend or family member who is dealing with a health problem.

As a qualified massage practitioner there are very few courses that will cover every medical condition that you will come across in your massage career, or you may have been taught to simply not massage a specific condition when in reality massage would be effective. Cancer is a good example of this; many colleges still teach that massage when someone has cancer is contraindicated, even though the medical research has moved on in this area. This book aims to fill in some of those gaps and to not only provide an easily accessible reference point for the condition but also discuss how to treat someone effectively and safely.

The book is also aimed at empowering individuals to give effective massage treatments to friends or family members. While in many cases individuals will feel happier going to see a qualified practitioner, there may be times when for reasons of finance, life circumstances, or simply client choice this is not possible, and it is perfectly fine to use massage in the home. So long as you are not charging for your services, which takes you into the professional arena, then it is possible to give safe and effective treatments.

There are some conditions that would benefit from daily massage to make a real difference. The tremors of Parkinson's disease will respond well to massage, but ideally this needs to be given daily and not many people can afford a daily professional massage. Twice daily massage to a child with cerebral palsy can have a real impact on the tone and spasticity of muscles but, again, not many people can afford this—but it can be integrated into the daily care routine given by a parent or carer. The book is therefore also aimed at empowering friends and family members to be able to treat conditions at home.

There are some caveats that need stating at this early stage.

- This book will not promise cures for medical conditions. Massage for serious medical conditions should be carried out in conjunction with conventional medicine and in collaboration with the client's doctor. Even if the massage makes a huge difference to the person's life and they want to start reducing medication, that must be under the supervision of the client's medical practitioner.

- The premise for all of this advice is to "first, do no harm." Some of the treatments in this book use deep massage techniques but that should never be at a level deeper than the client wants to work and is able to breathe through. Always err on the side of caution and if in doubt—don't.

- This book is not a replacement for professional massage training. While you can follow the instructions in the book to treat friends and family members, reading the book does not qualify you as a massage practitioner. There are ample courses, both short and long, that you can do to gain hands-on supervised experience. Using some of these techniques on friends and family may leave you wanting to do more, which is great, but go on to train with a school or college and get professional insurance to work professionally. The length of course needed will depend on the massage regulations where you live and these vary significantly around the world.

There are certain terms used in the book that need explaining at the start. A *contraindication* to massage refers to a reason why you should not massage; these are given for each condition in the book where they are applicable, but make sure you also read the whole of this introductory chapter where I discuss general contraindications for massage.

I refer in the book to the *client*. This is simply the person receiving the massage, be that a paying customer if you work professionally or the friend or family member receiving the massage.

A Little Bit of History

It can be useful to know a little of where massage has come from to understand what it is that we do. Massage has a long history across cultures, and in both traditional Eastern and more Western medicine. Although we loosely divide massage into Eastern and Western, especially in terms of history, there will doubtless have been crossover between them as travel across countries and continents developed.

Eastern Approaches

Eastern massage styles have been a part of everyday life for thousands of years, passing down the generations, people sometimes learning from each other at the parent's knee, and these were seen as an important and integral part of health care.

In China we have the first documented descriptions of massage, dating back around 5000 years to 3000 years BCE (before the Common Era). Chinese Taoist priests practiced "qigong," a meditative movement revealing and cultivating the vital life force. Traditional Chinese Medicine (TCM) is based on the principle that every illness, ailment, or discomfort in the body is due to an imbalance of "qi," or "ch'i."

Records in India also date back to at least 5000 years ago, and the unique form of medicine known as Ayurveda (the "art of living"), which, amongst other things, describes massage and herbal treatment for various conditions.

3000 years ago, around 1000 BCE, Japanese monks began to study Buddhism in China. They witnessed the healing methods of TCM and took them back to Japan. The Japanese not only adopted the Chinese style, but also began to add to it by introducing new combinations, eventually reaching a unique form called Shiatsu—"shi" meaning finger and "atsu" meaning pressure.

Traditional Thai massage, also called Thai yoga therapy, is a therapeutic style of massage therapy that dates back thousands of years. Its origins are unknown, but practitioners traditionally trace their lineage to Jivaka Komalaboat, also known as Shivago, who was a personal physician to the Sangha, a friend and physician to the Buddha and renowned as a healer in Buddhist tradition. Thai massage, like most oriental forms of massage, combines massage, stretching, and what we now refer to as chiropractic manipulations into one treatment. This is just a small sample of the longer-standing Eastern massage techniques, but massage has also had a long history in the West.

Western Traditions

Hippocrates (ca. 460 BCE–ca. 375 BCE), the "father of modern medicine" argued that massage was "one of the arts" with which a well-rounded physician should be familiar, believing that a real proficiency in massage only came with lots of practice. He suggested that massage could both firm up muscles or organs that were too lax, and relax muscles, joints, or other organs that were too stiff, rigid, or tense.

Hippocrates also reversed the traditional Eastern direction of massage. In cultures where the focus was on energy and, for some, negative entities, massage was conducted from the center of the body outward to the extremities, as this would draw stale, excess, or negative energy out from the body. Hippocrates established the principle instead that massage should work toward the heart in order to assist the heart and circulatory system in their work, and to transport and finally eliminate pathogenic wastes and toxins from the body.

This is a divide which still exists in massage today with, generally speaking, Western-based massage working toward the heart and Eastern-based massage working from the center outward.

Massage is still developing; for example, we are only just beginning to understand fascia and how this affects the body, but we are able to draw upon these various systems of massage and take what works and what makes sense to us and integrate them. Some people will argue for light-touch massage, others will argue only for deep massage. If we can learn anything from the history of massage then it is that all forms have their uses; one client might respond to one form of treatment and another to an entirely different approach. That doesn't mean that one is right and one is wrong; the diversity offered in massage is its strength. Provided you do not massage when it is contraindicated, work only to the depth that the client is happy to work to, and also go by the maxim "first, do no harm," then there is nothing to be lost from this focused application of touch that we call massage, but there may be a great deal to gain.

Using Massage Oil

For some parts of the massage treatments using a massage oil will help. There are lots of commercially produced massage oils, but you can use a good quality, simple oil such as grape-seed. Almond oil, holly oil, and a whole variety of other oils can be used—be careful with nut-based oils in case anyone has a nut allergy. There are also good quality preblended massage oils, which are base oils (such as grape-seed) mixed with essential oils. Essential oils are powerful oils derived mainly from flowers or plants and have "qualities"—some are calming, others are uplifting or are good for muscular aches and pains. A few chapters recommend specific oils, but if you are not experienced in blending oils then it is simpler, and possibly cheaper, to buy a preblended oil.

You should not need a great deal of oil but make sure that when you come to use it, you pour it onto your hands and then rub your hands together to warm the oil. As well as taking out the shock of having cold oil applied, it also spreads the oil more quickly, and not having a pool of oil on their skin will be much more pleasant for your clients! You only need enough oil so that your hands don't drag the client's skin, so apply it a little at a time; remember some massage doesn't need oil so don't apply it all of the time, just as needed and directed.

Contraindications

There are some times when it is not appropriate to massage; these are known as contraindications, and the details for these for each condition are given chapter by chapter. There are also times when it is generally not appropriate to massage someone in the usual way or when specific areas should be avoided, and these are listed below, along with the reasons.

- If someone is feeling sick or has a cold, flu, or fever, massage is contraindicated. The client would likely feel worse and their fever could intensify. If they are feeling sick, they are likely to be sick. As you are working in close proximity with that person and what they have may be contagious, you are also leaving yourself open to catching or becoming a carrier for that illness.

- Massage should never be carried out over, or close to, an area with varicose veins—this could cause the vein to burst, which would be a medical emergency.

- If a bone is broken, if a joint is swollen, or if an area of tissue is red and inflamed, massage should be avoided.

- Massage is contraindicated when the client has had recent alcohol intake—it is likely to heighten the effect of the alcohol in their system and make them nauseous.

- If a client has a burn, open sore or wound, or open eczema, massage should be avoided on that area. Not only would it be painful, but you are risking introducing infection into the area and inhibiting healing.

- If the client has had recent surgery it is best practice to wait a minimum of three months post surgery before massaging close to or on the area that has been operated on. This is to allow the time for the scar tissue to form and

for deeper-level healing to take place. In the case of abdominal surgery, wait six months before carrying out any abdominal massage. The client should have the "all clear" in their routine postoperative checkup and be signed off from their surgeon prior to commencing massage treatment.

Conditions not contraindicated but with special precautions not covered elsewhere in this book:

- Diabetes: Massage is not contraindicated for someone with diabetes but there are additional precautions that you need to take into account. Clients who are type 1 diabetic (reliant on insulin injections) will be used to regularly testing their blood sugar and should be asked to bring their blood-testing kit with them. Ask them to test before the treatment starts and have sugary snacks or drinks available if needed. You then need to ask them to test every 45 minutes during the treatment. Do not worry about disrupting the flow of the massage; it is more important to avoid what could be a potentially dangerous dip in blood sugar.

- Asthma: Ensure that clients have their inhaler with them and that you know where it is prior to commencing treatment so that it can be easily accessed if needed.

- Epilepsy: If clients have epilepsy, they are likely to know how well controlled it is. If they indicate that they think an attack is coming on, get them off the massage table onto the floor and clear the area so that they cannot hurt themselves during a fit. Most people with epilepsy will not need hospital treatment, but check how your clients would like you to respond if they do have a fit; do not try to restrain the client at all during a fit.

For other contraindications specific to individual conditions, please see the advice given in each chapter.

Breathing

Working with the client's breath is important to get the most out of massage treatments. Encourage your client to take deep, slow breaths and wait for their out breath before using deeper massage moves or working on more tender areas. Using the breath like this will help you pace your massage better so that you are not rushing in or rushing through a treatment. If clients are struggling to breathe in a deep and relaxed way ask them to place one hand on their belly and one on their chest and to breathe so that the hand on the belly comes up more than the hand on the chest. This may feel odd to begin with but it is a natural way to breathe—watch a baby or young child breathing and you will see this happen very naturally. Deep breathing will also slow breathing down; if your client is anxious or stressed this focus on breathing will start the relaxation process.

Massage Tables

Massage tables (also known as massage beds, or plinths) are soft, padded tables with a face hole or cradle at one end—this allows your clients to lie down in comfort and be able to breathe without needing to keep their head turned to one side. It is possible to do many aspects of massage without a massage table as the client can be either seated or lying toward the edge of a normal bed (even the dining-room table will do if you're pushed), but there are some moves that should not be done without a table as they are dangerous when the client's head is turned to one side—these are all identified in the descriptions of the individual treatments.

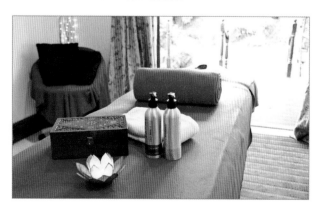

To get the correct height of your massage table, stand either barefoot or in the footwear you will massage in, and the table should be somewhere between the main part of your hand and your first knuckles. If your client is larger than average you may need to put the table down one level so that you can comfortably stretch over their back.

Buying a Massage Table

If you are going to be doing regular "at-home" massages on friends and family it is worth considering investing in a massage table, and you can often get a good second-hand table fairly cheaply. There are some things to keep in mind if you are going to do this. Firstly make sure it does have a face hole or an add-on face cradle; you can adapt all of the techniques here to a face hole or a face cradle, but tables with face holes can be more comfortable for your clients, especially if they have neck problems, and can feel more secure for you as the practitioner.

Secondly make sure that the table is height adjustable; there are a few different mechanisms for these, some are quicker to release than others and these are a matter mainly of personal preference. If you are working on a particular friend or family member then you will not need to change the height too often, but you do need to ensure that you can adjust it to the correct working height for you.

Finally check the weight-bearing ability of your table; if you will be working on heavier clients then tables with aluminum frames and legs will generally be stronger than wooden ones.

As with many things, you get what you pay for in a massage table and you may be better getting a good quality, strong second-hand table than a cheaper new one. All massage tables should be easy to wipe down with antibacterial wipes so buying a second-hand one should not be any compromise on health—just check it's not damaged and that all nuts, bolts, and screws are tight.

Water

After a massage treatment it is important to encourage your client to drink lots of water. This supports the body in its natural process of eliminating toxins; if someone gets a headache after massage they should be encouraged to drink water. Massage will help flush out both natural and chemical toxins from the body, but this process must be accompanied by hydration to allow the body to do its job. If clients' urine is very dark after a treatment they again should be encouraged to drink plenty of water to assist the process of healing.

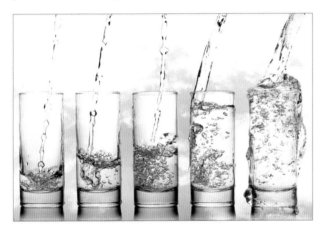

Rest

In busy lives it is tempting to squeeze a massage in when there is a small gap in a schedule; however, your clients will get the most out of a massage if they are able to rest after the treatment. Specifically, if clients are going to drive after a treatment and are in a deep state of relaxation they need to be given time to sit and sip water and gently "come round," rather than dashing out slightly dazed post treatment.

Hygiene

Good hygiene should be maintained at all times while you are giving a massage treatment. Careful hand washing should be done before a treatment starts—include the forearms and elbows in this as you may use these to massage, and if you sneeze, cough, or need to blow your nose then stop and rewash your hands before continuing.

You are not likely to catch any serious illness giving a treatment, but be sensible, and blood contact should be avoided at all times; if your client has a cut or open sore then you should not be massaging on or near that area. If you have a cut on your hand then this should be covered fully, either with a secure waterproof medical dressing or even with a thin glove.

Ensure that the area you are working in is clear and clean and that you have fresh towels for your massage table; if you are working on more than one friend or family member, these should be clean for each person. If you are working professionally then, naturally, full professional-clinic levels of hygiene apply.

If you are working at home, make sure that the television is switched off and the answerphone is switched on, so that both you and your client can fully focus on the treatment in hand.

Finally, enjoy giving your treatments. If you are relaxed giving a treatment, your client will be relaxed. To make a difference to someone's life by specific and focused touch is an incredible gift to be able to give, enjoy!

2 Hand Massage

Detailed Hand Massage

The hands are often the key to releasing lots of arm, shoulder, upper-back, and neck tension. Working these in detail can be of great benefit in a treatment and is something that can be done without needing a massage table or a separate treatment room. These techniques can be used for a wide range of conditions; start with this hand treatment and then return to the relevant chapter for the rest of the treatment details.

Begin by warming up the muscles in each hand; you can do this by holding the hand in yours and rubbing your thumb up across the whole palm of the hand. Always work upward from the ends of the fingers up toward the arm. Understanding something of the muscles in the hands will help.

You will see in the diagram below that the muscles in the hand become much more developed as they enter the palm. There has been a tendency in massage therapy to overlook the hands as a whole, but especially the fingers due to their lack of muscle.

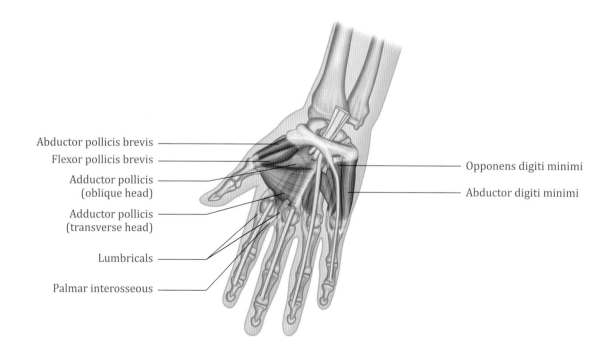

Abductor pollicis brevis

Flexor pollicis brevis

Adductor pollicis (oblique head)

Adductor pollicis (transverse head)

Lumbricals

Palmar interosseous

Opponens digiti minimi

Abductor digiti minimi

The connective tissue in the fingers is really important as it provides a link into the muscles of the hands and arms. If we are to understand the body truly holistically, then we cannot just give a cursory stroke to the hands and believe they have been massaged effectively.

The fingers are an important part of releasing tension in the rest of the hand, and from there into the arms and then into the whole upper body. We need to start hand massage at the ends of the fingers so that we are starting to release tension held in the whole structure of the body. Otherwise, we are missing this critical starting point of where tension is held.

Shoulder pain, neck pain, upper-back pain—all of this needs to be addressed by starting at the tips of the fingers. If we have a pain in the shoulders and only massage the shoulders we can provide temporary relief—much the same as if we have a dandelion pop up in the lawn we can make the lawn look pretty for a short while by lopping the head off the dandelion—but we will only ever really get rid of the weed by getting it out by its roots. In the same way, we need to dig out the root of the tension and pain by tracing it back to its origin and treating that first.

It is important therefore to start your hand massage by working the fingers in detail.

Which finger you start on does not matter greatly as you will need to work them all; initially warm the finger up by rolling it between your own thumb and forefinger, taking each "section" of each finger in turn. You may feel a crunching as you do this rolling movement: this is tiny acid crystals that build up in the capillaries.

The body will store lactic and uric acid in this form. Uric acid, left untreated, tends to build in joints where it can develop into gout. These tiny crystals feel like grains of sand under the skin; as you knead the fingers the graininess should start to diminish as the body flushes this excess into the bloodstream and out of the body. This is one of the key reasons that massage therapists recommend drinking plenty of water after a treatment so that the body is assisted in this cleansing process.

Work each finger in turn and, working upward from the tip of the little finger, you should find that the fingers become softer and more flexible—don't worry if they change color and turn red; this is because you are increasing the blood flow through the fingers, which is a good thing! As always, do not work too deeply, this should always be within your client's tolerance levels. Avoid the joints always skipping over the knuckles as you work.

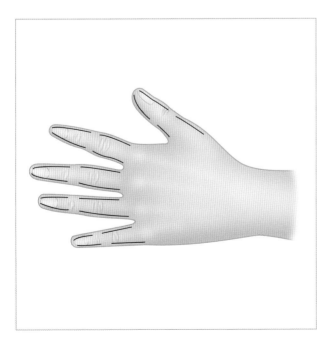
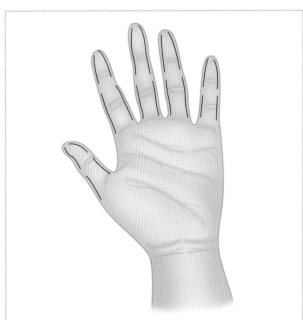

Once you have finished this soft tissue work on the fingers, go back and gently move the joints through their normal range of movement; never force them, just give them a gentle workout.

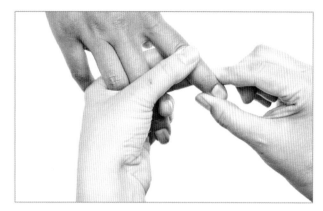

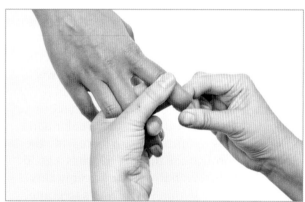

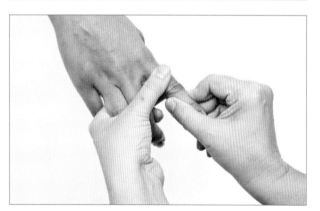

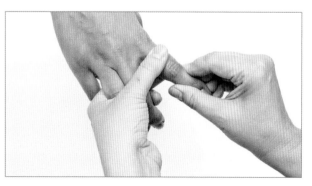

If the client has any form of arthritis be even more careful and gentle and miss out this joint movement.

Next you need to move into the palm of the hand and to the back of the hand. You can either do the fingers on both hands first or complete the massage on one hand first and then start again on the other; it does not matter which way you do it, so work on whatever is more comfortable for you and the person receiving the massage.

As you look at the diagram of the hand (page 14) you will see that the muscles go in a number of directions, and there are also muscles at different depths. Some you will be able to work on just under the skin level, while others you will need to work on much more deeply and move the hand around while you work.

There is no one set place for you to start but it is often useful to warm the muscles of the palm first; do this by supporting the back of the hand with your own hand and use your own thumb to stroke outward and upward across the whole of the palm.

Still supporting the hand in this way, place your thumb at the base of the first and second fingers just where the palm starts—you will feel a groove between the bottom finger knuckles in the palm just below the fingers.

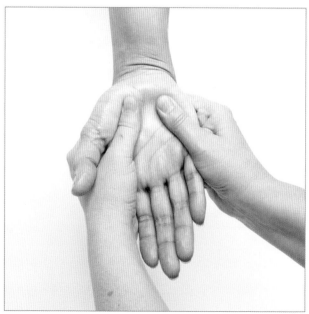

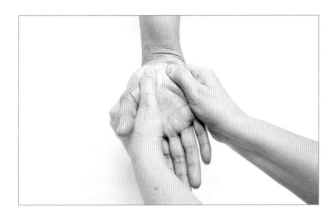

Press into this groove and slowly move your thumb or finger (whichever you are using to apply the pressure) upward until you reach the first crease in the palm; repeat this move three or four times and then move to the second and middle finger groove, repeating the moves there. Finally repeat the same move between the ring and little fingers.

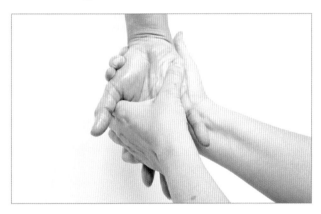

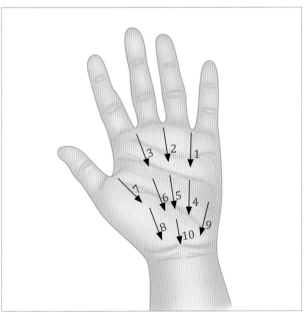

Next move into the belly of the palm; place your own thumb between the first finger and the thumb and then slide across the palm so that you cross the whole palm, finishing the move at the end of the palm that runs below the little finger. Keep repeating this move until you have worked the whole of the palm, ignoring for now the fleshy part of the palm connected to the thumb.

If you are working on someone whose hands are bigger or stronger than your own then you can use your knuckles to work this area; do not be afraid of experimenting to see what works best for you but be careful not to strain your own hands.

In the heel of the hand you may pick up more of the sand-like crystals—it can feel as though this area is full of crystals. If the person receiving the massage is muscular in this part of the hand then you can use your knuckles to knead this area to help break up the crystals. With an elderly client or child your thumb will give you sufficient pressure.

There are three areas of the hand that we still need to work: the side of the palm coming down from the little finger, the fleshy thumb area, and the back of the hand. Moving first to the side of the palm below the little finger, take your thumb and first finger and pinch the flesh just below and to the outside of the bottom finger knuckle; remember that you are trying to grasp the muscle—you are not just pinching the skin.

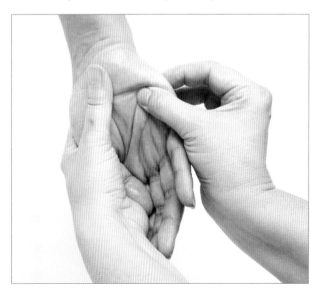

Roll this between your fingers backward and forward four or five times. You are working the skin, fascia, muscle, and connective tissue and, again, you may feel it softening in your hand. Once you have worked that area, move up a finger width so that you are working the area just above where you have just worked; continue up toward the wrist until you have covered the whole area, then go back and start again until you have worked it all two or three times.

Moving across to the thumb, you now need to work this fleshy part. If your client is pregnant do not work this area, this area is contraindicated for massage during pregnancy. It is known in Eastern practice as the "great eliminator" and massage here is reputed to be able to cause a miscarriage (see the section on pregnancy massage for more detail).

Assuming that your client is not pregnant and you are ok to work this area, try to feel for the inside of the bone that goes from the base of the thumb to the wrist. With your finger on the palm side and your hand on the upper hand side, roll this area between your thumb and finger.

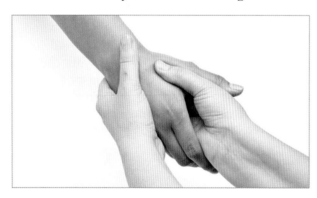

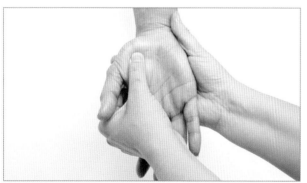

Work your way down so that you are working close to the bone and you will be working on both the muscle and the connective tissue. Move across the fleshy area at the base of the thumb to just below the lower knuckle of the first finger and repeat the same moves as before until you reach the V where the two bones come together. Roll this area all the way down two or three times, as you did for the previous moves. Now work on the fleshy part of the thumb and knead it gently, again always working upward toward the wrist.

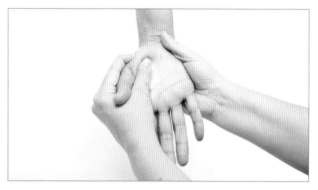

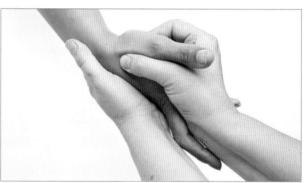

Finally, we move to the back of the hand. If your client is elderly, use a little oil or body moisturizer on the back of the hand so that you do not drag or tear delicate skin. Placing the person's hand flat on a cushion or your knee, place your four fingers just below the base of his or her fingers; you will feel the metacarpal bones either side of your fingers—you are working on the space between the bones, not on the bones themselves. Moving your fingers from side to side by just a tenth of an inch or less, work your way down the back of the hand, stopping when you feel those bones coming together into the wrist bones.

Do not lose contact with the skin during this movement and press just hard enough that you are moving the skin and underlying tissue rather than gliding across it. Repeat this whole process three or four times.

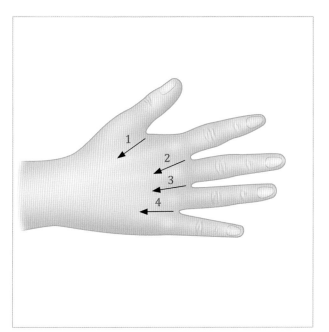

If you have worked one hand completely at this stage, ask the receiver to open and close their hand and gently move it about—they should be able to feel the difference between the worked and the nonworked hand. The worked hand should feel warmer, softer, lighter, and more flexible. The gift of hand massage is remarkable but, sadly, much overlooked.

Work both hands equally.

Some treatments described in this book will give specific instructions for massaging the rest of the arm; others will just say to also treat the arm. In the latter case, you can give the following massage treatment—these instructions are not for a detailed arm massage but are suitable for cases where you need a general arm massage.

Making sure the client's arm is supported, gently move the wrist through its normal range of movement; do not force any movement that is not free and natural and work slowly, rotating the hand three or four times in each direction.

Use massage oil to lubricate the skin as you work. Start by warming up the muscles on the inner forearm and then use your thumb to knead the muscles, working from just above the wrist to just below the elbow, and repeat this whole sequence four or five times.

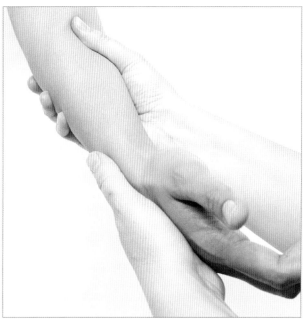

Next, using oil or cream, apply deep strokes up from the palm side of the thumb just above the wrist to just below the elbow. This is a powerful muscle and it can be tight and sore, only gradually deepen your pressue and you will feel the muscle soften as you release the tension from it. Next work with the same moves along the outside of the inner arm, following from just above the little-finger side of the wrist until just below the elbow.

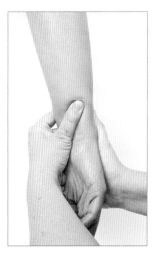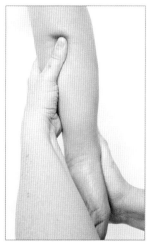

Turning the arm over, running up the center of the radius and ulna bones is the muscle that is primarily responsible for extending the arm. You can work this with your thumb and fingertips, either pressing and releasing the muscle as you move inch by inch up the center of the arm, or you can use oil or cream and slide up the muscle.

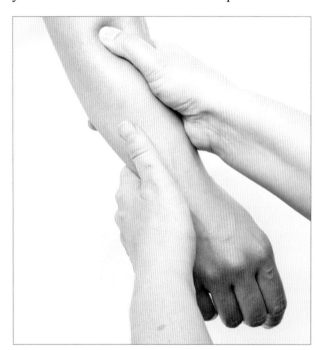

Be careful not to exert too much pressure as this can be a sensitive area. Now you are ready to move to the upper arm; avoid massaging over or behind the elbow. You may find that the upper arm is very tender to the touch, in which case work very gently at first. Use massage oil to lubricate the skin, and follow the direction of the muscles upward from just above the elbow to just below the shoulder, being careful not to work close to the joint and avoiding the armpit.

You can first warm up the muscles with long strokes, by slowly kneading the muscles with your hand or by gently pressing into the muscle with your thumb, holding that pressure for 30–60 seconds and then releasing, and repeating this around the arm until you have massaged the entire upper arm.

3 Foot Massage

Detailed Foot Massage

To massage the foot in detail, have your client sitting or lying in a comfortable position, and ensure that you are also in a comfortable working position as you will ideally be massaging the feet for a good 30 minutes. If you have a massage table with a face hole, then you may find it easier to work with the client facedown with a pillow placed underneath the lower legs to take any pressure off the back. It is not a problem if you do not have a massage table as you can also give a foot massage with your client seated on a sofa or chair, with you sitting on the floor and resting the foot on a cushion on your lap.

Your aim in giving a therapeutic foot treatment is to get rid of any residual tension that is held there. Start by looking at the feet with your client standing, if they are able to, and then seated or lying down. You need to be asking yourself if both feet look the same, and try to assess if there is any obvious tension in the foot. When a foot is relaxed the toes should be fairly "loose"—you should be able to lift them with a finger without feeling much resistance.

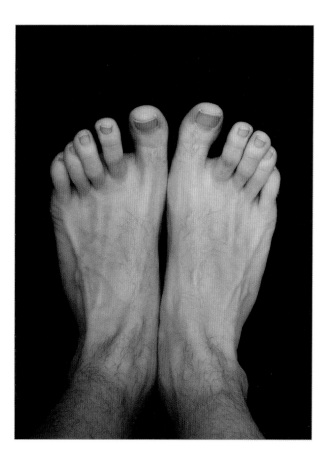

Toes should be reasonably straight; many people by the time they get to adulthood will have some deformation in the feet where toes may not be quite straight—this may be due to injury, ill-fitting shoes, or bad postural habits—but you are not aiming to try to correct any structural bending of the toes where the bend is sideways at a joint. What you are looking for is to see if the toes either pull up or pull under, as they do in these photographs.

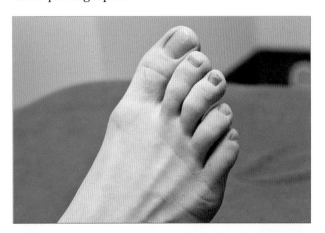

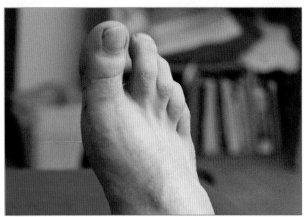

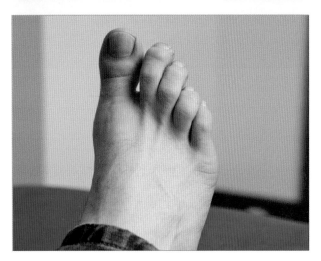

This indicates residual tension in the foot. Part of the aim of your treatment is to try to reduce this pulling of the toes either up or under.

As you are massaging you are working on all of the structure of the foot—muscles, fascia, and other connective tissue—so you need to start your work from where that tension will be embedded: at the end of the foot in the toes. You don't need to worry about what it is you are working on, with the exception that you should not be massaging over joints or bone. Your aim is to simply find any areas that are tight and, by your massage, help them to relax.

It does not matter which toe you start with, but work systematically so that you work each toe in turn.

Hold the end of the toe and gently roll the tip of the toe between your fingers; avoid putting pressure onto the nail bed. Work up each toe following the lines in the illustration.

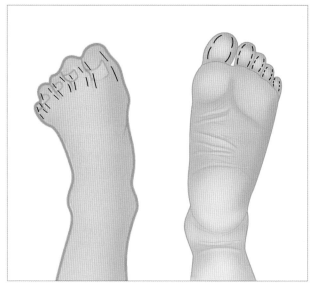

There are two key movements that you can use. By placing your fingers on opposite sides of the toe you can either gently squeeze, holding your pressure for around 5 seconds and then releasing it, or you can roll the toe in small movements between your fingers, applying pressure as you do.

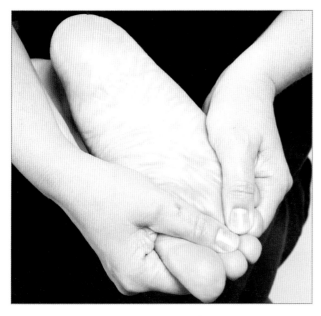

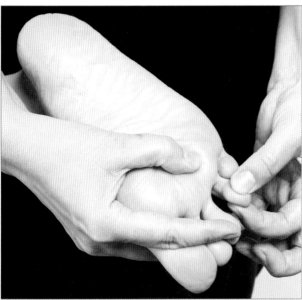

Make sure you then change your hand position so that you also work along all of the lines illustrated.

As you press or roll over these areas with your fingers, you may become aware of areas that are more resistant than others and, while this can be hard to feel in the toes, these are the areas that you need to work; even if you cannot feel anything specific, just massage this area with the gentle pressing or squeezing and you will begin to release any residual tension held there.

Do not use any oil when working on the toes or your fingers will slip off. Avoid working on the knuckles, but otherwise work your way up the toes, stopping just before you reach the webbing of the toes.

Repeat this for every toe of the first foot before moving into the sole of that foot. You are aiming to work all of one foot before moving to the other.

Having massaged each toe on the foot, you are now ready to work on the rest of it.

Begin by kneading the ball of the foot, just below the toes. You may be able to use your thumb here if you have strong hands, but if the client has thick skin here you can also use the knuckles of a flat fist, or if you are working professionally and can work with precision, you could use your elbow.

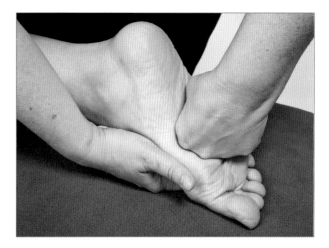

If you are using your knuckles or your elbow, support the client's foot in your hand so that you can always judge the pressure you are applying and to prevent any trauma to the small bones in the foot.

Next use your thumb to massage into the arch of the foot. Support the foot in one hand and massage with the other so that at all times you know that you are not applying too much pressure. Starting at the base of the toes and using just a little oil to help you slide across the skin, make long sweeping, stretching movements with your thumb from the base of the toes to the start of the heel.

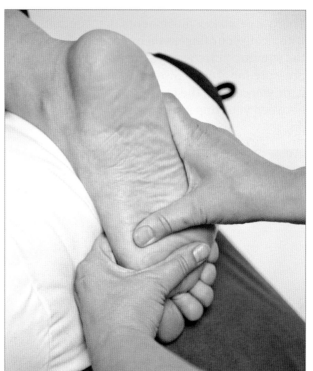

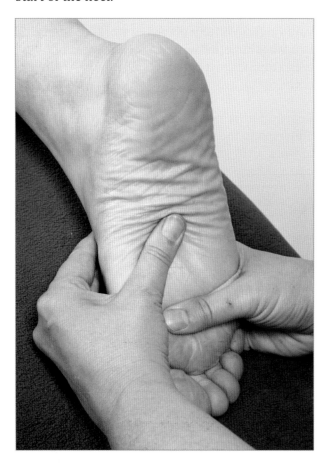

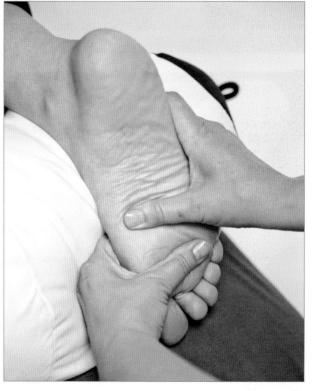

You can start at the outer or inner part of the foot, but be sure to repeat this move so that you cover the whole of the base of the foot. This area may be tender, so only work to a depth that is comfortable to your client, but press firmly enough that you are not tickling. If clients are very ticklish, you can work without oil through their socks rather than directly on the skin.

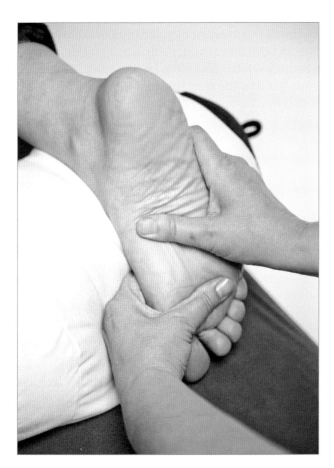

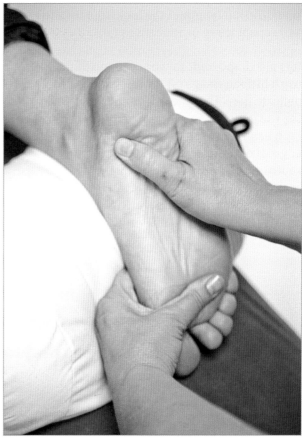

Repeat this four or five times across the whole foot, slowly increasing your depth each time but only to within your client's tolerance; this should feel like a good, relief-giving stretch, and should not be painful.

You can now work to the outside edge of the foot, an area that usually feels amazing when massaged. Supporting the foot in one hand, use either your thumb or the heel of your other hand to press into the edge of the foot, and make small circles with your thumb or hand so that you are moving the edge of your client's foot as you work.

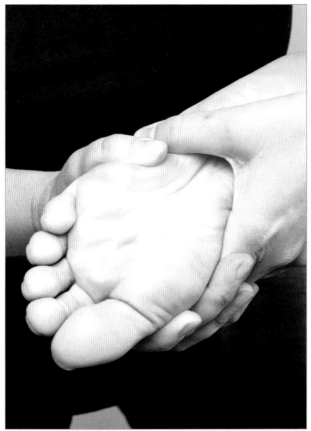

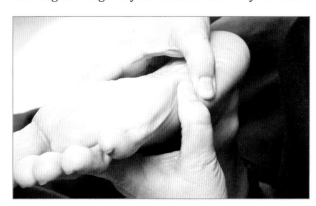

Work the full length of the foot from toes to heel, and repeat three or four times.

It is also important to work the top of the foot; use a little massage oil for this as the skin is more delicate here. Use one finger and start where the toe joins the foot—simply follow the groove between the metatarsal bones until you run out of groove as the bones join together in the foot; repeat three or four times. Which finger you use to do this will depend on the size of your hands compared to the client's foot; again, this should not be too uncomfortable for your client.

To finish this treatment you can take the whole foot in both hands and, using a little oil, squeeze gently down the foot from heel to toes, bringing your hand to the very tips of the toes and off the foot from the edge of the toes.

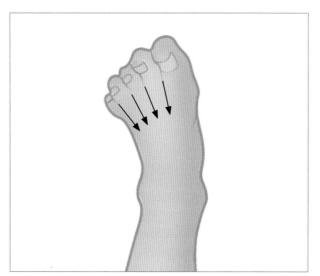

4 Head Massage

A head massage is one of the most relaxing massages to receive and it can be given on its own for general relaxation or as part of a wider treatment to help address specific problems.

Ideally your client should be lying down, facing upward. If you have a massage table this will be easy for both you and your client, and you should work seated behind your client. If you are working on friends or family members and don't have access to a massage table you can ask them to lie on their bed with their head at the bottom or side of the bed so that you can easily reach it by sitting or kneeling on the floor. If possible, try to avoid working with the client lying on the floor as this is likely to put pressure on your own back and shoulders as you are giving the treatment.

You may need a tiny amount of massage oil for when you are working on the forehead and face so that you do not drag the skin, but you can also use the client's own moisturizer if you do not have massage oil to hand. Try to work in a room that is softly lit and avoid using a room with overhead lights switched on.

Starting a treatment by relaxing the eyes can be very effective. Either use a folded towel to cover the eyes or gently cup your hands over the eyes (without pressing on the eyes) and hold for two minutes, and then release gently and slowly. You may find that the clients' vision is a little blurry immediately afterward; reassure them that this is normal, as the eye muscles have relaxed—it will quickly return to normal.

The scalp should be able to move around reasonably freely over the skull; if you place your fingers firmly on your own head and press in so that when you move your fingers you are moving the skin rather than just hair, you should find that you can move your fingers a few millimeters in all directions. A person who is very stressed or anxious or who is in pain is likely to have a very tight scalp, and this movement will be much reduced.

Place your hands so that your thumbs are at the center top of the head and your fingers are out toward, but not on, the ears.

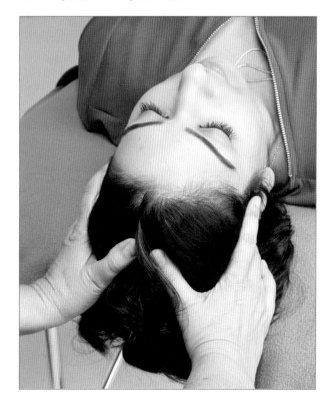

Starting at the hairline, imagine that there is a centerline on the head running down to the back; place one thumb on each side of this centerline and press down with both thumbs at the same time. Your pressure should be firm but it should not be uncomfortable for the recipient. Hold for three to four seconds and slowly lift your thumbs, move down this line a fraction toward the back of the head, and repeat.

The aim is to massage the whole of this centerline from the hairline down to where you can no longer reach with the client lying on their back. You need to work slowly and with a consistent pressure. This should feel good for your clients; they may report that one or two spots are more sensitive that others—this is normal.

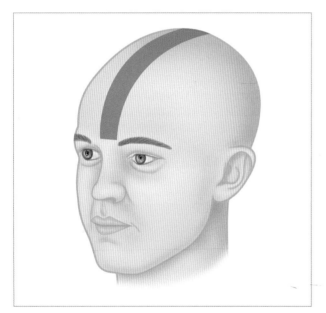

Next place your middle fingers together so that the pads of the fingertips are together in a line. Move back to your original starting point at the hairline, and this time make small circles with your finger pads; make sure that you work slowly—the aim is to relax, so slow and steady work is critical. Starting at the centerline make slow, small circles across the whole scalp, mirroring your movements at each side so that you are working both sides of the head at the same time. It is important to use a lighter pressure on the temple area—this is a delicate part of the scalp and is one area that you do not work deeply.

These two movements will take five to ten minutes; keep repeating them, alternating between the thumb pressure and the finger circles. Your client should already be feeling more relaxed.

Now you come to gently massage the face; the jaw and eyebrows can hold a lot of tension so it is important to release these areas.

Using your index and middle fingers together on each hand, find the center point between the eyebrows, apply gentle pressure downward, hold for three to four seconds, and release; lifting off the skin so that you do not drag it, move just half an inch out and reapply the pressure, repeating this until you reach the edge of the temples, where you should stop.

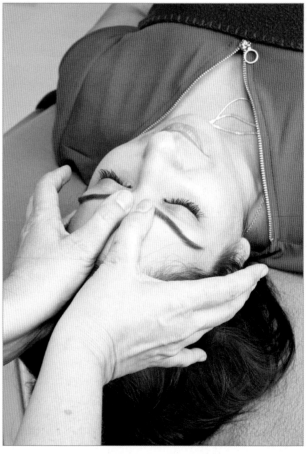

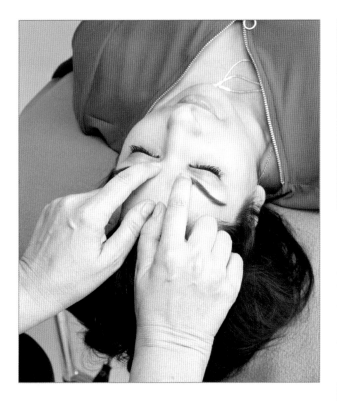

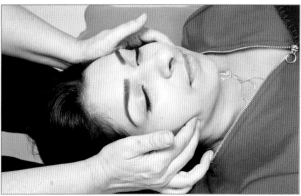

Place the index finger of each hand at the center of the jawline on the very tip of the chin. Use your thumbs on the very edge of the chin underneath but do not apply any pressure with your thumbs; there are lots of glands under the chin and you need to avoid pressing on these—the use of the thumb is just to keep the finger at the top steady.

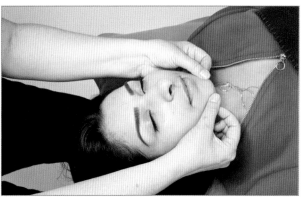

Move further up the forehead, starting again in the middle, and repeat this until you have reached the hairline. Repeat this whole process three or four times. Finish this section by gently stroking your fingers across the same area, applying just enough pressure for it not to be ticklish but stroking rather than prodding the area. If the recipient has very dry skin or is elderly, use a little massage oil or moisturizer for this work on the forehead to prevent dragging on the skin.

Next we come to work the area of the jaw; this can be incredibly tender so be aware of the pressure that you are using—you need to ensure that you are not pressing the cheek into the teeth. Place your middle three fingers together and very gently make circles across the cheeks from the corner of the lips and moving outward toward the jaw; repeat this two or three times. You may become aware of an increase in tension as you get toward the jaw and your clients may complain that it becomes very tender around this area; this may be because they have been gritting or grinding their teeth.

Using the same action as you did on the centerline of the head, press gently with your fingers following the line of the jaw, outward toward the jaw joint. Your client should be able to feel the pressure but it should not be unduly painful. However, as you get toward the jaw joint, it is likely to become more tender.

Placing your middle three fingers together, massage in small circles around the whole jaw joint area. You will feel the two lines of teeth as you massage; again, be careful not to press the cheek into the teeth and avoid pressing into the temples. You are applying a little more pressure here than elsewhere on the face as your aim is to begin to release the jaw tension. Ask your clients to open their mouth just a little so that the jaw joint is relaxed, and work with small circles into the joint.

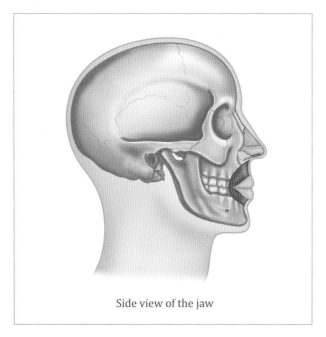

Side view of the jaw

The area immediately in front of the joint is likely to be more tender than most areas, but it is important not to avoid this area as working here is critical to releasing the tension. If you are working professionally, and if your client is not wearing dentures, you can apply moderate pressure here by holding the point on the cheeks just inside where the jaw has opened—hold for no more than four seconds as this will be a tender spot.

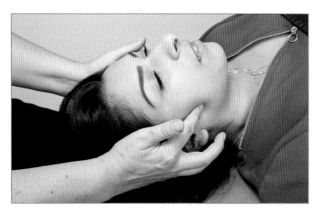

If the jaw area has been particularly painful, go back and repeat the forehead work; the tenderness in the jaw will be temporary and the result that is gained from relaxing the small but powerful muscles around this joint is worth any initial discomfort. You can repeat any of the scalp work at any time to help the client to relax.

If your client has medium-length or long hair then you can also pull the hair to help release the scalp; done well this feels like your scalp can breathe, but done badly it will take your client back to the school yard, so it is important to do this skillfully. Hold a small handful of hair between your fingers and pull straight out.

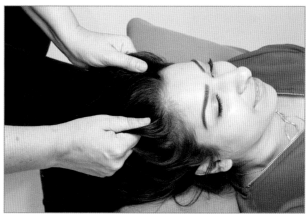

Make sure that you are not pulling one area more than another or this will hurt, and do make sure that you pull with equal pressure on both sides of the head at the same time. Get feedback from your clients—if they don't report something along the lines of it being "wonderful," stop and practice on yourself first. If this is good for your client, work all the way around the head with this technique.

You can finish this treatment by gently stroking over the lower forehead; start at the top of the nose where the eyebrows meet and move up just around an inch, moving slowly and gently for a minute or so, this may allow your client to drift off to sleep and should leave them feeling incredibly relaxed.

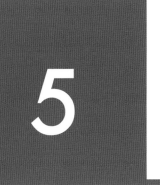

5 Back Massage

Introduction

For massage practitioners, a back massage is one of the most commonly requested treatments. It's an area we can become acutely aware of problems in—we may have a general backache or be unable to move freely because of pain and muscular tightness. However, if we only massage the back when it aches or feels stiff we are only really completing half a treatment as the root of that tension is often held elsewhere in the body, most frequently in the hands or head for upper-back pain and in the feet and legs for lower-back problems. It is important that, if you are following the instructions for massage of a particular condition, you do not omit the hand, head, or foot elements of the treatment recommended and go straight to the back. This back massage guide is given as a separate chapter here simply for ease of cross-referencing.

Specific Contraindications

You should be aware of the specific contraindications for the condition that you are treating. In addition:

- Do not ask a pregnant or breastfeeding client to lie facedown on the massage table.

- Do not carry out a back treatment if a client has had spinal surgery without first getting the all clear to massage from their doctor.

- Do not carry out a back treatment with the client facedown if the client has had abdominal surgery within the last six months.

- Do not carry out a back massage if your client has bone cancer unless you are working professionally in massage, have had specific oncology massage training, and are working with the client's medical team.

- Do not perform neck massage on a client with a history of strokes without the permission of their medical practitioner.

If you are working on friends or family members and do not have a massage table with a face hole or face cradle, do not apply pressure on the neck or upper back while clients are lying on their front and have their head turned to one side; instead, carry out this part of the treatment with the client seated facing forward on a chair.

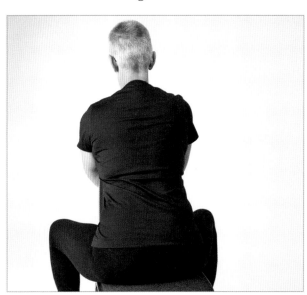

Massage Treatments

Make sure that you have completed the head massage detailed in Chapter 4 and the hand and arm massage in Chapter 2 before moving on to work on the back.

The muscles of the head and neck allow us to make some of the finest and fastest movements in the entire human body. They not only allow the movement of the head and neck, and chewing and swallowing, but are also integral to our speech, facial expressions, and eye movements.

There are some precautions to working on the neck: it contains some major arteries and veins, not least the carotid artery and the jugular vein, and the median nerve so you need to work gently and carefully. Never try to massage the front of the neck near the throat. If you feel a strong pulse where you are working, pull back from it and adjust your position. If your client complains of a numb arm or has pins and needles, you are touching a nerve so again pull back. You should never be working deeply enough, or quickly enough, to cause any damage to arteries, veins, and nerves. You do, however, need to work the neck gently and steadily to loosen these muscles and in turn to free the back, but talk to your clients as you work and use their feedback to guide you. To begin this treatment we are going to work at the sides and the back of the neck.

You will see from the diagram how complex the muscles of the neck are; this is because they carry out such diverse, complex, and detailed movements.

Remember that if you are massaging a family member or friend that you are aiming simply to loosen tight muscle, so try not to be put off by the technical detail of what you are doing.

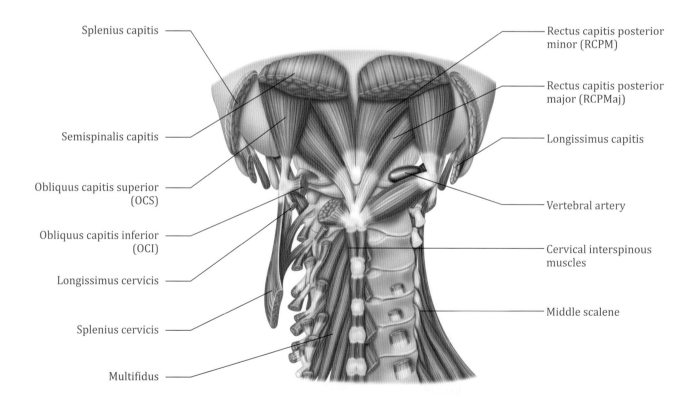

Splenius capitis

Semispinalis capitis

Obliquus capitis superior (OCS)

Obliquus capitis inferior (OCI)

Longissimus cervicis

Splenius cervicis

Multifidus

Rectus capitis posterior minor (RCPM)

Rectus capitis posterior major (RCPMaj)

Longissimus capitis

Vertebral artery

Cervical interspinous muscles

Middle scalene

Before beginning any detailed work, you need to warm up the muscles at the back of the neck; if your client has long hair move this out of the way. Warm some massage oil in your hands and stroke upward from the top of the shoulders to the base of the skull or hairline, without losing contact with the skin, then stroke back down from base of the skull to the top of the shoulders. Repeat this five or six times, being careful not to apply any pressure directly onto the spine.

You can start this next stage of the treatment at the base of the skull by treating the deeper suboccipital muscle group. Have your client lie faceup on the massage table. The suboccipitals (below) are a group of four muscles that are located on each side of the back of the neck, just below the base of the skull. These muscles connect the skull with the top two vertebrae of the neck. The suboccipitals are responsible for both turning and tipping your head.

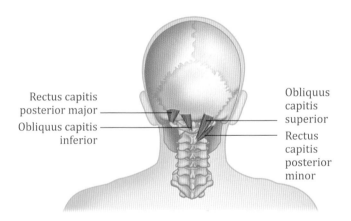

Rectus capitis posterior major
Obliquus capitis inferior
Obliquus capitis superior
Rectus capitis posterior minor

These muscles also have a strong connection to eye movement. You can experience this for yourself by placing your fingers underneath your skull toward the top of your neck. There are surface muscles that you need to work past, so gently roll your fingers into your neck either side of your spine; you will need to press in fairly hard but not so hard that you cause pain.

Keeping your fingers still, move your eyes as far as you can to the left and then to the right, then upward and downward; do this slowly and without moving your head, only your eyes should be moving, and you will feel movement

in these suboccipital muscles as your eyes move. These are deep but critical muscles; you need to use medium pressure and to work slowly. Quick movements will cause your client to pull away during treatment as the protective mechanism of all of the muscles in this region is a strong one, designed to protect the spine.

With your client lying facing upward, cradle the head in your hands so that your fingers are curving into the muscles just below the base of the skull, and warm up these muscles by gently stretching the neck, pulling the head toward yourself; this should be a pleasurable not a painful stretch.

Do not use this stretch if your client has had spinal fusion surgery in their neck or if they have Down syndrome. Release the stretch a little but still support the head and slowly tilt the head so that the chin moves toward the chest by no more than half an inch. Keep your fingers still, pressing gently onto the suboccipital muscles. Ask the client to look directly up at the ceiling and to relax; then without moving the head, look at his or her toes, and then to relax the gaze back up to the ceiling; then, again without moving the head, to look up to you, then back to the ceiling.

Ask the client to look to the left and back to the ceiling and then to the right and back to the ceiling, all only with eye movements and keeping the head still.

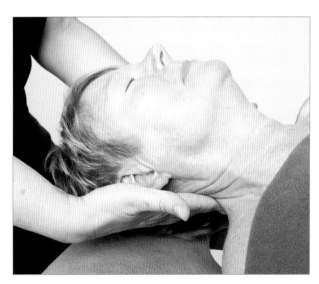

Securely lift the head by another half inch, keeping a firm contact with the suboccipital muscles, and repeat the looking down, up, left, and right movements, always returning to look at the ceiling between eye movements. This will help relax the muscles at the top of the back of the neck. Gently replace the client's head on the couch. This may cause some short-term eye strain and you can help to relieve this by gently cupping your hands over the client's eyes for 20–30 seconds—without making contact with the eyes. The eyes should return to normal within a few moments and you can reassure your client that this is normal.

Repeat the neck warm-up massage, stroking upward from the top of the shoulders to the base of the skull or hairline, without losing contact with the skin, then stroking back down from the base of the skull to the top of the shoulders, being very gentle as you get to the area you have just worked in more depth as this still may be a little tender to the touch.

Next ask your client to turn the head; it does not matter which direction this is in to start with as you will eventually work both sides. You will be able to feel a group of strong, ropey muscles that come down from behind the ear and go down toward the shoulder and collar bone. This is where we are now going to work, being careful not to slip forward to touch the throat.

Using a little massage oil so that you do not drag the skin, place the flat of your index finger so that you are gently pressing with the pad of your fingers on the top of the sternocleidomastoid (SCM) muscle (opposite), and slowly follow the muscle down to where it inserts toward the center of the collar bone.

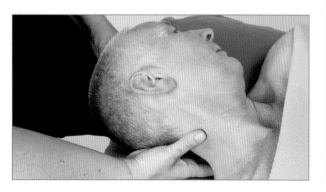

Repeat this move, slowly, three or four times. Always work downward from head to collar bone, never upward. If there are particular spots that are resistant to your touch and that the client reports are tender, simply hold your finger still on that point, maintaining (never deepening) your pressure, and you will feel the muscle relax under your touch.

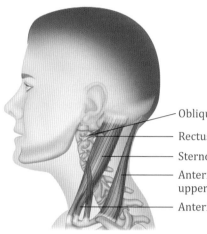

Obliquus capitis superior
Rectus capitis posterior minor
Sternocleidomastoid
Anterior portion of upper trapezius
Anterior scalene

Ask your client to return his or her head to center and then to turn it to the other side, and repeat the work to the SCM on the other side. Having completed that, again repeat the warm-up massage sequence; although you are no longer warming up the muscles you are applying massage over a wider area, and this is good practice having worked specific muscles within that overall muscle group.

Now you are coming to work on the levator scapulae (below). The levator scapulae muscle has the nickname "shrug muscle" because when it contracts you lift your shoulders up and shrug.

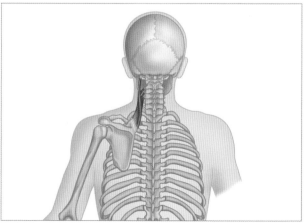

If you are very tense then your shoulders may feel like they are in a permanent upward shrug, and this shortens the levator scapulae. One of the things that we are likely to do when we have a headache is to pull our shoulders up and forward in a "protective hug," but in the long term this does not help the problem. The levator scapulae originates on the first four cervical vertebrae and inserts into the shoulder blade. When the muscle gets shortened, it pulls the four vertebrae down and to the side.

You can do this work with your client faceup or facedown. If you have a table with a face hole or face cradle, you will find it easier to work with the client facedown, but if not you can work with the client faceup and reach underneath to access these muscles.

Work all the way down this muscle using very small circles with two fingertips placed together. If your client is faceup, turn the head very slightly to reveal the muscle; once you have worked down the muscle three or four times you can then work a little more deeply but always within the client's tolerance—the area being massaged may feel tender but you should not be causing pain—if you feel your client tighten up against your touch, reduce your pressure. As you repeat the massage you will begin to feel the muscle soften to your touch.

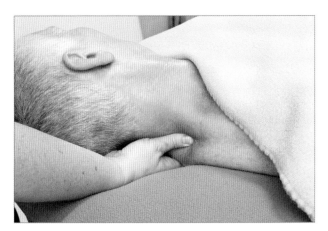

With the client facedown into a face hole or cradle, or sitting supported leaning on the chair, you can now carry on to work the rest of the back.

Using massage oil to lubricate the skin and with the flat of your thumbs either side of the spine, warm up the area up by gliding down the back, making sure you do not touch the spine itself. Work both sides of the spine at the same time.

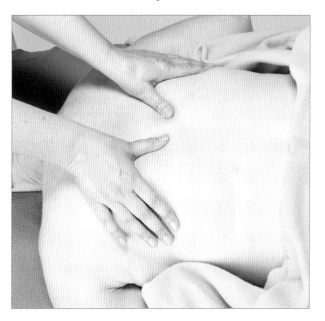

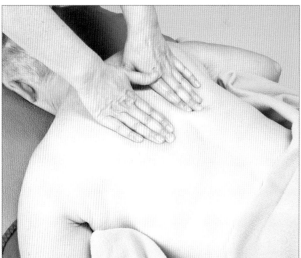

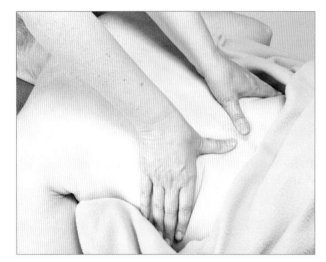

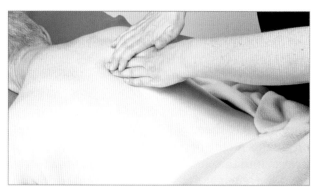

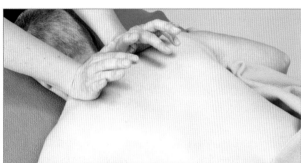

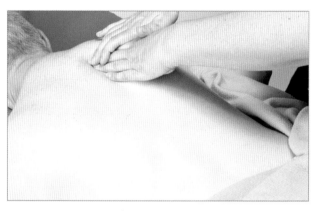

After you have warmed up the area with three or four strokes down both sides, you can begin deeper, detailed work on the back. After you have moved down the spine with your thumbs you can start to come back up with the outer sides of your hands.

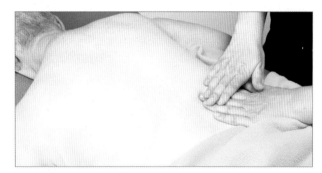

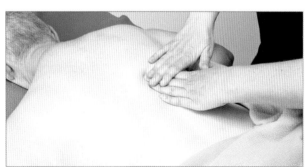

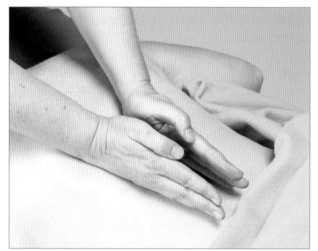

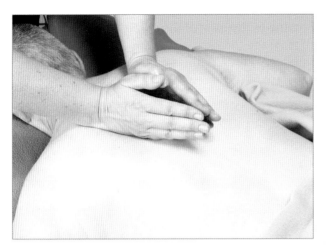

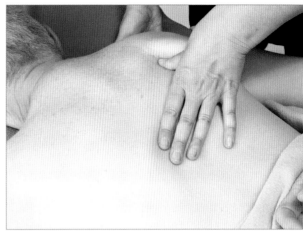

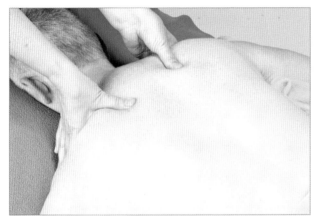

There are enormous natural variations in how much someone's shoulder blade will raise, so there is no right or wrong depth to work to; simply slide under it, hold until the muscle begins to relax, and then move further up so that you cover the whole area. Support the arm as it relaxes back to its original position.

You can now return to the shoulders and treat the top of the shoulders. This is easier with your client facedown, but you can adapt it to the client lying faceup by reaching underneath the shoulders, or you can work with the client seated.

Ensure that you work all the way down from the top of the shoulders to the sacrum at the base of the spine, but avoid placing your hands underneath the client's underwear. Repeat four or five times.

Now check if the area at the back of the shoulder blade is tight—ask your clients to put their hand behind their back so that the shoulder blade is a little raised. Use a pillow to support the arm so that the clients do not need to hold the arm up themselves. If you are working with people with multiple sclerosis or Down syndrome, always ask them to move their arm into this position themselves so that you do not overstretch by assisting them in the move. If clients cannot raise their arm up to their back you can simply ask them to place their arm on the massage table next to their body. You should be able to either see or feel the shoulder blade, and you will be working on the area inside this. Using the flat of your thumb, simply press down so that your thumb moves underneath the edge of the shoulder blade.

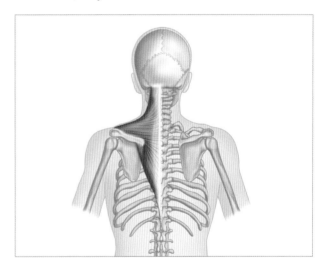

Start at the top of the shoulders at the center with your thumbs either side of the spine, and you can stroke outward and down across the trapezius muscles above; you can also use the palm of your hand or even your forearm to carry out these moves, being careful not to massage on the spine or the ribs.

While it is nice for the client if you start this work moving downward, once you have the muscles warmed up you can work in any direction; you may notice the skin redden—this is not a problem so long as you are not working too deeply for the client.

As you work, the muscle will start to soften. If you work on an area that your client reports is tender or that you can feel is tight you can press and hold on that spot, you may need to hold the pressure for one or two minutes for it to release; if you do use this technique always massage over the wider muscle again afterward.

To work the teres major and infraspinatus, positioned in the back just behind the armpit and shoulder, you should start by massaging inward from the outside of the body. For clients who lift weights, who drive a lot, or who spend long hours at a computer, this can be a very tender muscle; if this is the case working with the flat of your hand will be tolerated much better than working with thumb or fingers. Once you have warmed up this area you can again work in any direction.

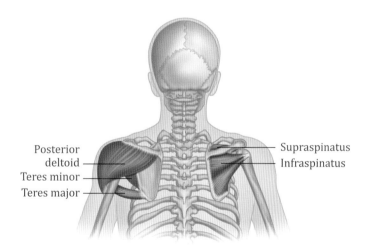

Posterior deltoid
Teres minor
Teres major
Supraspinatus
Infraspinatus

Moving to the base of the spine, we now need to massage the sacrum to complete the back massage. The sacrum is a flattened bony area at the base of the spine.

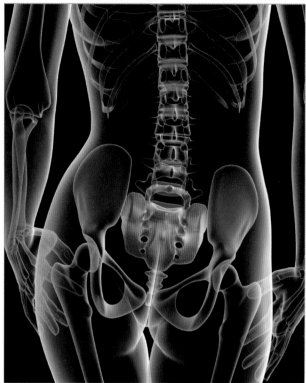

If you feel across it with your fingers you should be able to find the edges of the sacrum. It is safe to massage with gentle to medium pressure over this area; if you are new to massage only use gentle pressure. Using thumb pressure, work your way along and across the whole sacrum so that you cover the whole area with a press and release action; hold each press for five to ten seconds.

You should also be able to feel the bottom edges of the sacrum—these will be angular, coming from the base of the sacrum (the top of the intergluteal cleft), moving upward and outward in the direction of each hip. With the flat of your thumb, gently roll off the edge of the sacrum.

Finally you need to ask your client to turn over and to move the body so that it is more toward the edge of the massage table, and so that the shoulder joint slightly overhangs the table. Support the extended arm in your hand.

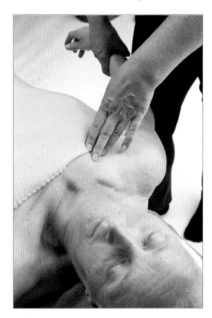

Place the flat of your closed fist or the flat of your fingers so that it is just inside the shoulder joint as shown in the photograph.

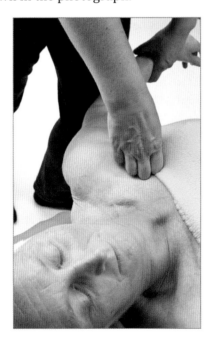

Anatomically, you are applying pressure towards the top of the pectoralis major, not the deltoid.

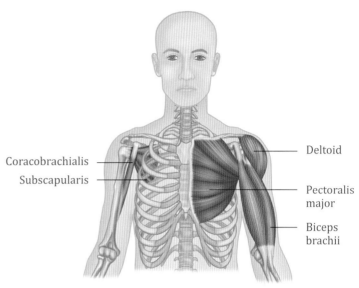

Coracobrachialis
Subscapularis
Deltoid
Pectoralis major
Biceps brachii

Press straight down to a depth that is good for your client and, with your other hand, move the client's arm backward and forward no more than an inch or so; this combination of pressure and movement can very quickly release the tension in the front of the shoulder, allowing the back of the shoulder to move backward and relax back onto the table.

Place your client's arm back across the body and ask him or her to move to the other side of the table, and repeat this process with the other arm. Although you are working on the front of the shoulder, this can complete a good release into the back of the shoulders, and is a good compliment to the back massage.

PART II
AN A–Z
OF MEDICAL
CONDITIONS

Ankylosing Spondylitis

Background to the Condition

Ankylosing spondylitis (AS) is "a painful, progressive form of inflammatory arthritis. It mainly affects the spine but can also affect other joints, tendons and ligaments."[1] Most often diagnosed in people between the ages of 18 and 30. Ankylosing is a Greek word meaning "fusing" and spondylitis refers to inflammation of the vertebrae.

Early symptoms of AS are pain and stiffness usually around the middle of the back, but the pain can start anywhere within the spine and can also affect other areas, and any joint can be affected. Knees may be swollen, hips and heels painful, and for a number of people their eyes will be impacted by the disease, with pain and/or photosensitivity experienced. For some people, the lungs, heart, or bowels can also be affected with the inflammation. Some people with AS will be at risk of osteoporosis, while others can develop a skin condition known as psoriasis.

There are ways of managing the symptoms of AS but, at present, there is no cure. Although genetic testing is now being introduced in early diagnosis, this is an area of ongoing research and is not yet fully understood. There is often an 8- to 11-year gap between developing the early symptoms and the effects of the AS showing on x-ray or other imaging. Some fusing of the spine usually takes place, but it is unusual for the whole spine to fuse.

It is useful for the massage practitioner to understand what takes place within the body in order to be able to treat a person with AS effectively. Massage is safe to use provided the practitioner acts with care and caution and all manipulative moves of joints are avoided.

AS is a progressive condition; some people will experience periods of remission where their symptoms settle down significantly, others will see no break in symptoms and, because of the nature of the disease, symptoms become progressively worse.

The first stage of degeneration occurs at the "entheses." Entheses are the areas in the body where tendons and ligaments meet the bone and it is this area that is the "primary target organ in a collection of rheumatic conditions, the best known of which is ankylosing spondylitis."[2] In AS, "inflammation [occurs] at tendon, ligament or joint capsule insertions."[3] Enthesitis is inflammation in the entheses—the point at which

---

[1] Ankylosing Spondylitis Guidebook, National Ankylosing Spondylitis Society (UK), October 2012.

[2] Where tendons and ligaments meet bone: attachment sites ('entheses') in relation to exercise and/or mechanical load, M Benjamin et al., *Journal of Anatomy*, 2006 April, 208(4): 471–490.

[3] http://www.arthritisresearchuk.org/health-professionals-and-students/reports/topical-reviews/topical-reviews-autumn-2009.aspx

the tendon or ligament joins to the bone becomes inflamed. This inflammation causes a knock-on effect where part of the bone will be eroded; once the inflammation begins to subside, the body's natural healing response takes place and the body lays down new bone. As this process is repeated with subsequent bouts of inflammation and healing, movement can be restricted as "bone replaces the elastic tissue of ligaments or tendons."[4] Eventually this can lead to the fusing of vertebrae and other joints.

AS is usually worse first thing in the morning or after sitting or working in one position for a long period of time, and pain will decrease as movement is reintroduced. People diagnosed with AS will be encouraged to exercise (with nonimpact exercise) and to be very careful about their posture. A physiotherapist will be able to guide the individual client as to the exercise that is best suited for that individual, and massage can be very beneficial, helping to keep movement and restore correct posture from bad postural habits.

As the body stores tension, so massage releases that tension. Massage works on the skin, fascia, and muscles and their attending ligaments and tendons, which then has an impact on the skeletal structure. Massage can free up the body to move as best it can within the confines of its individual structure. Massaging someone with AS will not cure the AS, you will never unfuse a fused bone, but you can help that person to gain the best movement that is possible within the limits of their condition, and you will release tension and, therefore, pain in the muscles impacted by the condition.

As the mid and lower back are both affected by AS, it is important to work with your client both on the upper and the lower body—only massaging one of these will restrict the outcome.

Specific Contraindications

Some AS sufferers may be able to tolerate deeper massage, but for others this will be too painful and you will need to work gently, at least at first, until the muscles begin to release and relax.

You need to work closely with your client to first of all establish their comfort on the table, additional folded towels or pillows may be needed for support for joints already affected by the AS, and you will need to be in dialogue with your client throughout the treatment as to the appropriate depth that you work to.

Massage Treatments

It may be best to start with lower-body work, as the sacrum is an area that is often first affected by AS; in order to do this you should work from the feet upward. Begin the treatment by following the protocol for the foot massage in Chapter 3.

When working up from the foot, be careful to work all around the ankle by gently pressing and releasing all of the tissue around the ankle joint; this is done by applying static gentle pressure all around the outskirts of the ankle bone, pressing in with your thumb, holding for 20–30 seconds, releasing, and then moving around the ankle so that you cover the whole of the ankle area, but without dragging the skin.

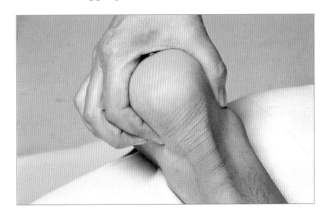

---

[4] Ankylosing Spondylitis Guidebook, National Ankylosing Spondylitis Society (UK), October 2012.

Then you can gently rotate the ankle, supporting the foot as shown in the photograph. As you do this rotation you are simply moving the foot through its natural rotation—do not manipulate or overextend the joint.

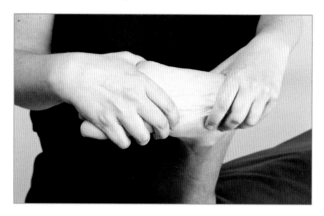

Once you have fully worked the foot and ankle you can move up the leg into the muscles of the calf and the front of the leg, being careful not to apply any pressure on the area behind the knee joints.

Work up the leg, in the direction of the heart, in medium-length strokes so that you are covering around six inches of muscle in any one stroke. If your client can take deep pressure, work up to this so that you first free up the fascia and the surface layers before working more deeply.

Once the muscles of the lower leg have released and are softer to the touch, you can move up to the larger muscles in the upper leg. Using the heel of your hand will be more comfortable for your client than using your thumb (and will protect your thumb from damage) and you can also use your forearm or the side of your hand so that you are working up these muscles with a larger surface area; this will also help to protect your client from unnecessary bruising. Ask your client to turn over so that you can also work the front side of the thighs, concentrating your treatment on the outer thigh muscles.

Stretching is very important in treating AS so, after you have finished working each limb, finish treating that area with long stretching strokes up the full length of the muscles, making sure that you stretch all of the areas you have been working on.

You should work in the same way up both legs before you do any work into the hips. While most massage work would include the sacrum in lower-body work, for the client with AS you should leave the sacrum work until toward the end of the treatment, when you will have also worked the upper body, so that all areas of muscle that impact on the sacrum and sacroiliac joint have been worked prior to you treating this area.

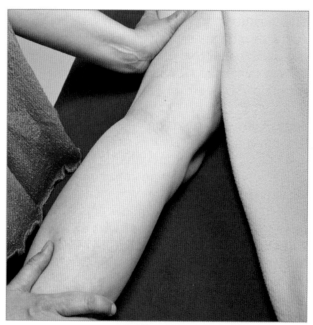

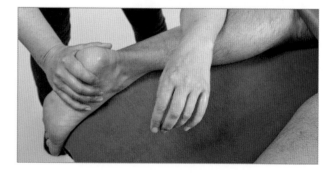

Now that you have completed this lower-body work you can begin again on the hands and arms; follow the protocol in Chapter 2 for this massage work, to start the release of the upper body.

With your client faceup you can then follow the instructions in Chapter 4 on how to give a massage treatment to the head; do not omit the jaw massage from this unless any of the specific contraindications listed in that chapter apply.

The muscles of the back should also be stretched by long massage strokes as part of this treatment. Some AS sufferers will have restriction of the ribs, so special care should be taken around the intercostal muscles, the muscles between the ribs, to ensure that stretching of muscle takes place but that there is no direct pressure put on bones where there may have been skeletal fusion. You can do this by using one continuous stroke, starting at the top of the shoulders and stroking all the way down to the sacrum; use your thumbs either side of the spine for this, being careful not to press on the spine or the ribs either side of these muscles.

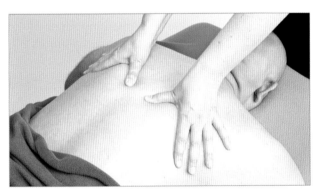

The muscles surrounding the spine are designed to allow it to flex in different directions, but AS can result in a permanent "looking down" as it "sets up a serious tug of war between the spine and the muscles that move it, and the increased flexing of the spine causes chronic shortening of the flexor muscles, which cause the extensors to have to compensate by increasing contraction to maintain as upright posture as they can".[5] The aim for AS massage is to lengthen the spinal flexor muscles while at the same time relaxing the spinal extensor muscles (see below).

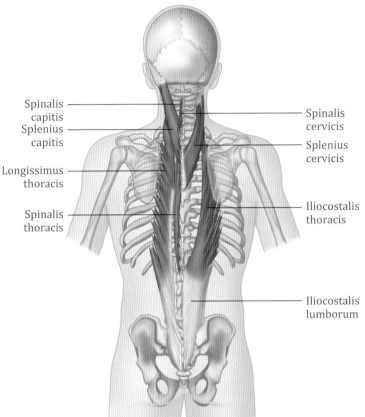

Spinalis capitis — Splenius capitis — Longissimus thoracis — Spinalis thoracis — Spinalis cervicis — Splenius cervicis — Iliocostalis thoracis — Iliocostalis lumborum

Stretching the erector spinae muscles and working in detail down the spine toward the sacrum are critical in achieving this. Long movements that start at shoulder level and extend all the way down to the sacrum will provide this stretch. At all times be very careful with your pressure and get constant feedback from your client so that you know you are working at a comfortable depth for the client, and follow the massage below for the sacral work.

[5] http://www.sacramentomassagecenter.com/massage-ankylosing-spondylitis/

The erector spinae muscles embed into the sacrum so it is key to work all the way down to, and then carefully across, the sacrum. The role of the sacrum in AS is pivotal; according to the National Institute of Arthritis and Musculoskeletal and Skin Diseases in the US, "the hallmark of ankylosing spondylitis is "sacroiliitis," or inflammation of the sacroiliac (SI) joints, where the spine joins the pelvis."[6]

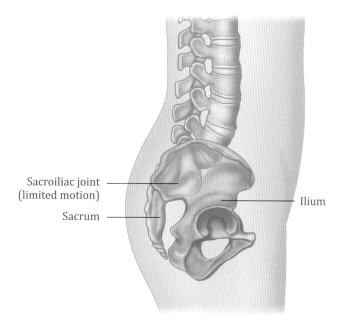

Sacroiliac joint (limited motion)

Sacrum

Ilium

The sacrum is a key player in both the stability and the strength of the body; it allows the pelvis to move without twisting, whilst at the same time providing stability between the spine and the lower limbs. The sacrum is the attaching point for a number of muscles including the gluteus muscles, the stabilizing muscles of the lower back, the piriformis, and the hamstrings. Tightness in any of these muscles will put pressure on the sacrum and cause a knock-on effect of tightness elsewhere in the body, often tilting the pelvis and having a marked effect on gait, which in turn can cause problems in the hips, knees, and ankles. Add to this that AS often causes a fusing of the SI joint. The SI joint is a

major stabilizing joint, yet it has a very small range of movement—but even small movements have an effect on the spine, and on the rest of the body.

While massage will not free the SI joint when it has fused, massaging all of the areas that lead into it will help to eliminate the uneven "pull" on the SI that tight muscles can lead to. Usually, as massage practitioners, we would avoid massaging onto bone as this will be painful and unhelpful, but the sacrum is the one exception.

This massage should, however, be done slowly and carefully. Ask your client to lie facedown with a pillow placed under the ankles to prevent the spine being stretched uncomfortably while you work. Using the flat of one of two fingers, gently press and hold the skin above the sacrum—the client should feel the pressure but there should not be any sharp pain. Hold each press for 10–15 seconds, lift the fingers and replace them a little further along the sacrum; the aim is to massage the entire sacrum. The sacrum is usually easy to find and you will feel the edges at a wide V from the center of the lower back. Working the whole of this area can provide an immediate sense of relief and it will also encourage healthy blood flow to the area.

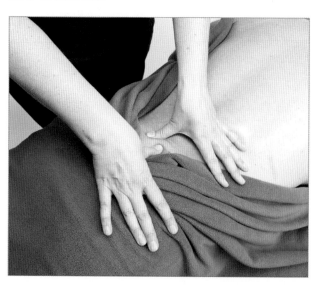

[6] http://www.niams.nih.gov/Health_Info/Ankylosing_Spondylitis/

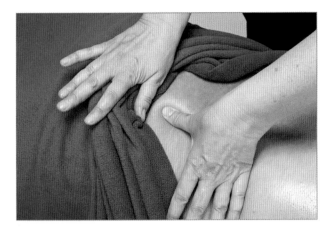

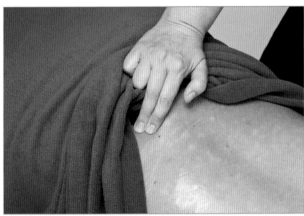

The raised leg should be fully supported so that you are not putting any undue pressure on the hips or sacrum as you work this area. The pressure that you can place on the hips will depend on the development of the AS, so be very careful to check often that your client does not find the pressure too much.

Place your hand at the top of the femur (you will be able to feel the head of this bone on most clients) so that your middle finger is continuing on the same line as the femur. Spread your fingers, and your three middle fingers will be approximately on the three points in the hip that you need to work. It will vary depending on the size of your hands and the size of your client, but this is a good guide. Using three or four fingers together, feel around this area—you should find three points in the hip (roughly adjacent to the spread of the three fingers) where, when you press gently into the hip, there is more resistance than in the other areas of the hip. These are the three areas that you need to press into to help the hip to release.

Having completed this work you are able to do some deeper hip work. If your client is able, ask him or her to lie in the side position, supporting both the raised knee and the client's head with pillows.

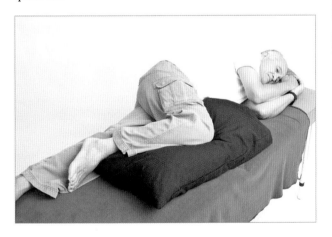

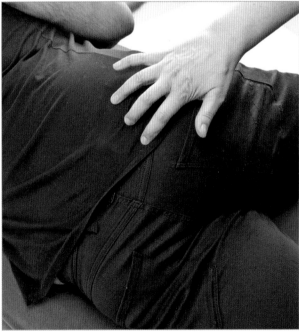

If you are a trained massage professional then you can, if you were trained to do so and are confident in your ability, use your elbow to apply the pressure here. If you do not have this level of training then use either the heel of your hand or two or three fingers forming an open fist.

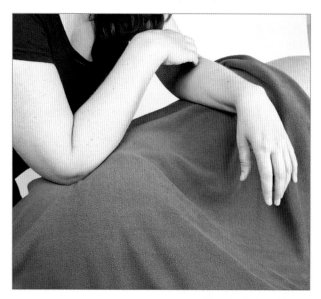

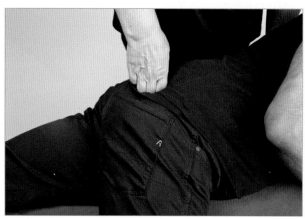

It is vital that you work with your client's breath for this move; you can apply pressure on the out breath. The client should not feel any pressure on the hip joint or sacrum—the pressure is within the muscle. The hip may roll forward, and you should encourage your client to allow this to happen. As you first go into this move, ask your client to rate the depth: one being a feeling of light pressure and ten being very painful—aim for five or six out of ten if your client is happy to work to that depth and if you feel confident in what you are doing, otherwise aim for a three or four (or to your client's maximum if that is lower), and now hold that pressure. You may need to hold this for up to a minute, but as you do the client will report that the pressure feels like it is dropping. When they get to the point where it just feels like you are leaning on them, you have achieved your goal. As you have not released the pressure until this point, it is the tightness in the muscle that has released. Release slowly from this position.

Repeat this process for all three points on both hips, being careful to support the client's leg and hip with the pillow at all times. This move will also stretch out the muscles that hold the hip tight, and will begin to gently stretch the muscles around the sacrum and SI joint.

Massage can give symptomatic relief of AS and help the individual to maintain muscle movement; it can also encourage lymphatic flow, which itself can help the body to deal with inflammation. Massage will also help to increase circulation and bring much-needed oxygen to the damaged tissues. As with any medical condition, if you are in doubt as to whether an area should be treated, ask the client's doctor or specialist and work within the bounds of your training. If you are massaging to assist a friend or family member, work with caution and get constant feedback from the person you are working with. As time progresses you will be more confident in what you do, and the person receiving the treatment will be able to direct you to areas that need attention. There may be times that you want to seek the professional guidance of a massage practitioner, but you can also ask your practitioner for guidance in how to complete self-care for your loved one.

Anxiety Disorders

Background to the Condition

An estimated 57 million people worldwide suffer with an anxiety disorder and, of these, two-thirds are women.[7] While many of us will suffer moments of anxiety, a generalized anxiety is often only defined as a disorder when it has gone on for longer than six months,[8] so the number of people suffering from some form of anxiety may be much higher.

The medical world generally accepts that there are different levels and subcategories for anxiety, these include:

- Generalized anxiety disorder

- Panic attacks

- Phobias

- Post-traumatic stress disorder

- Obsessive–compulsive disorder

- Social anxiety disorder.

All share some common symptoms, and the impact on the life of the sufferer can be anything from significant to catastrophic and life changing. This chapter will focus on the generalized anxiety disorder (referred to from here on as simply anxiety), but the massage treatments used for this can be applied across all forms of anxiety. It is useful to understand what happens during an anxiety attack, or when the anxiety is heightened.

From our evolutionary roots our bodies come equipped with a "flight or fight" mode, designed to allow us either to run away—fast—or fight for our lives. This mode gives us extra adrenalin, also known as epinephrine, to be able to face up to the challenge ahead. When a threat, real or imagined, occurs, the sympathetic nervous system signals to the adrenal glands (located above the kidneys) to release adrenalin, which along with other hormones increases breathing, heart rate, and blood pressure.

The increase in these three processes moves oxygen-rich blood more quickly to the brain and muscles, and glucose and fatty acids quickly into the bloodstream, increasing muscle strength ready for the impending flight or fight.

[7] Harvard Health Publications, Harvard Medical School, July 2008.
http://www.health.harvard.edu/newsletters/Harvard_Womens_Health_Watch/2008/July/Anxiety_and_physical_illness

[8] http://www.nhs.uk/Conditions/Anxiety/Pages/Diagnosis.aspx

Muscles tighten as joints and ligaments are prepared to run away or to fight. Ready for this fight, our senses become keener and we become less sensitive to pain. In our evolutionary past, when the source of this stress was a dinosaur looking at us as its dinner, this adrenalin would be used up instantly—we would fight or run. When the source of our stress now is an overdemanding boss, an impossible work deadline that is suddenly dropped on us, office politics, or a very difficult social setting, fighting or running away is never a particularly good career move.

If the threat, or perceived threat, persists, then the body also begins to release cortisol. Again, this is a critical function, cortisol being responsible for helping to regulate blood pressure and the immune system, and assisting balancing insulin to keep the blood sugar level normal, and generally helping the body to respond to stress.

However, cortisol can also interfere with the function of neurotransmitters, the chemicals used by brain cells to communicate with each other. Too much cortisol can impair long-term memory, and people who have been in very stressful situations may have "gaps" in what happened, as the brain has been overwhelmed and has not been able to fully lay down the long-term memories.

Our bodies are equipped to deal with all of this in short bursts: as the sympathetic nervous system releases the fight or flight response, so the parasympathetic nervous system will calm it down. However, the release of adrenalin is a much more effective and faster response than the calming effect of the parasympathetic nervous system.

Where in days of old we would have used up most of the adrenalin or hidden in a cave while the rest of it wore off and we could return to a state of calm, in modern-day life we can go from one stressful situation to the next, so the parasympathetic nervous system never gets a chance to catch up. Exercise and consciously taking time out to relax will help, but for someone whose stress levels are very high and whose body is constantly releasing adrenalin and related hormones, there is never a chance to get to that point of balance where the body can self-regulate.

Most people will suffer some form of stress during their lives; stress in itself is not always a bad thing, it can heighten our senses and enable us to perform, do a particularly good job, or to get through a specific situation. It is only when the stress continues for a longer period of time that the stress hormones within the body start to accumulate.

Sleep can become elusive as the brain refuses to "be quiet" and people can wake with a sense of doom and foreboding. Blood pressure can be increased, and headaches and muscle tensions—particularly in the shoulders and neck—can be painful.

As a tight muscle is impaired in its functioning, the person suffering may also feel permanently weak; add this to lack of sleep and the fear of something going wrong, and it is easy for this to become a downward spiral. The anxiety sufferer will often report an increasing cycle of attacks; they may be reluctant to leave the house and fear a panic attack if they are in a crowded or public place. Feeling trapped in a social situation is part of the flight or fight reaction, where a clear exit is needed to be able to flee from the situation. The fear of an anxiety or full-blown panic attack then causes the release of the stress hormones, and so the whole situation cycles downward.

If you are supporting someone with an anxiety problem it is easy to get frustrated, but telling someone not to worry or to "get a grip" is not helpful—they are in the middle of a situation which is both physical and psychological.

There are, however, very positive things that can be done to help. Professional help by way of counseling, cognitive behavior therapy, or

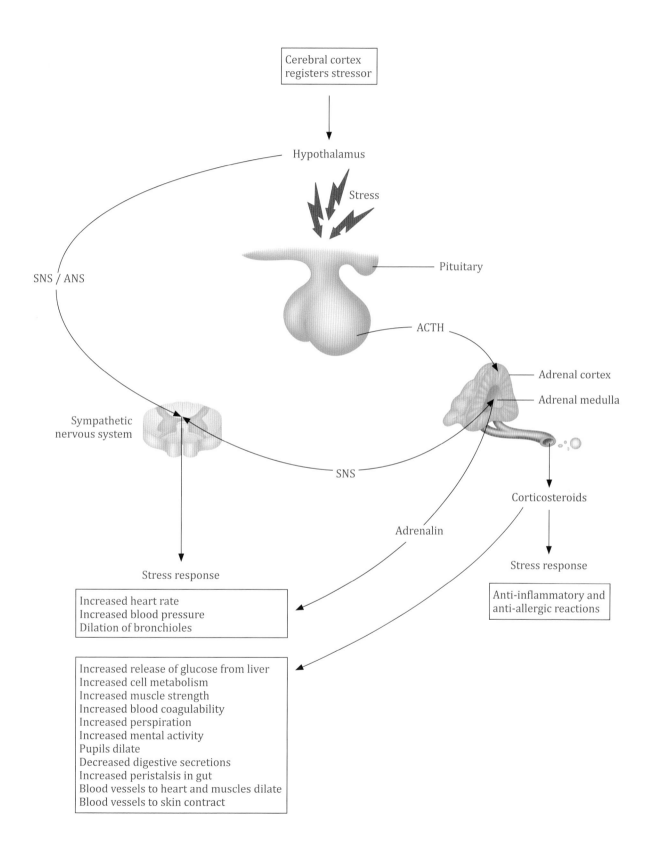

Cerebral cortex
registers stressor

Hypothalamus

Stress

Pituitary

ACTH

SNS / ANS

Adrenal cortex

Adrenal medulla

Sympathetic
nervous system

SNS

Corticosteroids

Adrenalin

Stress response

Stress response

Increased heart rate
Increased blood pressure
Dilation of bronchioles

Anti-inflammatory and
anti-allergic reactions

Increased release of glucose from liver
Increased cell metabolism
Increased muscle strength
Increased blood coagulability
Increased perspiration
Increased mental activity
Pupils dilate
Decreased digestive secretions
Increased peristalsis in gut
Blood vessels to heart and muscles dilate
Blood vessels to skin contract

neurolinguistic programming can help with the psychological aspects and in regaining a sense of control. For example, the stomach-churning feeling that gives that sense of doom can also be reinterpreted as an excited stomach churn that releases endorphins, the "happy hormones," and endorphins will help the body counter the negative effects of stress. This process may take time and, along with professional help, there are self-help guides available that can assist with this process. Not least, these techniques allow the person suffering from anxiety to realize that they can regain control of their stress and this need not be a permanently downward spiral—this knowledge in itself can aid recovery.

Before we move on to look at the specific massage techniques that can be used to assist the person struggling with anxiety, we also need to discuss the importance of proper breathing. Breathing deeply though the massage will also help increase the positive effects of the massage, but learning to breathe deeply on its own will also be beneficial.

Find a place where the client you are working with feel safe, secure, and warm and ask them to lie down on their back, close their eyes if they are comfortable to do so, and to place one hand on their chest and one on their belly just below the belly button. Ask them to take slow, deep breaths, trying to make the hand on the belly rise higher than the hand on the chest.

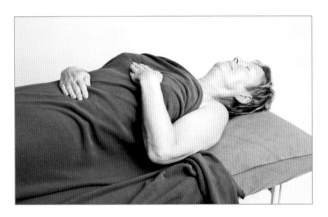

During an anxiety episode breathing will become quick and shallow, so you are trying to achieve the opposite of this: slow, deep breathing. You can either talk them through this, put gentle music on in the background, or use one of the guided breathing meditations available on download or CD. As they relax further the breathing should slow down and naturally deepen; if exhausted from their anxiety, they may fall asleep. Again, this is an important part of the healing process and the deep breathing learnt in this setting can also be applied in the middle of a shopping mall when anxiety strikes.

A person suffering with anxiety will often complain about having sore shoulders, a stiff neck, and maybe headaches: these are all physical manifestations of the anxiety. Massaging these areas will assist the person in recovery and relaxation. The various medications that are available for anxiety work on the chemical messages from the brain and body, but most are for short-term use only. Both benzodiazepines and the "Z drugs"[9] are highly addictive and the body soon develops tolerance to them, so more are needed to achieve the same effect. These can be good short-term solutions during a major crisis that overwhelms, but they do not address the underlying causes of anxiety and are not a long-term solution.

While the drugs switch off the brain side of the flight–fight response, massage can help to break the same cycle in the body, relaxing the muscles and allowing the body to relax—which in turn allows the brain to relax as the sense of danger recedes.

[9] Medicines with the names zaleplon, zolpidem, and zopiclone for the treatment of anxiety are commonly called the Z drugs as a generic name.

Specific Contraindications

There are no specific contraindications for treatment, but please see below for suggestions to make your client feel more relaxed and comfortable during the massage.

Massage Treatments

Have your clients lie faceup on the table; this way they can see what is around them if they are feeling anxious and need to know their exit. It can be good to offer the clients the option to stay fully clothed to begin with to again allow a sense of control (they can leave straight away if they need to) and start your work on their head. While the term "client" is being used here, there is nothing in this massage that cannot be done by a friend or family member, but if you are in doubt on the pressure, err on the side of gentleness. The head massage described here is slightly different to the main head massage protocol, so is given in detail.

The scalp should normally be able to move around over the skull; place your fingers firmly on your own head and press in so that when you move your fingers you are moving the skin rather than just hair. You should be able to move your fingers an eighth of an inch or so in all directions. The person who is very stressed or anxious is likely to have a very tight scalp and this movement will be much reduced.

Place your hands so that your thumbs are at the center of the head and your fingers are out toward, but not on, the ears. Starting at the hairline, imagine that there is a centerline on the head running down to the back; place one thumb each side of this centerline and press down with both thumbs at the same time. Your pressure should be firm but it should not be uncomfortable for the recipient. Hold for three to four seconds and slowly lift your thumbs,

move back down the line by just the depth of your thumbs, and repeat. The aim is work the whole of this centerline from the hairline down to where you can no longer reach with the client lying on their back. You need to work slowly and with a consistent pressure. This should feel good for your clients, they may report that one or two spots are more sensitive than others and this is normal.

Next place your middle fingers together so that the pads of the fingertips are together in a line. Move back to your original starting point at the hairline and this time make small circles with your finger pads; make sure that you work slowly, the aim is to relax so slow and steady work is critical. Starting at the centerline, make slow, small circles right across the whole scalp, mirroring your movements at each side so that you are working both sides of the head at the same time. Be very gentle in your work over the temples.

These two movements will take five to ten minutes; keep repeating them, alternating between the thumb pressure and the finger circles. Your client should already be feeling more relaxed. Next you are coming to work on the forehead and face.

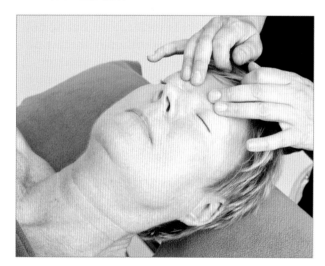

Using your ring and middle fingers together on each hand, find the center point between the eyebrows, apply gentle pressure downward, hold for three to four seconds, and release; lift off the skin so that you do not drag it, move just half an inch out, and reapply the pressure, repeating this until you reach the edge of the temples where you should stop.

Move further up the forehead, starting again in the middle, and repeat this until you have reached the hairline. Repeat this whole process three or four times. Finish this section by gently stroking your fingers across the same area, applying just enough pressure for it not to be ticklish but stroking rather than prodding the area! If the recipient has very dry skin or is elderly, use a little massage oil for this work on the forehead to prevent dragging on the skin.

Place your middle three fingers together and very gently make circles across the cheeks, moving outward toward the jaw; repeat this two or three times. You may become aware of an increase in tension as you get toward the jaw and your client may complain that it is very tender here; this is most likely to be because of gritting or grinding of the teeth. Using the index finger of each hand, place your fingers at the center of the jawline on the very tip of the chin. Use your thumb on the very edge of the chin underneath, but do not apply any pressure with your thumb; there are lots of glands under the chin and you need to avoid pressing on these—the use of the thumb is just to keep the finger at the top steady.

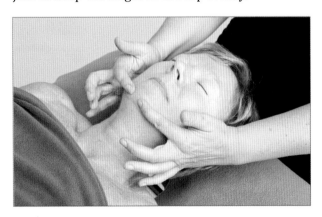

Press gently with your fingers following the line of the jaw, outward toward the jaw joint. Your client should be able to feel the pressure but it should not be unduly painful. However, as you get toward the jaw joint, it is likely to become more tender. Placing your middle three fingers together, massage in small circles around the whole jaw joint area. You will feel the two lines of teeth as you massage, just be careful not to press the cheek into the teeth and avoid pressing into the temples. You are applying a little more pressure here than elsewhere on the face as your aim is to begin to release the jaw tension.

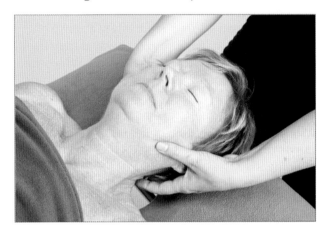

Ask your client to open the mouth just a little so that the jaw joint is relaxed, and work with small circles into the joint. The area immediately behind the joint is likely to be more tender than most areas but it is important not to avoid this area as working here is critical to releasing the tension. If that has been particularly painful, go back and repeat the forehead work; the tenderness in the jaw will be temporary and the result that is gained from relaxing the small but powerful muscles around this joint are worth any initial discomfort. You can repeat any of the scalp work at any time, this will help the client to relax.

By this stage your clients should be feeling less anxious about the treatments and it would be useful for them to remove the clothing from their upper body so that you can access their shoulders and neck easily, but you can do the whole of the treatment with your clients clothed if they prefer. Make sure that you have a large towel, blanket, or sarong (depending on your climate) so that the clients can feel covered and secure during the treatment.

Ask your clients to lie facedown; if you do not have a treatment couch with a face hole then use a small pillow or cushion so that the clients can place their forehead on it and still be able to breathe freely. At this stage the neck should be straight rather than turned to one side.

Using some warmed massage oil, lavender oil will be good for this as the properties of the oil will also aid relaxation, apply the oil by stroking downward from the nape of the neck across the shoulders.

You need to massage the back and shoulders in detail and you can follow the protocol for back massage in Chapter 5 for this, but with one addition if you are able—try when you are massaging to never break the contact with the client so that even as you change position to massage a different area, you always maintain some contact. Try to work smoothly and slowly and keep your massage flowing—this will allow your client to relax into the massage more.

Having completed the full back and shoulder massage as detailed in Chapter 5, there is one additional technique to add to this treatment. Ask your client to roll over so that they are laying face up. Place your hands so that you are supporting the client's head in your hands with your fingers placed at the base of the skull; you should feel the edge of the bone, and with equal pressure on both hands, pull your fingers upward with gentle pressure. Gently and slowly rock the head from side to side, moving just half an inch, as this will help you deepen the pressure safely and without the need to press more. Hold this for one to two minutes and gently place the head back down.

You can repeat any of the scalp and forehead work to finish; ending a treatment with gentle forehead work is very relaxing for clients and you may find that they drift off to sleep for a few minutes. If they do this, leave them to sleep, and when it is time to bring them round (if you cannot just leave them to sleep) do so gently and softly so as not to cause alarm and retrigger the flight or fight reaction!

If a person has full-blown panic attacks there is another technique you can use, which, along with the professional help and breathing treatments, is emergency first aid massage. A vigorous scalp massage can help to break into a panic attack and stop it developing further. If you have short nails you can use these so long as you do not press on too deeply; using the tips of your fingers work quickly across the scalp in small but strong movements.

If you are on your own and you cannot do this to yourself (for example if you are in a work setting and can feel the panic rising) then press hard right in the middle of the top of your head and make small circles with just one or two fingers. You won't go deep enough to do any harm as it will hurt too much, but this action can interrupt the thought processes that are leading to the panic attack, which then gives you time to focus on your breathing and take longer, deeper breaths and to be able to refocus your thoughts onto more positive thoughts of being in control, breaking that downward cycle.

Asthma

Background to the Condition

The treatments offered here are to be used only as a supplement to asthma medication and are not meant as a replacement. Asthma is a serious medical condition that if untreated can be fatal—this is a complementary, not an alternative, treatment.

Asthma is a chronic (long-term) lung condition in which the airways are inflamed and narrowed, making it harder to breathe normally.[10] When people with asthma come into contact with one of their asthma triggers (something that irritates their airways), the muscles around the walls of the airways tighten so that the airways become narrower and the lining of the airways becomes inflamed and starts to swell.

Sometimes, sticky mucus or phlegm builds up, which can further narrow the airways.[11]

These reactions make it difficult to breathe and can cause a cough, wheezing, a tight chest, and breathlessness. Globally it is estimated that 250,000 people die each year from asthma, and the World Health Organization (WHO) estimates that 235 million people currently suffer from asthma.[12] In the UK alone there are 3 deaths from asthma each day,[13] and in the USA it is 9 a day.[14] Most of these deaths are preventable, with asthma being a severely underdiagnosed and undertreated illness.[15]

There is no known single cause of asthma but certain factors make someone more likely to develop it. A family history is a strong indicator; the child of a parent with asthma or a lot of allergies is more likely to develop asthma than a child neither of whose parents has asthma or allergies. There is a strong link between having an atopic condition such as eczema, hay fever, or a food allergy and developing asthma.

If your mother smoked during pregnancy or if you were exposed to tobacco smoke as a child then you are more likely to develop asthma. If you had a low birth weight or were born early and needed a ventilator as a baby then you are more susceptible to developing asthma, as you are if you had lung infections as a child. For some people asthma starts in infancy but it can develop at any time of life, including in old age. Environmental factors—such as exposure to allergens, including pets, cleaning products, and dust—can increase the likelihood of developing asthma. Air pollution and chemical irritants can trigger asthma, and some medications—including aspirin, beta blockers, and nonsteroidal anti-inflammatory drugs—can

---

[10] http://www.blf.org.uk/conditions/detail/asthma

[11] http://www.asthma.org.uk/knowledge-basics

[12] http://www.who.int/mediacentre/factsheets/fs307/en/index.html

[13] http://www.asthma.org.uk/asthma-facts-and-statistics

[14] http://www.aafa.org/display.cfm?id=8&sub=42

[15] Ibid.

cause an attack. Some sufferers will have an asthma attack triggered by extreme cold, whilst extreme emotions—fear, grief, and even extreme excitement—can be the trigger for other people.

Asthma can be well managed and there are both short-term and long-term drugs available. An individual with asthma, or who suspects they may have asthma, should be under the regular care of their medical practitioner and be working together with them to manage their asthma on both a daily and a long-term basis. An acute asthma attack is a medical emergency and must be treated as such.

The symptoms of asthma can be so severe that some massage practitioners will view asthma as a contraindication to massage. We need to be clear that massage is not a suitable treatment for someone in the middle of an asthma attack; they need to use their inhalers or take other medications, and if the symptoms do not resolve or improve quickly, seek urgent medical help. Massage is not a cure for asthma, but it can be helpful in a number of ways and there are several factors to take into account.

Specific Contraindications

Do not use this treatment as an emergency procedure. Someone having an asthma attack needs medical treatment.

It is tempting when massaging to fill the room with scented candles or to burn incense, but these should be avoided when treating someone with asthma. If you are giving a massage and are asthmatic yourself then check how these things may affect your asthma. Good massage oils will be made up of a base oil and essential oils; either of these could be an irritant. Grape-seed is a very low allergen and can usually used safely, but if you have someone who is highly allergic, you can use their own moisturizer instead of massage oil to be very sure. Almond oil is the base for many pre-blended oils, but can cause allergic reactions

that could trigger the asthma so use it only with caution. The essential oils that are used in the base oil are plant or flower based and, again, this can be a problem so unscented oil may be best, at least to start with until you can check someone's reaction to the oil. Be careful with the cleaning materials that you use prior to the client arriving and the detergent that you use on your linens and towels. If these are a problem for allergic clients, invite them to bring their own linens and clean your surfaces with hot water just before a treatment starts.

It is very important that clients bring their inhalers with them when they come for a treatment; most asthmatics will be very good at carrying these at all times, but check prior to a treatment and check where they carry the inhaler so that you can recover one from a bag if it is needed quickly.

Massage Treatments

There has been little medical research around the subject of massage and asthma. There is anecdotal evidence that reducing stress through massage has helped some people reduce their asthma medication, but most asthma help web pages carry some kind of warning that there is little medical evidence to support the idea that massage will help asthma. There is, however, a growing body of evidence that links postural problems and asthma. Gonzalez and Manns have led some of this research, and report that "patients with asthma present an increase in lower airway resistance and hyperinflation. The maintenance of hyperinflation could lead to a flattening in the dome of the diaphragm and shortening of the accessory inspiratory muscles.

The consequence of overuse of the primary and secondary respiratory muscles may lead to the development of head and cervical spine postural changes."[16] Put simply, the person with asthma is likely to have extremely tight breathing muscles and so the diaphragm and the intercostal and

[16] Gonzalez, HE & Manns, A (1996) Forward head posture: its structural and functional influence on the stomatognathic system: a conceptual study. Cranio, 14: 71-80.

scalene muscles will likely benefit from massage. If people with asthma can feel more in control of their breathing and feel that they are less constricted in their chest, and therefore more in control of their own bodies, this is likely to reduce stress levels, which will in turn help with their posture. It is, however, important to note that if someone is struggling to breathe and is having an asthma attack then urgent medical attention is necessary—giving a massage is not the solution and could cause a dangerous delay in getting treatment.

Massage for stress reduction for the asthmatic will be beneficial; the chapter on anxiety will give clear guidance for how to do this, but there are also specific techniques and areas for massage to consider in order to assist the person with asthma. Just to repeat this again to be clear: this is massage for between asthma attacks, not during an asthma attack when medication should be used.

The diaphragm is the dome-shaped sheet of muscle that separates the chest from the abdomen; it is attached to the spine, ribs, and sternum and is the main muscle involved in breathing.

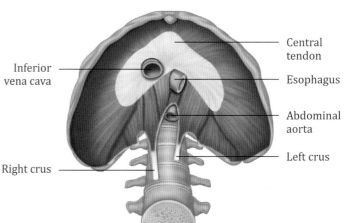

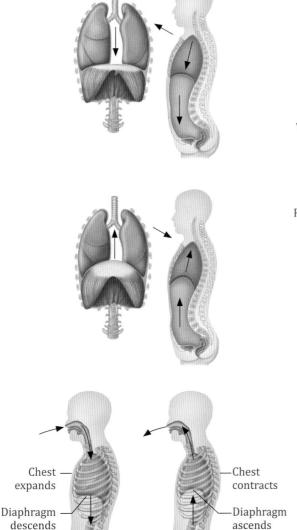

Chest expands

Diaphragm descends

Chest contracts

Diaphragm ascends

Breathing in   Breathing out

When you breathe in, your diaphragm contracts (tightens) and moves downward. This increases the space in your chest cavity, allowing your lungs to expand. At the same time the intercostal muscles between your ribs (the muscles that connect your ribs to each other) contract to pull the rib cage outward and upward, further enlarging the chest cavity. With the out breath the opposite happens—the ribs lower and come in and the diaphragm moves upward.

The intercostal muscles may be very tender to the touch so be gentle as you work. Make sure that you provide blankets or sheets so that the recipient feels safe and secure in how he or she is covered. Ask your client to lie faceup; in women you will be restricted in where you can work as you need to avoid massaging breast tissue—you can work below the breast and to the side, but never attempt to massage the intercostals through breast tissue. You can carry out this treatment through a thin blanket or sheet if your client is more comfortable that way; when working on women, even if you are working directly on the skin, the breasts should always be fully draped. In men, just avoid the area immediately around the nipple as this will be hypersensitive to touch. Use warmed massage oil to avoid pulling on the skin and make sure your own hands are warm!

Start by placing the tip of a finger between the eighth and ninth ribs; to get your starting position imagine the arm was stretched upward and you are following a line down from the arm—you do not go on the inside of the line into the abdominal cavity. Using the flat of your finger, feel for the intercostal muscle between the ribs, gently apply pressure downward, and follow the muscle as it runs between the ribs; go as far toward the back of the body as you can—only while you can feel the intercostal muscles between the ribs—then move back to the starting position, but one rib higher, and repeat the same movement.

Continue as far up as you can (until the breasts in women—do not massage on breast tissue); so long as you can feel the muscle between the ribs, you should be able to feel rib bone either side of your thumb. If your thumbs are too big, use a finger so that you are not rubbing onto the actual rib bones. When you have finished one side, repeat on the other. If as you work one area feels particularly tight you can stop on that point, hold a consistent pressure—do not press harder—and ask your client to tell you when the pain subsides, then move on. For clients having gall bladder treatment this work may be extra tender for them on the outer right-hand side; ask your client for

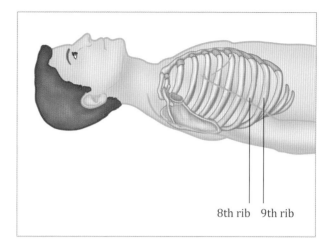

8th rib   9th rib

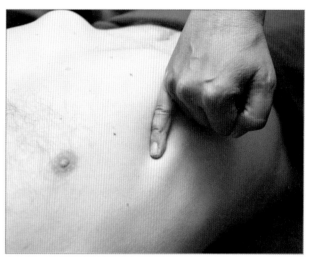

feedback and adjust the depth of your treatment accordingly to lighten your touch.

If this is too tender to work or if your client wants to remain clothed you can use the pressure of their own breathing to assist the massage. This move can also be done in conjunction with the detailed intercostal work described above. Ask your client to lie faceup and to raise the arm above their head. Place a flat hand on the rib cage toward the side of the body, ask the client to take a deep breath and then to exhale fully, with the out breath apply a gentle pressure onto the ribs, and maintain this pressure as the client breathes in again.

The pressure you apply through your hand does not increase; you are simply trying to maintain the ribs at their "breathed out" position—the intercostal muscles will need to work harder to try to lift your hand, giving a supported resistance movement. Simply maintain your hand position—you do not press down—and make sure that your hand is flat so that you are not placing more pressure on one area of the ribs than another. As the client breathes out, raise your hand to release your pressure. Repeat three or four times and then swap to the other side and repeat the whole process.

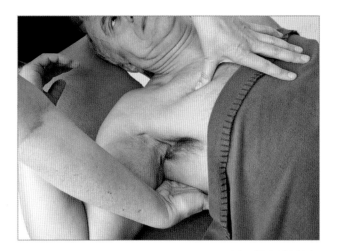

Next you need to work on the upper intercostal muscles. These are harder to reach for massage but, again, ask your client to lie faceup and to raise one arm above the head and stand above the client at the head. Place one hand underneath the client so that you are holding the outer ribs adjacent to the armpit, as shown in the photographs.

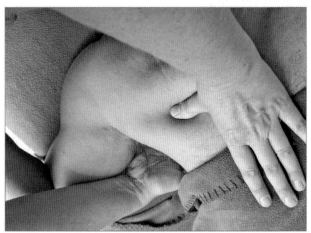

Place the other hand on top of the client's ribs at the very top of the chest, just above the main area of breast tissue on a woman, and with the heel of your hand placed below the scapula. If a woman is large breasted you can ask her to place her opposite hand on the top of the breast so that the breast tissue can be moved downwards by the client and held out of the way allowing you to be free to work on the chest area above the breast.

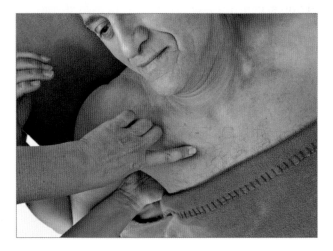

With the client taking slow, deep breaths, pull the hand that is underneath the client upward toward yourself (and toward the client's head). Your hand should not be raised off the table—you are aiming to pull the back of the ribs upward toward the shoulder, not up off the table. At the same time press gently with the hand that is on the top of the ribs. Hold this move for five to ten deep breaths and you should feel the ribcage begin to relax. Repeat the whole process on the other side.

Once you have completed this, ask your client to raise the knees; support the knees with a pillow if needed, or have your client with the knees bent and feet flat on the massage table. Ask the client to raise the arms up toward the chest; this treatment can be given through clothes if preferred—if not, ensure that your client is fully draped. Feel for the bottom of the ribcage and on the client's out breath gently and slowly place your fingers so they are curled just underneath the ribs. This is the area of the diaphragm. For two or three breaths, as the client breathes out gently tease out tension in this area, moving your fingers very minimally (up to around an eighth of an inch or so) underneath the rib cage.

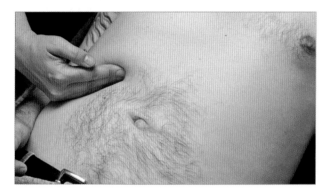

If you are professionally trained in massage, on the last of these breaths you can keep your fingers in place and ask your client to breathe in and hold his or her breath. You fingers will have sunk a little into the belly underneath the rib cage; move your fingers no more than half an inch as you apply very gentle friction massage to this area. When the client needs to breathe again, release your pressure. This should not cause your client any pain so stop immediately if this occurs, you should not be working deeply in this area. Depending on the size of the client and of your hand you may need to repeat this action two or three times to cover the whole length of the bottom front of the ribs, before repeating the whole process on the other side. If your client is large and has a lot of belly fat you may not be able to see the ribs to know where to place your hand; in this case ask the client to roll onto one side, supporting the head with a pillow and with the legs in recovery position, and the belly will drop away from the upper side so you can work that area, asking the client to turn over to access the other side.

Whether you are working professionally or on a friend or family member you can then finish the treatment and, with your client clothed or fully draped and lying on their back, ask him or her to place one hand on the lower belly, between the belly button and the pubic bone, and the other hand on the chest. You now want to encourage your client to breathe freely and deeply so that they begin to breathe abdominally. If you watch babies breathe, their whole belly will rise and fall naturally as they do; this is the most efficient way to get a deep breath and it's something that, as we grow older, we often forget. The hand that is placed on the belly should rise and fall more than the hand on the chest.

Cancer

Background to the Condition

For many years, having or having had cancer was seen as a contraindication to massage, unless it was end-stage cancer where the benefits of massage have always been recognized. Even when someone had finished treatment and had been discharged from the care of the oncologist, massage could be denied.

This reserve and misconception is still evident in some of the available publications; for example. "Cancer can spread through the lymphatic system, and because massage increases lymphatic circulation, it may potentially spread the disease as well."[17] A number of spas and clinics will not massage people who have, or have a history of, cancer. However, this is a view not now supported by the main cancer bodies and support groups.

The organization Cancer Research UK says "Some people worry that having a massage when you have cancer may make the cancer cells travel to other parts of the body. No research has proved this to be true."[18]

Macmillan Cancer Support says something very similar: "Some people worry that massage could cause cancer cells to spread to other parts of their body, but research has not found any evidence of this."[19]

Massage Today magazine states "Most massage therapy schools taught that cancer was a contraindication for massage. The two main concerns of how massage therapy could spread cancer involved its effects on circulation and the cancerous tumours. Research continues to dispute the original concerns that massage therapy can spread cancer. The support to dispute this myth grows each year through credible experts and numerous studies."[20]

The Cancer Council of New South Wales explains this further: "Cancer may spread (metastasize) into the lymphatic system via the lymph nodes, or it may start in the lymphatic system itself. However, the circulation of lymph—from massage or other movement—does not cause cancer to spread. Researchers have shown that cancer develops and spreads because of changes to a cell's DNA (genetic mutations) and other processes in the body."[21]

---

[17] http://www.dummies.com/how-to/content/knowing-when-not-to-massage.html

[18] http://www.cancerresearchuk.org/cancer-help/about-cancer/treatment/complementary-alternative/therapies/massage-therapy

[19] http://www.macmillan.org.uk/Cancerinformation/Cancertreatment/Complementarytherapies/Typesoftherapies/Massagetherapy.aspx

[20] http://www.massagetoday.com/mpacms/mt/article.php?id=13542

[21] http://www.cancercouncil.com.au/17958/b1000/massage-and-cancer-42/massage-and-cancer-benefits-of-touch/

Not only is correctly applied massage for someone with cancer not harmful, it can be incredibly helpful. Having a diagnosis of cancer is for most people a traumatic and isolating time. They may feel that they have no control over their body, that their body has let them down, and despite the very caring and careful work by oncology units, cancer treatments are "given" or "done to" the body. High-tech and potent medical treatments can dominate life, while the worry about the outcome of both the disease and the treatments can take over the mind and cause extreme stress and anxiety. Massage can provide a profoundly therapeutic touch during this time. The Cancer Council of New South Wales reports that receiving massage during cancer can have real positive benefits, including making the person feel "whole again." It allows people to share feelings in an informal setting; it can help people feel more positive about their body and rebuild hope.[22]

A large American study looked at the effects of massage therapy on almost 1300 individuals with cancer over a three-year period. People in hospital had a 20-minute massage, and others treated as outpatients had a 60-minute massage session. The study found that, overall, massage therapy reduced pain, nausea, fatigue, anxiety, and depression. The benefits lasted longer in the patients who had the 60-minute session.[23]

Many health care professionals recognize massage to be a useful noninvasive addition to standard medical treatments. Therapeutic massage is most often given by trained massage therapists, although caregivers can also be trained in safe massage techniques.[24]

Before looking at the specific contraindications for massage for someone with cancer, it is worth first talking more about what cancer is and how it spreads. Our bodies are made up of more than a hundred million million (100,000,000,000,000)

cells.[25] The different parts of the body—organs, bones, muscles, skin, blood—are each made up of different types of specialized cells. At the heart of each cell is the nucleus, which has within it thousands of genes made from DNA. DNA is what defines us physically—human DNA is different to dog DNA or plant DNA. The DNA takes the form of a double helix; it is this DNA that carries the hereditary information that means we inherit features from our parents, grandparents, and down through the generations.

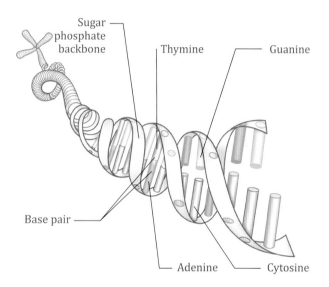

DNA has the ability to copy or duplicate itself; when cells divide to create new cells, each new cell has an exact copy of the DNA present in the old cell.[26] The human body has within it an amazing capacity to reproduce; most of our cells are replaced with new, duplicate, cells when they get old, worn out, or damaged. The blood is a good example of this as the human body makes millions of new red blood cells every single day; the old ones are broken down by the body and are flushed away. Our bodies are in a constant state of renewal and healing. Sometimes this process goes wrong, and a cell becomes abnormal when one or more genes within the cell get damaged or changed. The reasons for this can be complex—it may be something that the gene is

[22] Ibid.

[23] Ibid.

[24] http://www.cancer.org/treatment/treatmentsandsideeffects/complementaryandalternativemedicine/manualhealingandphysicaltouch/massage

[25] http://www.cancerresearchuk.org/about-cancer/what-is-cancer/how-cancer-starts

[26] http://ghr.nlm.nih.gov/handbook/basics/dna

predisposed to and this can produce cancers that repeat across generations, but in other cases it is an environmental factor such as smoking that introduces the change. If the abnormal cell also has this capacity to divide and reproduce, a group of abnormal cells forms; as this continues to develop, the group of cells becomes a tumor. Not all tumors are malignant (cancerous), but we are focused here specifically on cancerous tumors. The tumor then grows and spreads, damaging and invading other tissue around it.

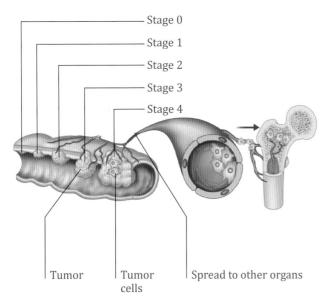

Stage 0
Stage 1
Stage 2
Stage 3
Stage 4

Tumor   Tumor   Spread to other organs
         cells

Most, if not all, solid tumors also shed cells into the lymphatic system and the blood system; understanding of this is still developing within the surgical world,[27] but a small number of these cells may then embed and cause a new tumor—this is the process known as metastasis. Research into understanding this in the medical world is an ongoing process and a critical part of the fight against cancer, but we know that many thousands, if not millions, of cells may be shed from a tumor as part of the tumor's growth.

Not all cancers will form a solid tumor; for example, with leukemia the cancer cells build up in the blood and sometimes the bone marrow rather than forming a solid mass.

Specific Contraindications

There are some clear contraindications for massage during and after cancer that the practitioner or friend or family member needs to be aware of in order to provide a safe and effective treatment.

Massage over and immediately around the area containing the tumor should be avoided. We know that cancer cells can shed from a tumor, and this happens naturally once a tumor has its own blood supply. There is clinical evidence that during some cancer surgeries additional cells may be released from the tumor site, and where this is a risk factor for a particular surgery, it is dealt with as part of the overall treatment.[28] What we do not know is if direct pressure on the tumor can also increase the rate of shedding, so we must always act with caution and avoid any pressure at all directly onto a tumor. While most tumors would be too deep to reach with hand pressure from massage—for example, if they are in the liver, pancreas, or brain then these are areas we would not access through massage anyway—but other tumors in the skin, skeletal muscles, bone, or bowel could be accessible, and so we must act with the utmost caution. This is worth repeating: there should be no pressure applied directly over a tumor during a massage treatment.

If an area is suspected to contain a tumor but this is not yet confirmed, treat the area as though it does until a tumor is ruled out.

If the location of a tumor is unclear then only the lightest of pressure should be used for a massage treatment.

For anyone whose cancer has spread to the bones, or who has osteoporosis or any other bone-thinning condition, there is an overriding requirement to avoid any deep pressure. If the cancer has spread to the bones then the bones can be weakened, there could be lesions on the

---

[27] http://www.sciencedaily.com/releases/2012/05/120507210137.htm

[28] http://www.cancertreatmentwatch.org/general/biopsies.shtml

bones, and growth might be uneven within the bone. Massage should be light, avoiding deep pressure or any joint manipulations as this could lead to bone fractures. By "light," I mean the massage should only be as strong a touch as you might use to apply a moisturizer or sunscreen to the skin.

If someone's vital organs have been affected by the cancer or the cancer treatment then massage should be very light touch—the same "applying moisturiser" principle as above. The organs to be concerned about are the brain, heart, lungs, liver, and kidneys; if any of these organs has been affected then use gentle massage so that you are not adding any additional challenges to the body.

Care needs to be taken with the type of massage oil used during radiation and/or chemotherapy treatment as the skin can become very sensitive. Using a pure base oil, a prescribed lotion, or the client's own moisturizer can be a better option than aromatherapy oils. If you are in any doubt about this, speak with, or ask your client to speak with, their oncologist about the best lotion or oil to use during treatment.

Massage on or immediately around areas treated by radiotherapy should be avoided for the duration of the treatment and until a few weeks after the radiotherapy has finished; even if the tumor is too deep to be accessed by massage the skin will be affected by the treatment, so work on this area is contraindicated.

For clients undergoing chemotherapy, consult with their oncologist as to when in their treatment cycle a massage would be most appropriate. This will not be the same for all forms of chemotherapy or all clients so this should be checked on a case-by-case basis. If the chemotherapy drugs used change during their treatment, recheck that the massage timings you have established are still appropriate. During chemotherapy treatment the client will come to

what is referred to as the "nadir period" (a nadir is the lowest point of anything). At this point the blood cell counts are at their lowest. While chemotherapy directly targets cancer cells, it also affects healthy blood cells in the process. Red blood cells, white blood cells, and platelets are cells that are manufactured in the bone marrow, and as bone marrow activity may be decreased, this may result in lowered blood cell counts within the body.[29] Again, check the timing of massages with your client's oncologist.

People taking blood-thinning medication, or whose platelet count is low as a side effect of chemotherapy, may be very susceptible to bruising, so specific medical consent should be sought for these clients prior to massage.

If there are any intravenous lines in place as part of the treatment these must be avoided for massage.

If blood clots are considered a risk, massage should be avoided. A doctor may permit massage on unaffected limbs, but it is essential to check with the client's specialist first.

Lymphedema can be a problem after surgery, either because of postsurgical swelling or because surgery has removed lymph nodes. If this is the case, deep massage to that area must be avoided but specific massage for lymphatic drainage can be very beneficial. A description of how to do this is included later in this chapter and many hospitals will offer this as a free treatment; specialist training is also both available and recommended in manual lymphatic drainage.

As massage involves skin-to-skin contact, it is critical that massage practitioners ensure that they are not at risk of introducing any kind of infection, either by having a cold or other illness themselves, or having come into contact with anyone else who may have, within their clinic.

---

[29] http://cancer.about.com/od/chemother3/a/nadir.htm

The hygiene of the practitioner, their linens, and their clinic are critical, with extra care being required when treating someone undergoing cancer treatments.

Chemotherapy can affect the digestive system. Sickness, nausea, constipation, and diarrhea can all be experienced and abdominal massage is generally contraindicated. Chemotherapy can also affect the skin, hair, and nails. Skin can become dry or inflamed, hair and nail loss can occur, and it is important for the massage practitioner to avoid any areas of inflammation and take particular care not to massage over any areas of broken skin or where nails have come away.

Peripheral neuropathy can also occur with chemotherapy; there is a separate chapter on this condition, but it's worth saying here that it is important to only work very gently and take into account all other factors around cancer and chemotherapy in treating this.

While this is a frightening list of side effects and contraindications, it is important to note that not everyone experiences the same side effects or even to the same degree. Massage during chemotherapy should be in consultation with the client's oncologist, doctor, or nurse and will need to be reviewed before each treatment. If treatment is not appropriate for that individual during chemotherapy treatment, then the massage can be booked ahead so that the client has something else to look forward to on completion of their treatment.

Once clients have finished their treatment they should then check again with their oncologist whether there are any areas that should be avoided for future massage, and you may be able to increase your pressure as the body recovers from the side effects of the treatments.

Specialist Massage or Friend and Family Massage?

It is critical when massaging someone with cancer for there to be an ongoing client consultation so that you can assess needs as they develop, but it will depend on where you are working as to how you access this information. In much of Europe the expectation would be that the client liaises with the oncologist and it would be rare to find an oncologist speaking directly to the massage practitioner. In some US states there would be an expectation that oncologist and massage practitioner would have a direct relationship. There is no worldwide consensus or mode of working for this.

There is a growth in specialist oncology massage training and in some places this training would be a requirement to be able to treat someone professionally, but that is not the case everywhere. It is the view of this author that massage, essential touch, is a great gift that we can give both professionally and to friends and family. If you are working professionally then, even if it is not a legal requirement for specialist training where you are based, it is best practice to obtain this training. Of course, not everyone can afford to pay for professional massage treatments and one of the gifts we have to give to each other as human beings is the gift of touch; don't be afraid to massage a friend or family member in need—but do so mindfully and cautiously so that you "first, do no harm."

Massage Treatments

How then can massage be safely practiced for someone with cancer? Taking into account the contraindications and special concerns raised above, then massage can usually be given, but it should be lighter. If the person has neck tension then working the hands, arms, head, shoulders, neck, back and the top of the chest, as detailed in the relevant chapters, will be effective in eliminating that tension in the same way as it would for someone without cancer. If someone with cancer develops Dupuytren's contracture then you can safely follow the directions for treating this specific condition—just take into account the contraindications.

We can treat individuals for their ongoing conditions and injuries just taking into account these specific ways of working. While cancer treatments might dominate someone's life for a while, it does not need to define the person. Many people undergoing chemotherapy might need to rest for the whole period and be treated very gently but others might take the opportunity to take on new challenges and physical tests—the case study given below illustrates this point.

Case in Point: Ben Ashworth

Ben is a long-term client of mine who was diagnosed with stage 4 bowel cancer in 2012. In 2013 he was given a terminal prognosis, and at the age of 35 was given 6–12 months to live. The youngest of his 3 daughters was just 5 months old at the time. Ben started treatment and was given an innovative targeted drug that the specialists hoped would buy him extra time with his family, alongside a more traditional chemotherapy drug.

Having always wanted to run a marathon, Ben decided it was time to get training and he started running.

Three years on he is going strong and has smashed his aim to run one marathon by averaging one a month for the last 24 months; he has completed 24 marathons in 24 months while undergoing a heavy and debilitating regime of fortnightly chemotherapy.

Ben has visited me for massage on regular occasions during training and before or after a marathon. We do not do any abdominal massage. If he has upper body tension we avoid the area of his arm where his pic line is fitted for him to receive his treatment and I go light on his back in the area in which his liver lies behind. I use a neutral massage oil which I know will not interfere with his chemotherapy drugs and we try to time the massage so that he has his treatment from me 2–3 days before he has his chemotherapy. His oncologist is delighted that he runs and very happy for him to have his massage treatment. With these precautions, I massage him as I would any other runner. At times he has incredibly tight feet and calves and I am sure that Ben would not say that I worked gently on them.

Ben, pictured here with his wife Louise when they had both just finished this year's London Marathon is one of the most positive people I know and does everything he can to raise awareness of bowel cancer. He pushes his body to the maximum and he is defying the odds of his diagnosis—I am very privileged to be part of his journey.

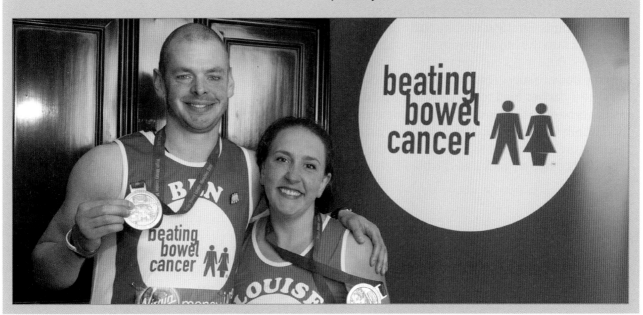

Manual Lymphatic Drainage

One additional massage treatment to consider as part of this chapter is manual lymphatic drainage (MLD) massage. MLD is used in cancer care to assist with lymphedema. Lymphedema is a chronic swelling in the tissues and MLD is used to help to drain the excessive fluid; the most common cause is lymph nodes having been removed as part of cancer treatment.

MLD is not a cancer-specific massage; the lymphatic system may be compromised for a number of reasons (for example injury, infection, or genetic condition) and it is essential to know the underlying cause before determining if massage is appropriate. Critically, not all chronic swelling is due to lymphedema—it could be due to heart failure, kidney disease, or injury—so it is vital to establish the cause of the swelling prior to treatment and this should be in consultation with the client's oncologist.

Before explaining how to carry out lymphatic drainage massage it is helpful to know what the lymphatic system does. The lymphatic system is a network of thin tubes running throughout the body, the tubes are known as lymph vessels or lymphatic vessels, and also involves various organs including the spleen, thymus, tonsils, and adenoids.

The lymphatic vessels carry a colorless liquid called lymph. The lymphatic system has four main functions. Firstly it continuously drains fluid back into the blood system; as the blood circulates, fluid leaks out from the blood vessels into the body tissues. This fluid is important because it carries food to the cells and waste products back to the bloodstream. The leaked fluid drains into the lymph vessels and is carried through the lymph vessels to the base of the neck, where it is emptied back into the bloodstream.[30]

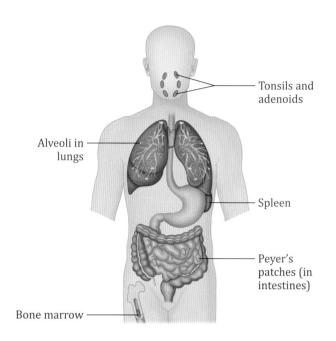

Tonsils and adenoids

Alveoli in lungs

Spleen

Peyer's patches (in intestines)

Bone marrow

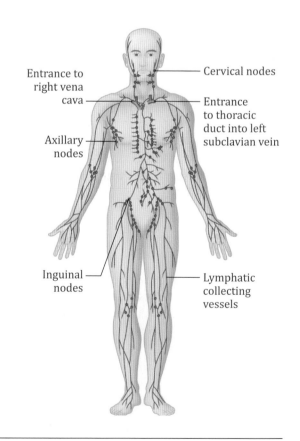

Entrance to right vena cava

Cervical nodes

Entrance to thoracic duct into left subclavian vein

Axillary nodes

Inguinal nodes

Lymphatic collecting vessels

---

[30] http://www.cancerresearchuk.org/cancer-help/about-cancer/what-is-cancer/body/the-lymphatic-system

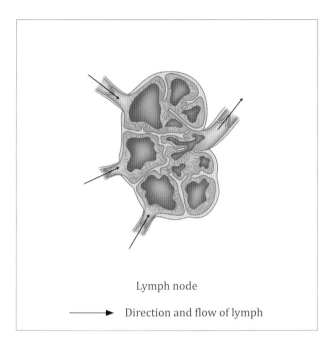

Lymph node

→ Direction and flow of lymph

these are the cells that produce antibodies—and the lymphatic system also detects and destroys foreign bodies.

Removing part of this system can result in swelling and fluid retention in the area affected. This can sometimes show itself as a soft puffiness under the skin but in other cases the skin will be sore and stretched as the fluid builds up to a high level; this can impair movement and cause a lot of pain and is known as lymphedema. The whole system of lymphatic flow and drainage can be compromised when an area of lymph nodes has been removed as part of surgery to remove a tumor or prevent the cancer from spreading.

There are specialist massage practitioners who will give lymphatic drainage treatments, and train individuals in how to encourage lymph flow, particularly when all of the lymph nodes have been removed. It is also safe to do a version of lymphatic drainage massage at home, either on friends or family members, or as part of a self-care regime. There are different terms in use for this; when done professionally it can be referred to as lymphatic drainage therapy, and the terms manual and simple lymphatic drainage are more often used when the treatment is self-given or given to friends or family. Regardless of the terminology, the aim of the treatment is to increase the flow of the lymphatic fluid through the lymph system.

The second role of the lymphatic system is to filter the lymph fluid as it passes through the lymph nodes. In terms of cancer, lymph nodes are checked by oncologists because when cancer cells break away from a tumor they will often get trapped in the nearest lymph nodes, so checking lymph nodes indicates if a cancer has spread. The third role of the lymphatic system is the filtering of the blood; this takes place in the spleen. The spleen filters the blood, taking out all the old, worn out red blood cells and then destroying them. They are replaced by new red blood cells that are made in the bone marrow.

The spleen also filters out bacteria, viruses, and other foreign particles found in the blood. White blood cells in the spleen attack bacteria and viruses as they pass through.[31] Lastly the lymphatic system fights infection. The lymphatic system, though described as a system in its own right, is actually part of the body's immune system. The lymphatic system has a critical part in white blood cell (lymphocyte) production—

Lymphatic massage is a gentle, light-touch massage. The lymph system is very close to the surface of the body and it is surface work that will have the positive impact. We are used to, in most Western massage, always working upward toward the heart, but lymphatic drainage massage is different this massage starts by working outward and then comes back in.

---

[31] Ibid.

Firstly you are opening up and clearing the system, then coming back in you are rinsing it—all the time working with the body's natural flow. The lymphatic system does not have a pump of its own, as the heart is to the circulatory system, so the massage helps to stimulate the natural flow It is worth repeating that lymphatic massage is very gentle; there is no deep or even moderate pressure. Sometimes just stroking the skin is enough.

The three main moves to practice on yourself before working on someone else are gentle skin stroking, gentle pumping, and gentle pulling upward. The skin stroking is literally a surface stroke. There is no need to use massage oil anywhere for this with the exception of the face, where the skin is very thin, and there you can choose to use it or not, depending on what your client wants. The second technique is a very gentle pumping action with the flat of your fingertips; practice this on your own hand first—work on one pump every one to two seconds where you are pressing down and slightly forward (a half to three-quarters of an inch maximum), but only at a depth where you are moving the skin. You should not be working on the muscle apart from on the very surface of it—the aim is to work just the skin.

Finally, practice a gentle pulling-upward motion; this can be easiest to master when you are seated by hooking your fingers underneath the inside of your leg and pulling your fingers gently upward, again so that you are just moving the skin, not the underlying muscle. As the aim is to stimulate the lymphatic system and to move lymph you do not want to be encouraging blood flow by also moving the muscles.

You can treat just the area affected, if it is localized to one site, or the whole body. Whichever part of the body you are working on, or if you do treat everything, you should always both start and finish a treatment with the vital neck work detailed below. Of the 6–800 lymph nodes we all have, a third are in the area of the head and neck.

Macmillan Cancer Support, as well as massage practitioners, encourages deep abdominal breathing at both the start and end of a treatment; this comes before the neck work at the beginning and again afterward at the end. This breathing helps to encourage lymphatic drainage by stimulating the deep areas of the lymphatic system. Make sure that your client is breathing into the abdomen. With one hand on the chest and one on the belly, the belly hand should lift up first with the in breath, followed by the chest hand. Breathing out, the belly hand should sink back down first. This is also the breathing that will help to quell panic or anxiety, so is a great technique to learn in itself.

The nodes underneath the clavicle (collar bone) are the key to opening up the whole lymphatic system, and this is where a full treatment would start. With your client lying down, or with you lying down if you are self-treating, use a small pillow or folded up towel to ensure that the forehead is raised higher than the chin; this then allows gravity to help in the process. Whichever area you are working on with MLD should be raised, so use pillows and cushions and adjust your client's position as needed as you work.

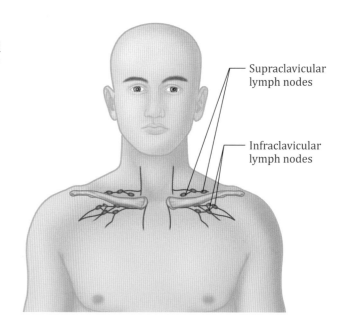

Supraclavicular lymph nodes

Infraclavicular lymph nodes

Begin by gently pumping the area just above the clavicle on both sides so that you are pumping downward into the area just beneath it—only a feather-light touch should be needed for this. Repeat these pumps between 30 and 50 times around one second apart; it should not be at all uncomfortable for your client. Move up the side of the neck by a half to three-quarters of an inch, and use your index and middle fingers together to do 10–15 pumps on that spot before moving another half to three-quarters of an inch and repeating the process until you have worked all the way up the neck. You may feel the thick ropey muscle of the sternocleidomastoid muscle (SCM) in the neck; you are not working on this muscle but you are following its line, so it is a helpful guide as to where to work.

Then move your fingers to the back of the neck and gently pull down the back of the neck. If your client has a long neck do this in two or three sections, starting closest to your shoulders and pulling downward, then moving up to the next section and pulling downward, until you have worked the whole neck. If you are splitting this neck work into two or three sections, do approximately 20 pull downs per section. If you can work the whole of the back of the neck in one go then do 50–60 repeats of this very gentle movement.

Next make a V with your fingers so that your little finger and ring finger are together, as are your index and middle fingers, place this V either side of your ears, and use a downward gentle movement to stroke from the top of the ear to the top of the neck. Repeat 50 or 60 times.

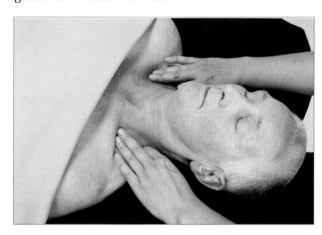

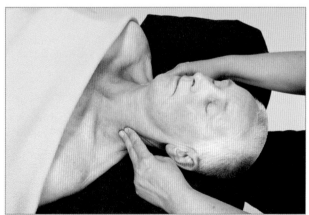

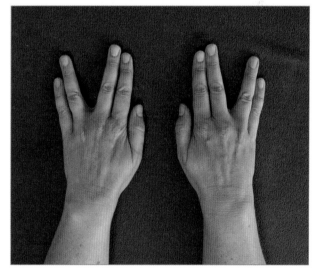

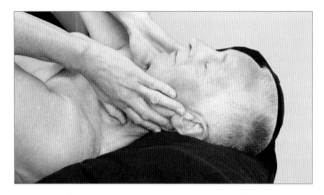

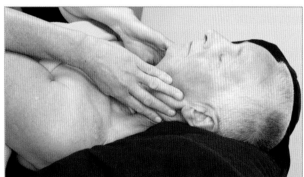

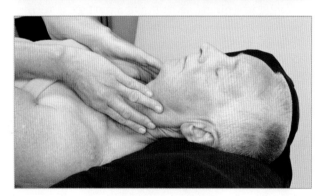

The lymph system is a liquid system and, as with clearing any liquid, as you clear it from one area it will allow the fluid built up behind it to flow down and create a suction or vacuum to draw the fluid down. This means that treating the part of the lymphatic system closest to the lymph nodes can also have a beneficial effect in clearing the rest of that area. Working the neck as above will also drain the face without needing to specifically work on the face itself.

A whole quadrant of the body can be affected by the removal of lymph nodes; for example, if the nodes in the left armpit have been removed, the lymphatic flow in the whole of this left side of the body may be compromised as a result. Likewise if the nodes in the right groin are removed, the lower right quarter of the body will be affected (image below).

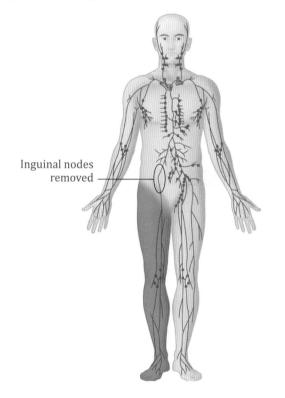

Inguinal nodes removed

After you have done this V work, repeat the work on the back of the neck 50–60 times, followed by repeating the side of the neck work 50–60 times, then repeat the move you started at the front of the neck above the clavicle. Remember that with lymphatic work you are clearing up and rinsing down, so it is always important to work back down with the same moves that you have worked upward.

You may find during this neck work that your client needs to swallow or feels that they have a tickle in the throat; these are good signs that the massage is working and are nothing to be concerned about.

To release lymphedema in the arms, start with the neck work and then, ideally supporting the arm so that the elbow is above the shoulder to allow gravity to assist, curl your fingers into the curve of the armpit. Relax the arm; you should not be using enough pressure to hurt even this delicate and sensitive area, and if the client is ticklish simply work through the clothes.

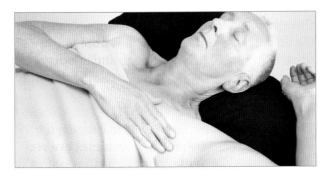

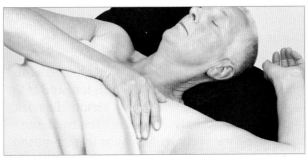

Pump upward with your fingers at least 50 times at a speed of just one pump per second. After that move to the inside of the elbow close to the body in the elbow crease, and simultaneously both pump and pull upward.

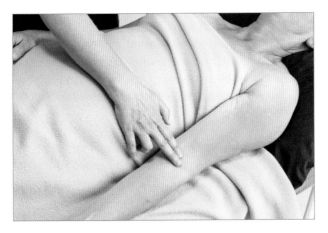

This draws fluid from the forearm and hand. Repeat the combined pump and pull 50 times before returning to the armpit and repeating that work, and then finishing by repeating the all-important neck work.

To drain fluid built up in the legs you need your client to be seated in a reclined position, with the back somewhere between lying down and sitting down. The legs should be supported with pillows to allow for gravity to assist the drainage process.

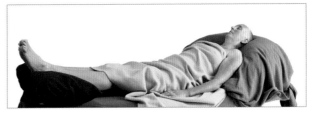

Ensure that the ankles are above hip height. The main lymphatic draining area for the lower body is in the crease between legs and torso and then up into the torso, so this is where we start the massage. Remember again that this is very light work so you are not applying much pressure at all in these moves, and it is different in both nature and application than the abdominal work mentioned elsewhere in this book.

Begin by placing your hand approximately one hand's width below the belly button in the center of the belly, and with a flat or cupped hand pump up and down into the belly (barely pressing the belly in, you are working at a surface level) at a speed of around one pump per one to two seconds, and repeating this 10–15 times.

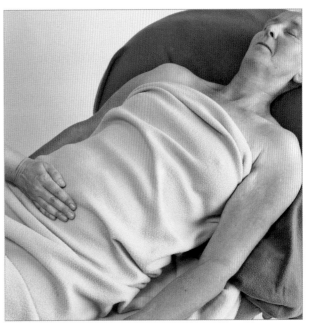

Next move your hand out toward the hip so that your hand is partway between the belly button and the hip, and repeat the light pumping 10–15 times, and repeat on the other side. Move down one hand's width and repeat.

Then place your hand on the inner thigh just below the crease between the belly and the leg and just above the midline of the leg, so that you are just below the groin area on the leg.

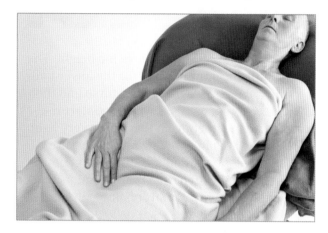

Repeat the pumping motions slowly, around 30–50 times. Repeat this pumping one hand's width down, and continue with this for as many hand pumps as it takes you to reach the top of the knee. Then repeat this whole process, working down to the knee another two times. On the second time, continue down across the inside of the knee, stopping as you get below the knee.

Cup your hand underneath the back of the leg, just above the inside of the knee, and gently pull in an upward motion 15—20 times.

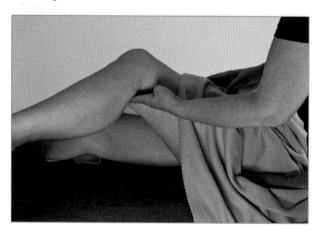

Once you have done that, repeat this motion up the entire leg, working just one hand's width at a time. Repeat this two or three times before going back to the abdominal pumping, and repeat that action as above.

This is a very simple and gentle massage but very effective—even if the foot and lower leg are very swollen, then doing this work above the knee will help to drain it without you having to work directly on the swollen and probably tender area that is affected by the swelling.

To summarize the order of treatment, start with the breathing, then the neck work, followed by arm or leg (or both) work, then back to the neck, and finally back to the breathing. The treatment has a nice flow to it so once you start to get used to this way of working it should be a relaxing treatment for both the person receiving the massage and the person giving it.

There are other specific and specialized techniques for lymphatic drainage massage that may be pertinent to your or your client's case. Working with a professional massage practitioner trained in lymphatic massage can be of great benefit, and some oncology departments will have someone on hand to assist with this and to teach self-massage techniques for individual problems.

The techniques described here can be of great benefit and, once mastered, are simple and effective for at-home treatments.

Cerebral Palsy

Background to the Condition

Cerebral palsy is a condition that affects muscle control and movement. The word cerebral means relating to the brain, and palsy refers to a complete or partial loss of the ability to move a body part. So cerebral palsy means loss of ability to move a body part because of a problem with the brain.[32] It is usually caused by an injury to the brain before, during, or (more rarely) after birth.[33] The main causes of cerebral palsy include a lack of oxygen to the brain, an infection in early pregnancy, abnormal brain development, and, very rarely, trauma to the brain in early infancy.

There are four classifications of the condition: spastic, athetoid, ataxic, and mixed. Spastic cerebral palsy accounts for around 70% of all people with the condition; the muscles will be very stiff and can be permanently shortened and this can make movements very jerky.

Athetoid (or dyskinetic) cerebral palsy occurs in approximately 20% of cases. Some people with this type of cerebral palsy have slow, writhing movements of the hands, arms, feet, or legs. Some people have sudden muscle spasms. These movements cannot be controlled. Sometimes the tongue or facial muscles are affected.[34]

Ataxic cerebral palsy occurs in less than 10% of cases. People with ataxic cerebral palsy have difficulties with balance and fine movement. This can mean loss of balance or being unsteady when walking. It can also make doing fine tasks with the hands, such as writing, difficult. The muscle tone is usually decreased rather than stiff.[35]

The fourth classification is mixed cerebral palsy, which is combination of the first three. Cerebral palsy ranges from mild to severe. Mild cases may result in an usual gait and some unsteadiness; severe cases may leave the individual needing full support in daily living or needing to use a wheelchair.

The massage techniques here can be adapted as needed; some people will not need all aspects of them and you can select those that are more useful based on individual need.

Cerebral palsy is not progressive in terms of the initial brain injury; the brain injury itself does not progress, but as the person grows up the impact of the injury becomes more apparent and as the muscle spasticity continues then joints can be pulled out of place. Massage can give symptomatic relief for the muscle tightness and pain.

---

[32] http://www.patient.co.uk/health/Cerebral-Palsy.htm

[33] http://www.scope.org.uk/help-and-information/cerebral-palsy

[34] http://www.patient.co.uk/health/Cerebral-Palsy.htm

[35] Ibid.

The younger the person with cerebral palsy is, the more effective the massage will be, but at any age some relief can be given to ease the muscles. In a study at the University of Miami School of Medicine, massage was given twice weekly to 20 young children with cerebral palsy with an average age of 32 months. The results concluded that the children receiving massage therapy showed fewer physical symptoms, including reduced spasticity, less rigid muscle tone overall, and improved fine and gross motor functioning.[36]

Massage also has a social role to play for clients who have cerebral palsy; most will have many routine hospital checks and physiotherapy, some will need assistance with daily living, so much of the contact with people outside immediate family is more akin to being handled rather than touched. Massage offers a chance for gentle and caring touch in a supportive environment.

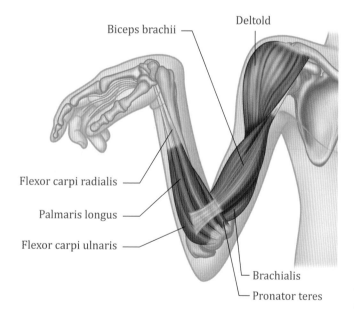

Biceps brachii

Deltold

Flexor carpi radialis

Palmaris longus

Flexor carpi ulnaris

Brachialis

Pronator teres

Specific Contraindications

If you are treating an adult with mild cerebral palsy, you can treat the person as you would for any other massage—if they have plantar fasciitis, a sore neck, etc., then treat for that. There are no barriers to treatment for people who are affected mildly. The instructions for massage below are targeted to those with more severe cerebral palsy and to treating children when the extent of the impact is not yet fully known.

The only contraindication to massage for clients with cerebral palsy is if the client cannot speak to express their wishes and to comment on depth. It is important then for the practitioner to be sensitive to the verbal and nonverbal cues given by the client and to respond accordingly. If the client and the person administering the massage do not know each other, it is important for the client's sense of security to have someone they do know present so that they can feel safe during the massage. If you are a parent or carer giving massage as part of everyday home care, it can become a part of the daily routine.

Massage Treatments

It is important to work gently, and use small stroking movements both up and across the muscles. Try to make the massage quite mobile, so that as you work you are gently moving the part of the body you are working on—this helps to introduce movement without resistance from the muscles.

If the client is a wheelchair user who has uncontrolled limb movements, it will be safer to carry out the treatment with the client in the wheelchair; being lain on a massage table runs the risk of the client falling off, and client safety must always be paramount. If the client prefers, the massage could take place on their bed, with bed buffers in place to avoid any risk of falling.

[36] http://www.hawaii.edu/hivandaids/Cerebral_Palsy_Symptoms_in_Children_Decreased_Following_Massage_Therapy.pdf

Using essential oils in a massage can enhance the experience for a client. Whether you are qualified in aromatherapy and blend your own oils or are buying pre-blended oils, allow your client to select the oil that they like the smell of that day.

For this massage you are working from the extremities inward. It can be relaxing to start with the head, although if you need to establish a new client–practitioner relationship then starting on the hands can be less intrusive and threatening, and you can then move to the head when you have established a relationship of trust.

Begin by working the fingers. The spasticity of the muscles may pull the fingers straight and inward toward the palm. Hold the client's hand in yours as you begin at the top of the fingers, gently roll each section of the finger between your own fingers, and then work all around the fingers one section (the area between the knuckles) at a time, stroking downward from the fingertip to just below the knuckle all around the finger.

Move down to between the next two knuckles and again stroke downward all around the finger, and do the same between the last knuckle and where the fingers join the palms. Do this for all fingers and thumbs, working one hand at a time.

After you have worked the fingers, use your thumb to stroke upward across the palm toward the wrist. Pay particular attention to the side of the hand down from the little finger and to the muscle between the base of the thumb and the palm. Work both up and across the palm so that you are making a series of crosses (if the client is a young loved one then you are making kisses!) on their palms. Turn the client's hand over and use your fingers to stroke up in the grooves between the carpal bones, working up the hand toward the wrist and stopping when the bones come together and the groove runs out.

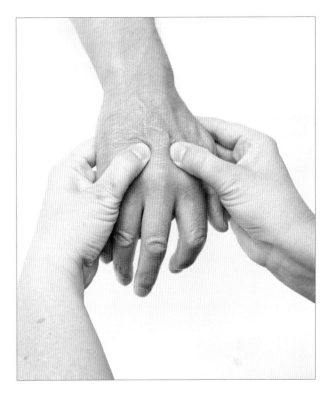

Having worked the hands you are now ready to work the client's forearm. The muscles here are likely to be very small and will feel hard to the touch. Use your middle three fingers together to warm up the muscle by applying gentle cross friction up the forearm. The muscle runs from wrist to inner elbow, so to begin with you are working from left to right across the muscle. Once you have done this three or four times you can follow the direction of the muscle and use gentle strokes to stretch out the muscle. Make sure you do not miss the muscles that run up the outside of the arm, coming up from the little finger, first working across and then up the muscle. Do the same up the outside of the forearm, working just in the space between the bones.

Avoid the elbow and the delicate area inside the elbow, and move to the upper arm. You will be able to work this in four parts: the inner, outer, front, and back of the arm. You will see from the diagrams below that there are a lot of different muscles involved here; do not worry too much about which muscles you are working when—by working the arm in quarters you will work all of them.

You can start working on any quarter and use the same gentle cross-frictional work you have done on the lower arm. Work all around the arm so that you cover all four quarters, and then repeat with the longer strokes up the length of the arm. Make sure you do not massage into the armpit, and stop as you get to the bones at the tip of the shoulders. Using a massage oil will help to lubricate the skin and will make for a more pleasant massage for the recipient.

The same massage techniques can now be used for the feet and legs. Start at the toes, work inward up the feet, up the calf, avoiding the knees as you did the elbows, but when you get to visually dividing the legs into quarters, do not work all the way to the top of the inner thigh, to afford your client privacy. If you are a parent working on a young child you can work higher while the child is comfortable with this.

Having worked the feet and legs and the hands and arms, you can now turn your attention to the head and neck; if you are working with a client you don't know you can opt to leave the head and neck work out for the first few treatments until you have established a good working relationship with your client. The detail about how to do head massage is included in Chapter 4. You can follow this in detail but avoid the detailed jaw work for clients with cerebral palsy as this may be too intrusive.

If your client is lying down, you can work the neck by starting with your oiled hands placed at the back of the body at the top of the shoulders and stroking upward toward the base of the skull—this will gently stretch the neck. If your client is seated, work downward from the neck to the shoulders. Varying the pressure on each finger as you work upward will help the muscles to relax and should help prevent the client tightening the muscles you are working on. This should still be gentle work, particularly for children; after three or four upward strokes you can deepen your pressure a little more and you should start to feel the muscle soften to your touch.

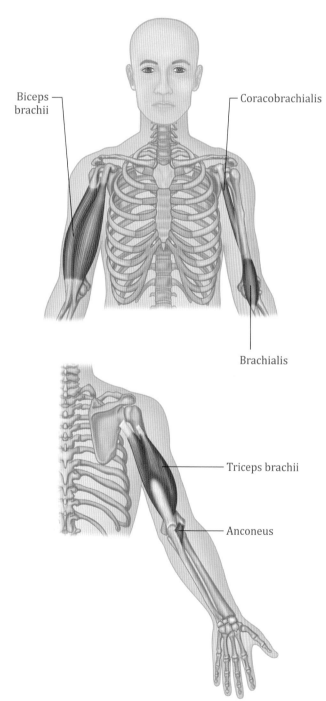

Biceps brachii

Coracobrachialis

Brachialis

Triceps brachii

Anconeus

Posterior view

If your client is lying down, hold the client's head in your hands; you can gently stretch the neck with your fingers, putting gentle pressure under the base of the skull—omit this stretch if your client is seated.

Working the shoulders with your client seated can be challenging, depending on whether your client is able to sit upright unaided. If he or she can, you can work the shoulders together; if not, simply work each shoulder in turn. Start where the neck joins the shoulders and work down and outward toward the shoulder tip, but avoiding pressing onto the bone at the shoulder tip—this would be painful and not beneficial. You can also gently squeeze and rock the muscle backward and forward at the top of the shoulder by rolling your thumb over it. If you have a massage table with a face hole and your client is comfortable and able to lie facedown, then you can do this work with the client lying down.

If the client is seated you will be limited as to how far down the back you can work—just be careful to follow the muscles either side of the spine and be aware that the spine may curve. You should be aiming to stroke down from top to bottom; you can use your thumbs for this—one thumb either side of the spine in one flowing movement. If you are working on a baby or young child who can lie on their front, you can also gently work the sacrum with small circular movements with your fingers across the whole lower back. The whole of this massage can be adapted to children by using a fingertip where thumbs would otherwise be used.

Finish the massage by returning to the hands and repeating the work of earlier. This is a calming, gentle, and nonintrusive way to finish. Treatment should ideally be carried out every day and be a part of daily routine for children or those severely affected; when this is not possible, then twice weekly, or at least weekly. The massage can be carried out by a professional practitioner but it can also be done safely a parent or carer. For a condition where parents often feel helpless looking at the enormity of the needs of their child, this is one practical treatment that can help the child and provide bonding between parent and child. The focus here has been upon more severe cases of cerebral palsy but the same treatments can be given to people with mild cases, and some techniques could be self-administered.

Cervical & Thoracic Spondylosis

Background to the Condition

Spondylosis, while sounding similar to ankylosing spondylitis, is a very different condition. Ankylosing spondylitis is a form of inflammatory arthritis and is covered in its own chapter; spondylosis is a medical term for both osteoarthritis of the spine and the general wear and tear that occurs in the joints and bones of the spine as people age.[37]

The term can be used to describe degeneration in the neck—when this occurs it is referred to as cervical spondylosis. Lower-back spondylosis is called lumbar spondylosis; when it occurs in the middle back it is referred to as thoracic spondylosis. Lumbar spondylosis is discussed later—here we will deal with cervical and thoracic.

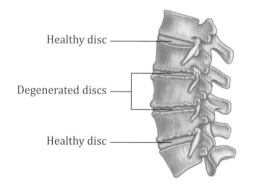

Healthy disc

Degenerated discs

Healthy disc

Cervical Spondylosis

The most common symptoms of cervical spondylosis are neck pain, stiffness, and headaches. There may be a headache that originates in the neck, shoulder, arms, or chest, and a grinding noise or sensation when the neck is turned. Symptoms of cervical spondylosis tend to improve with rest. Symptoms are generally most severe in the morning and again at the end of the day.

As we age, the discs of the cervical spine in the neck gradually break down, lose fluid, and become stiffer. From age 50 onward, the discs between the vertebrae become less spongy and provide less of a cushion. Bones and ligaments get thicker, encroaching on the space of the spinal canal; by the time they reach their 60s, around 90% of the population will have some degree of cervical spondylosis.[38]

Posture, employment, lifestyle choices, and certain exercise regimes can also have an impact on the development and severity of cervical spondylosis.

---

[37] http://www.webmd.boots.com/osteoarthritis/guide/cervical-spondylosis

[38] http://www.nhs.uk/conditions/cervical-spondylosis/Pages/Introduction.aspx

If cervical spondylosis results in pressure on the spinal cord (cervical stenosis), it can damage nerves—a condition called cervical myelopathy—leading to pain and/or pins and needles in the arms and legs, a loss of feeling in the hands and legs, a loss of coordination and difficulty walking, muscle spasms, and abnormal reflexes.

Cervical spondylosis is usually diagnosed through a physical examination, X rays, CT scans, and MRI. Most problems caused by cervical spondylosis will settle down, although they may reoccur at a later stage.

Treatment may include the use of nonsteroidal anti-inflammatory drugs, corticosteroid injections, the short-term use of cervical collars, physiotherapy or chiropractic treatment, hot and cold therapy, exercise, and firm pillow support. Massage can help in reducing pain, to allow the muscles to settle back to normal functioning, and to prevent the problem spreading to other areas as the individual stiffens up in response to pain and overcompensates by using a different set of muscles in order to protect their neck.

In a small number of cases where conservative treatments have failed then surgery may be recommended, and in around one in ten cases a person can go on to develop long-term (chronic) neck pain.[39]

Thoracic Spondylosis

As the thoracic spine doesn't work as hard as the lumbar or cervical spine, degeneration tends to begin elsewhere before affecting the thoracic spine. However, that is not always the case, as spondylosis can affect any part of the spine. Common symptoms of thoracic spondylosis include: pain and stiffness in the mid-back, particularly in the morning after getting out of bed; tingling or numbness in the legs, arms, hands, or feet; muscle weakness; and a loss of coordination or difficulty walking.[40]

For cases of thoracic spondylosis, treatment is usually conservative. Rest, lifestyle or work-habit changes, pain-relieving medications, physiotherapy, chiropractic or acupuncture treatments, and massage are usually effective. Only in the most severe cases would surgery be indicated.

Specific Contraindications

If symptoms come on suddenly and are accompanied by shortness of breath, refer to emergency medical treatment to rule out heart problems.

A possible complication of cervical spondylosis is cervical radiculopathy, when changes in bone structure, for example formation of bone spurs, cause pressure on nerves as they exit the bones of the spinal column.[41] Pain shooting down into one or both arms is the most common symptom.

If any of these symptoms occurs, clients should see their medical practitioner, as these conditions can need more immediate intervention to prevent longer-term nerve damage, and massage would be contraindicated until more serious spinal problems had been ruled out.

---

[39] http://www.nhs.uk/conditions/cervical-spondylosis/Pages/Introduction.aspx

[40] https://www.laserspineinstitute.com/backproblems/spondylosis/bloracic/

[41] http://www.webmd.boots.com/osteoarthritis/guide/cervical-spondylosis

Massage Treatments

Massage treatment is safe to carry out provided there are none of the complications listed above. A SpineUniverse survey in early 2008 showed that back pain patients are very satisfied with massage as a treatment option. It actually had the second highest patient satisfaction rating,[42] coming second only to prescription medication[43] in the perceived effectiveness of getting rid of pain. In spondylosis, the muscles surrounding the spine often become very tense, adding to the pain of the condition. Massage can help release that tension, reducing muscle inflammation and pain. Massage treatment for each of these two conditions will be discussed in turn.

Cervical Spondylosis

As the spine is in some way compromised in cervical spondylosis, massage treatment should be gentle and without any manipulations or sudden movements of the neck. The muscles can be softened and relaxed layer by layer. If you are working on a friend or family member and do not have a massage table with a face hole or face cradle, then only follow the instructions for working with your client faceup, as working with the neck twisted would put too much pressure on the neck and may cause further damage. You will still give pain relief from only doing the work with the client faceup.

Begin with your client faceup and start with a massage of the head, scalp, and face as detailed in Chapter 4. After this, and only if you are able to work with your client facedown, use a little massage oil and begin by warming up the back of the neck, top of the back, and shoulders. Use sweeping motions moving out from the edge of the spine down across the top of the shoulders, and then moving from the center out and down toward the shoulder blades.

Work both sides at once, being careful not to apply any pressure on the spine itself.

As you work you will find tender spots and some areas that feel firmer than others—these are the areas where the muscle tension is held. Don't be tempted to ignore these areas because they're tender; instead, once you have spent three or four minutes with the sweeping and warming-up motions, bring your attention to these tender and resistant areas and give them extra attention, but work slowly and gently so that you gradually release them.

There are two key ways that you can do this safely and effectively. The first is to find the individual tender or tight spots and, only working these one at a time, simply press onto that point in the muscle and hold your static pressure there until you feel the muscle soften and release under your pressure. You can use your finger or thumb, but in order to protect yourself place another finger or your other thumb on top of the first one to give it some added support—this will help to ensure you don't cause damage to yourself while you are trying to help someone else. You may need to hold this pressure for one or two minutes.

Move slowly around all of the tight and tender spots around the back of the neck, top of the shoulders, and upper back. The other technique is to gently shake the muscle; again, find that tight and tender spot and, using your first two fingers, apply moderate pressure so that you are not simply moving the skin, and then move quickly back and forth across the muscle. You should work the opposite way from how the muscle normally lies. Most of the muscles in the neck run up and down the body, so moving across them left to right and back should be effective.

---

[42] http://www.spineuniverse.com/conditions/spondylosis/alternative-treatments-spondylosis

[43] http://www.spineuniverse.com/conditions/back-pain/what-really-gets-rid-back-pain

Continue the shaking for up to a minute before moving on to the next tight area. Don't worry if the skin on the area appears a little red—this simply happens as you encourage blood flow to the area and it is a positive part of the treatment. After you have worked all of the tender and tight areas, finish this part of the treatment by repeating the earlier long stroking movements downward, moving with the flow of the muscle.

If you do not have a massage table and cannot do this initial part of the treatment, you can do an adapted version with the client lying face upward. The client should lie as flat as is comfortable for their neck, with long hair pulled out of the way to the side or top of the table. Warming a little massage oil in your hands, slide your fingers down the side of the spine sweeping outward toward the shoulders; you should be able to do at least two sweeps—one down the outside of the neck and across the top of the shoulders and the other lower down so that your hands slide underneath the shoulders.

People with cervical spondylosis will often have some kind of shoulder tension that will draw their shoulders forward, and this will allow you to get into the shoulders at the upper back more; you do not have to worry about applying additional pressure here as the weight of the body against your hands will give adequate pressure. This may not feel like you are giving a particularly smooth treatment, as the flow will be interrupted by needing to withdraw your hands toward the edge of the shoulders and then replace them close in to the neck after each move, but this is better than compromising the neck by working with the client facedown without the face hole or cradle. You will find that some areas of muscle are more tender for your client or feel more resistant to you. Again, these are the areas to give special attention to; you won't be able to shake the muscle out from this position but you can curl one or two fingers up slightly and hold that position—that alone should be enough to help the muscle to release.

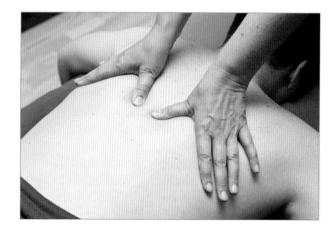

With that initial, but important, work completed in whichever position is possible for you, you can then move to the next stage. You will have already warmed up the head and scalp in your initial massage; now you need to do some deeper treatment to the area at the base of the skull and specific work to some of the muscles that support the neck. You will see on the diagrams below the position of the suboccipital muscles (top diagram, below), the nuchal ligament, levator scapulae, rhomboids, and trapezuis.

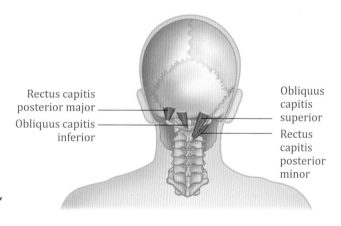

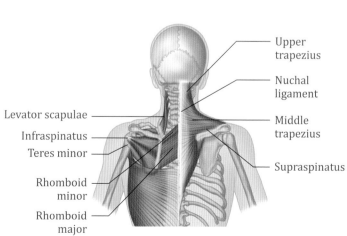

This is where you now need to work. Begin by cradling the client's head in your hands so that your fingers rest underneath the curve of the base of the skull; this is likely to be a tender area and your client will know that you are working there. (Note that you should not do this particular move for a client with Down syndrome.)

Gently curl your fingers upward and hold that upward pressure, encouraging your client to rest their head back in your hands. Heads are heavy so your hands should feel weighed down by the pressure of the client's head. Hold this position for around one minute, and then slowly and gently rock your client's head in your hands—the range of motion for the rock is no more than half an inch in each direction, and work very slowly with this move. Release the client's head and then repeat this part of the treatment, but this time raising the client's head no more than half an inch higher than you did the first time.

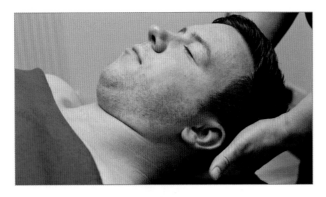

This allows the whole area very gently and naturally to stretch, but without putting any pressure on the neck, remembering that while the cervical spondylosis symptoms are present the neck is vulnerable and painful. When you have finished this move, gently place the client's head back down; do not let it drop back.

Now you are going to work on the splenius capitis muscles—these are the muscles that come either side to the back of the neck, as shown in the diagram below.

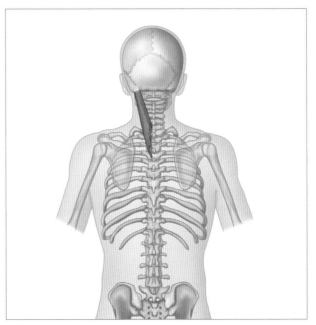

To do this, place your thumbs (with a little massage oil on them) either side of the spine about an inch below where the shoulders start to move out from the neck. Position your hands so that your thumbs are pointing inward toward, but not touching, the spine and then pull your thumbs gently upward toward the bottom of the skull. Your thumbs should move outward slightly as you follow the flow of these powerful muscles; you will find yourself heading toward the outer edge of the skull—stop when you reach the skull and repeat four or five times. If it is too awkward to use your thumbs you can use your middle three fingers, positioning them close to the spine just below the shoulders with your palms pointing upward.

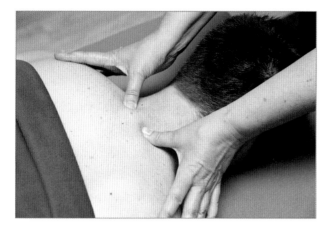

You can also mix and match using thumbs or fingers to ensure that you don't tire your own body. Finally bring your thumbs so that they are parallel with the bottom of your client's ear and move them to the back of the neck, just slightly out from the area you have just been working; you should be on the levator scapulae muscles—these are shown on the diagram (page 83). For these muscles you want to work downward from that starting point going straight down, curling out slightly as you reach underneath the shoulders—repeat this move four or five times.

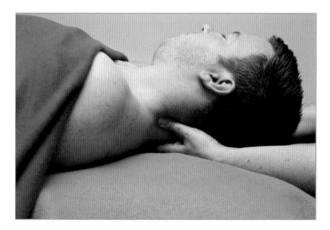

Your client should now be reporting how wonderful his or her neck feels as the muscles have been gently stretched and freed from tension! You can repeat this treatment daily to help alleviate symptoms; allowing the muscles to relax is not only good for relieving pain but will also aid quicker recovery as a relaxed muscle is also a stronger muscle.

Thoracic Spondylosis

Massage treatment should start as for cervical spondylosis, but adds in work on another two important muscles. As the thoracic spine is affected by tension coming up from the arms, massage treatments should also include work on the hands, arms, and shoulders—detailed in Chapter 2. People who do manual jobs that include a lot of lifting, those who spend long hours at a computer or carrying arms full of documents, and those involved in manual therapies (including massage practitioners) are liable to get problems with their thoracic spine as they lean forward using these muscles.

After you have worked down from the neck and inward from the arms, pay particular attention to the trapezius and rhomboid muscles (see diagram page 83) as these are likely to be both tender and tight. With the client lying facedown, start from the spine and work upward and outward into the trapezius and outward and down into the rhomboids. Begin with the warming-up sweeping motions and follow this up with the muscle shaking and static pressure work detailed above. You can also include the lower-body work as detailed in the chapter on lumbar spondylosis if you and your client wish—this gives a more holistic approach to the treatment.

Treatments for both of these conditions are effective, gentle, and safe and can either be carried out by a qualified professional, who may also add in other moves to the treatment, or they can be carried out at home. Ideally these treatments should be performed daily, and you should find that they make a significant positive difference to both the pain levels and the mobility of your client.

Chronic Fatigue Syndrome / Myalgic Encephalopathy

Background to the Condition

Chronic fatigue syndrome (CFS) causes persistent disabling fatigue or extreme tiredness (exhaustion) that is so bad it affects everyday life.[44] It does not go away with either sleep or rest. CFS is also known as ME, which stands for myalgic encephalomyelitis or myalgic encephalopathy.[45] Myalgia means muscle pain and encephalomyelitis means inflammation of the brain and spinal cord. Encephalopathy refers to a disease damage or malfunction of the brain.

There are a number of separate but similar conditions which come underneath this heading and research is ongoing.[44] CFS is sometimes also called chronic fatigue, or post-viral fatigue syndrome, or immune dysfunction syndrome. Along with the extreme tiredness there can also be muscular pains, joint pains, disturbed sleep patterns, poor concentration, and headaches. The term preferred by patient groups is ME, as "fatigue" sounds a little vague; ME will therefore be the term used in this chapter.

There is still no clear medical evidence or agreement as to why some people develop ME, but some of the factors that are thought to contribute include: an inherited genetic predisposition to developing the illness, viral infections such as glandular fever;

Legionnaires' disease; exhaustion and mental stress; depression; or a traumatic event such as bereavement, divorce, or redundancy. In addition, there are factors that are thought to make the condition worse, which include recurring viral or bacterial infections, not being active enough or being are too active, stress, poor diet, being socially isolated and/or feeling frustrated and depressed, and possibly environmental pollution.[45] Some research suggests developing ME could be linked to disorders of the immune or hormonal systems. Many people who develop ME were previously fit and active.[46] Research is ongoing.

There is no one test for ME so its diagnosis tends to be by the elimination of other illnesses that may give similar symptoms, when extreme tiredness has persisted for six months of more. Symptoms may vary from mild to severe, but even mild symptoms can mean carrying out the activities of daily life and holding down a job are extremely difficult. Those with severe symptoms may need to use a wheelchair to get around and may have difficulty even brushing their own hair. Those with ME, which was originally nicknamed "yuppie flu," can have a hard time having their symptoms taken seriously and may have to battle for a diagnosis. Treatment is often symptomatic: painkillers to help with muscle aches and pains, antihistamines for allergies, and sleeping

---

[44] http://www.nhs.uk/conditions/Chronic-fatigue-syndrome/Pages/Introduction.aspx

[45] http://www.patient.co.uk/health/chronic-fatigue-syndrome-me

[46] http://www.bupa.co.uk/individuals/health-information/directory/c/hi-chronic-fatigue-syndrome#textBlock201827

tablets for the insomnia that can accompany such extreme tiredness. Some people find that massage can help and it certainly has fewer side effects than long-term use of some medications.

Raymond Perrin, a UK-based osteopath, is conducting research into the role of the lymphatic system and recovery from ME. The work is still controversial owing to the lack of trials to date, but a number of patients have given good, positive feedback. Massage as a treatment stimulates the lymphatic system and, while some argue that alternative treatments shouldn't be used as they are expensive and unproven. Massage can be given by a massage practitioner or freely performed by friends or family members.

Specific Contraindications

There are no specific contraindications for working with a client with ME but, for some sufferers, ME and fibromyalgia may present together, and even without this added complication, the nature of the illness and the painful effect it has on the body would urge for gentleness and caution with treatment. As we are working with the lymphatic system it is important to work upward and inward in this treatment—always work up limbs and toward the heart. This works with the body's lymphatic system, encouraging the natural cleansing mechanism of the body. You can also carry out the lymphatic drainage massage described in the chapter on massage and cancer. It is vital with any treatment, but even more so for someone with ME, that the client is encouraged to drink lots of water following a treatment to facilitate this natural process. If a client gets a headache or has dark urine following a treatment, they need to drink more water.

Massage Treatments

You can begin a treatment at any part of the body and it may be nice to break treatments down into upper and lower body so as not to overwhelm clients or their system. Use a little massage oil, warmed in your hands, and start with either the hands or the feet, following the massage protocol in the relevant chapters, and use your fingers to perform stroking movements up the hand or foot. Make sure that you massage both sides and remember that you are not pressing so deeply that the person is in pain—you will exhaust the client by working too deeply or too quickly, but you also want to work deeply enough that you are working on the muscles and not just the skin.

Use long stroking movements up the legs or arms, covering all areas at the front and back of the body, you can use any of the treatments described in this book for individual massages but just use gentle pressure and slow movements. Once you have worked the hands and arms you can continue to work the shoulders and back. Try to get a flow and rhythm to your treatment, this will help the client to drift off; although ME leaves the person feeling tired it can be very difficult to "switch off," so that is one of the aims of your treatment. Both starting and finishing your treatment with the head massage detailed in Chapter 4 can help the client to do this, and you could consider giving a head massage as a treatment in its own right.

There are some very useful acupressure points that can be called into use during this massage. If your client is interested in following this route more fully then a consultation with a qualified and registered acupuncturist may give much better results, following very specific and individualized treatments; however, you can use some of these points and integrate them into your massage. In acupuncture and traditional Chinese medicine there would be an assessment of the person to treat their individual needs; however, these points are common to most treatments for ME:[47] ST 36, Du 20, and PC 6.

---

[47] http://www.acupuncturetoday.com/archives2005/aug/08wang.html

ST 36 is a point on the stomach meridian and is used to eliminate fatigue. It is located on the shin about a hand's length below the kneecap, just outside the prominent tibia bone. Pressing onto this point can be very powerful and it is much used in acupressure as an energizing point. Simply hold the point, applying pressure with your thumb or knuckle.

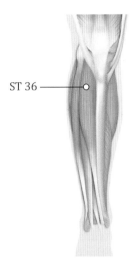

ST 36

Du 20, on the governing vessel meridian, is used to treat a variety of conditions including vertigo, dizziness, and insomnia. In traditional Chinese medicine it is an important crossing point within the energy system; its Chinese name Baihui translates in English to mean "hundred meetings" or "hundred convergences." This point can be found in the center of the top of the head by following up from the apex of the ears in a straight line to the midpoint of the head, as shown in the diagram. This is a very relaxing point to hold as part of a head massage, and the client may also report feeling the tension from that point going into the jaw—working the jaw will help to release that, which can help to ease headaches, but pressing on Du 20 alone can be powerful.

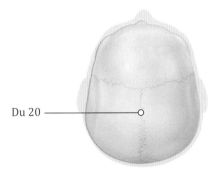

Du 20

Finally PC 6, on the pericardium meridian, is found on the inner wrist; amongst other things this point opens and relaxes the chest, helping alleviate chest tightness and insomnia, while also being useful in treating nervousness, stress, and poor memory. It can be found two of the client's thumb widths above the crease of the wrist, in the middle of the large strong tendons you will be able to feel in front of the wrist; again, applying pressure here during treatments will give some people relief and will do no harm.

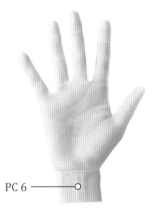

PC 6

One factor to bear in mind when treating ME with massage is that any massage can give rise to what is termed a "healing crisis;" this is where someone may feel worse before they feel better. For someone with ME this might make an almost bearable day unbearable, so it is important to work slowly and gently in short sessions until both practitioner and client know how the client will respond to the massage. Building length of treatment and depth with time is a good and safe way to work.

ME is a long-term condition and it would be incorrect to look to massage for a miracle cure from a long, deep session; indeed, this could make things worse. Instead build slowly; only deepen the treatment with time and constantly evaluate both how the client was after the last session and how the symptoms are on the day the treatment is planned. Finally: water, water, water.

If your client is going to support their lymphatic system, drinking plenty of water after a treatment is crucial.

Constipation

Background to the Condition

Constipation can be an annoyance for most people at some stage in life, but for some people it can be a chronic (long-term) condition that causes significant pain and discomfort and affects quality of life.[48] How many people this affects varies according to age, social demographics, and country, but one study where people self-reported being constipated found that 5% of Germans considered themselves to be constipated, against 18% of people in the USA.[49]

Constipation is not an illness in itself; rather it's a symptom of another illness or condition. This can be as simple as being dehydrated, or a diet too rich in processed food that doesn't include enough fiber. Stress and depression can have an effect on digestion, making bowel movements sluggish, and some medications cause constipation as a side effect.

Being too sedentary or ignoring the urge to go to the toilet can also cause constipation, as can severe trauma or poor childhood toilet training. In rare cases there may be a serious underlying illness that needs further investigation.

Specific Contraindications

- If someone has blood in their stools or unexplained weight loss, then massage is contraindicated and a medical practitioner should be consulted.

- Do not use this massage on a client who is pregnant

- Do not use this massage on a client who has had recent abdominal surgery (within six months)

- Do not use this massage on a client who has Crohn's disease or a leaky gut

- If the constipation goes on for longer than three weeks, despite making sure you are properly hydrated, eating roughage, and moving around, then a medical practitioner should be consulted.

---

[48] http://www.nhs.uk/Conditions/Constipation/Pages/Introduction.aspx

[49] http://www.medscape.com/viewarticle/560953_5

Massage Treatments

Technically, two things happen during abdominal massage for constipation relief: it gently increases pressure in the abdomen, which encourages rectal loading, and it stimulates peristalsis (the movement of food, liquids, and waste through the intestines). Gentle abdominal massage is very effective in relieving constipation and is safe to use with children, adults, and the elderly. It can be a treatment given by someone else or can be self-administered.

It is important to work with the natural flow of the bowel (clockwise) and to work both the small and large intestines. Although they share a name, the small and large intestines have very different functions. In the small intestine nutrients are broken down for the body to use; in the large intestine (made up of four sections: the cecum, colon, rectum, and anal canal) some B vitamins and vitamin K are produced, some water, vitamins, and salts or ions are absorbed,[50] and the leftover food is made into stools for elimination. The junction between the small and large intestines is the ileocecal valve; this prevents fecal matter from returning to the small intestine.

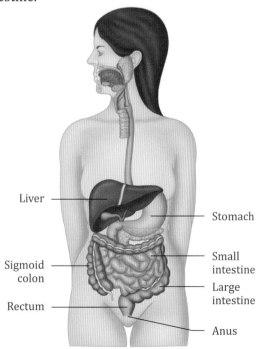

Liver

Stomach

Sigmoid colon

Small intestine

Large intestine

Rectum

Anus

Begin your massage by placing your hand with the navel at the center of the palm, gently shaking the belly for three to four seconds—repeat three or four times. Then begin the detailed massage by working on the small intestine. You can either work through clothes or directly onto the belly; if you are working directly use a small amount of warmed oil to lubricate the skin and do make sure you warm your hands too! Starting at the bottom right, about an inch below the belly button (about half that for children), make clockwise circles around the belly button; you do not need to press hard, just press firmly enough that the skin gently indents as you massage over it.

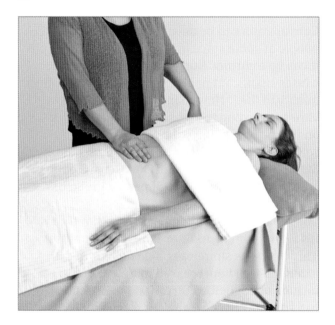

After you have worked the small intestine, move outward to the large intestine. Start at the bottom right of the client's belly, just to the inside of the hip bone. If you place a towel parallel with the top of the hip bones, that is the lowest you should work, and you only work as high as the start of the ribs. Begin by working in a large circle so that you move upward toward the ribs, across to the left-hand side, down the left-hand side, and then back across the lower belly to your starting point. Work in these smooth, large circles five or six times with the flat of your hand, gently pressing into the belly.

[50] http://commondigestivedisorders.blogspot.co.uk/2009/09/difference-between-small-and-large.html

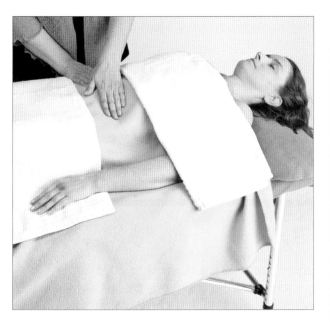

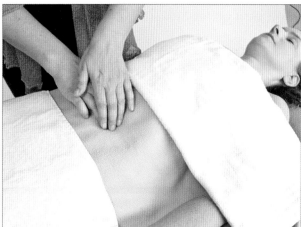

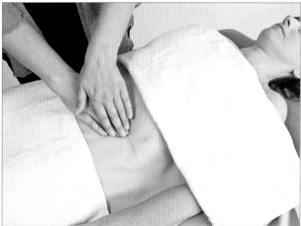

Having completed this warm up work for the large intestine you can begin to work a little more deeply. It is important to work with the client's breath for this movement, pressing in only on their out breath and releasing all pressure when they need to breathe in again. Using the flattened tips of your three middle fingers, start again at the lower right of the client's belly and gently press so that your fingers begin to depress the skin; ask for feedback—the client should feel your pressure and it may be a little uncomfortable but it should not be painful. Press in and move your fingers gently from side to side, moving no more than half an inch at a time and then release when your client needs to breathe in again.

Repeat all the way up until just before you reach the ribs. Now repeat the same movements, working along the belly from right to left toward the left ribs, again stopping just before the ribs. Using the same movements, work downward toward the inside of the left hip.

Finally work along the bottom of the belly; you stay above the pubic bone until you return to the starting position. Repeat this process three times around the belly and then return to the initial circling movements around the large intestine.

Relief should be fairly quick following this, and passing wind during a treatment is quite normal, but treatment can be repeated as needed and if one treatment does not give relief then it can be repeated an hour later. Encourage clients to drink water after a treatment to ensure that they are well hydrated. If you are working with a child, the treatment can be made into a game or, for persistent childhood constipation that has no underlying condition, then gentle abdominal massage can be a part of the nighttime routine.

This massage is also good for irritable bowel syndrome.

Cramp

Background to the Condition

Cramp is an involuntary spasm of the muscle caused when an already shortened muscle shortens further. It is a very painful condition and very common. The calf is the area most affected but foot cramps are also fairly common.

The majority of cramps occur at night. Known as nocturnal cramps, these are remarkably common, with 60% of the adult population reporting suffering from this at some point.[51] Most sufferers will wake as a result of the cramp, leading to fatigue for them and, usually, anyone they are sharing a bed with, as they leap out of bed shouting "I've got cramp." Cramp is usually short-lived, anything from 30 seconds to 10 minutes, but the muscle may be painful for 24 hours after the initial cramp subsides.

The propensity to suffer from cramp seems to increase with age, with around a third of the over-60 population and half of the over-80 population reporting regular leg cramps.[52] Pregnant women, children, athletes, and those with physical jobs are also more at risk than the rest of the population.

When a muscle is already shortened it is at greater risk from cramping, which is why most cramps occur at night—the foot relaxes and, for most people, the top of the foot will elongate, which puts the calf in a shortened position. Dehydration, working in heat, or not stretching after exercise all increase the likelihood of cramp.

Specific Contraindications

There are no specific contraindications for massaging for cramp.

Massage Treatments

Massage can help alleviate the acute cramp when it happens and regular treatment, combined with self-help stretching, can help to prevent cramp occurring. Massage during an acute cramp attack needs to be gentle as the muscle will already be painful. Self-massage of the affected area is also possible, although it can be easier if someone else does the massage.

[51] RE Allen and KA Kirby, Nocturnal leg cramps. *American Family Physician*, 2012, Aug 15;86(4): 350–355.

[52] http://www.patient.co.uk/health/cramps-in-the-leg & http://www.patient.co.uk/doctor/muscle-cramps

If the cramp is in the calf, gently shake the calf muscle—it will be very tight so even gentle work will be intense for the person receiving the treatment. Shake the muscle for 10–20 seconds and then stretch the calf out by holding the foot firmly on the bottom half of the foot, so that you are grasping the base of the toes and not just the toes, and stretch the toes upward toward the front of the body.

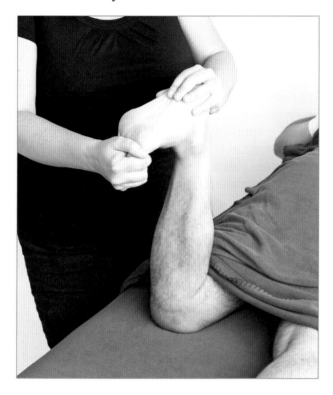

Work with your client so that you stretch within their tolerance; hold the stretch for 30 seconds, release it, and shake the muscle again—it should start to feel looser. Repeat the shaking and stretching until the sufferer reports that the cramp has gone. Then, using some oil or body lotion/moisturizer (assuming this massage is likely to take place in the middle of the night rather than in a clinical setting), stroke upward from the ankle to about an inch below the knee. Stroke up the outer side of the calf and then more gently up the inner calf. The inner calf will be tender so you need to use about half as much pressure as on the outer calf. After a few strokes on both sides, repeat the shaking of the muscle and the calf stretch that you did in the initial stages. Repeat this calf stroking, shaking, and stretching three or four times. Finish by

massaging the sole of the foot, by placing your thumbs at the base of the toes and move both thumbs upward and outward, moving rapidly and working up toward the heel; repeat three or four times.

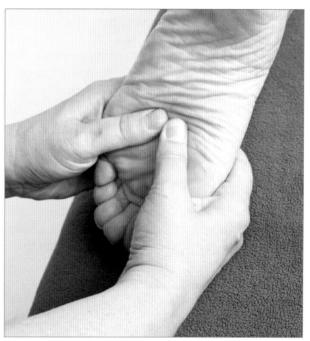

This whole treatment should not need to last more than 10 minutes and it should shorten the length of the cramp episode.

If the cramp is in the foot you need to work on first releasing the contracted muscle. The muscle in the arch of the foot is the usual culprit, so holding the toes firmly at their base and stretching the foot upward toward the front of the body will give some initial release. Next try to work out which toe is affected the most—usually it will be the big toe. Hold the big toe below the knuckle so that you are not putting any pressure on the joint and stretch the toe upward toward the front of the body. Hold both of these stretches for 20–30 seconds and alternate between the two stretches. Shaking the muscle out is difficult as they are very small muscles, but by placing one or two fingers firmly on the affected muscle and quickly moving the fingers in the opposite direction to the muscle, across the width of the foot and so that you are not sliding across the skin, you will be able to move the skin and muscle as a whole.

If the cramp is in the back of the thigh, shake out the muscle using your whole hand to go across the width of the leg in quick motions, making sure you are moving the skin and muscle and not just sliding across the surface of the skin. As this is a much bigger muscle you can also slide up the length of the muscle. Using the heel of your palm, place the hand one to one and a half inches above the knee joint and use long stroking movements up the full length of the muscle, stopping one to one and a half inches below the buttock.

The stretching needs to be done by the person with the cramp rather than you. There are a different ways to do this: first, with the person standing, the affected leg should be put out in front so that the only heel of the foot is touching and then he or she should lean inward. Care needs to be taken not to put pressure on the knee joint, but just a gentle lean in will be enough to stretch out the thigh. Secondly, standing with feet approximately hip width apart in front of a wall and with both hands on the wall, the person should lean into the wall so that the back of the leg is stretched outward.

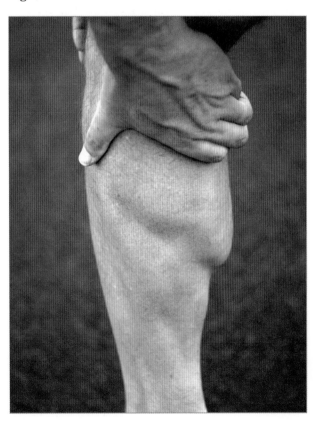

Repeat the shaking, stroking, and stretching until the initial cramp subsides. You can then ask the person to lie on his or her front and, using a little oil or moisturizer, use the flat of your hand or the heel of your hand to stroke the muscle from just above the knee to just below the buttock.

Be careful to never put any pressure on the back of the knee joint. Work all around the muscle, starting at the outside and moving inside. How many times you need to do this will depend on the thickness of the person's calf, but repeat all of the strokes three or four times.

This advice so far has been for night cramps, when the back of the leg is the most affected area. For sports people or for people in physical jobs cramp can be elsewhere in the body, but the same principles apply. The cramping muscle will have become shortened so you need to stretch it out by stretching in the opposite direction: if the cramp is in the back of the arm, stretch out the front of the arm; if it is in the buttock, then raise the knee as far as possible so that the muscles are stretched out. The shaking and stroking principles apply to any area of the body.

If you are working with someone who regularly suffers from cramp then you can direct your massage to help to prevent cramp. Your focus in these treatments needs to be releasing the tight and shortened muscles—these will usually be in the legs and that is the detail discussed here, but you can adapt the treatment to other areas of the body.

If someone is suffering from repeated cramps in the legs then it is important not to treat just the legs—this is where the symptoms of the muscular tightness are felt, but the cause of that tightness may lie further down in the feet so, for preventative or remedial work for leg cramps, the feet should be worked in detail and you can follow the instructions in Chapter 3 for this treatment.

Having completed the detailed foot massage you can then move on to work into the calf.

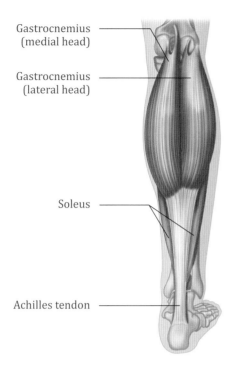

Gastrocnemius (medial head)

Gastrocnemius (lateral head)

Soleus

Achilles tendon

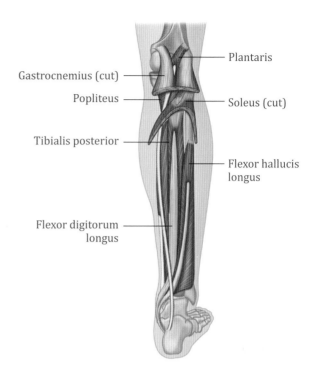

Gastrocnemius (cut)

Popliteus

Tibialis posterior

Plantaris

Soleus (cut)

Flexor hallucis longus

Flexor digitorum longus

Gentle warm-up work with long strokes and shaking out of the muscle will start to release the fascia and the surface layers of muscle. Once this work is completed you can begin to move more deeply to work on both the surface and deep muscles. Work each side in turn and avoid going directly in depth at the midpoint in the calf—working too deeply here without freeing the surrounding muscle will be very painful for your client.

Working up the outside of the leg first and starting just above the ankle working up to just below the knee, you can begin to knead these muscles using either your thumb or the ball of your hand; as the muscles start to release you can use the side of your forearm to be able to get greater depth. As always, work to the depth that your client can tolerate. After you have worked this area, work the inner calf; you will need to work more gently on this area, which is usually quite tender and can easily bruise. Follow the same pattern with deep strokes and kneading. Only once these muscles have been worked should you focus on the middle of the calf.

Placing your thumbs together either side of the Achilles tendon, work up the center of the

calf in smooth, long strokes, which can deepen with repetition. As you get to the midpoint of the leg you will reach the "belly" of the calf, and at this point separate your thumbs so that you stroke outward across the top half of the lower leg (the soleus muscles). Repeat these moves five or six times until you can feel the muscles soften. Coming back to the center point on the upper half of the lower leg, you come to work the gastrocnemius muscle, the big surface muscle at the top of the calf, and this can be worked with quick rhythmic moves; again, always working upward but stopping one to one and a half inches below the back of the knee.

As you will be deepening your massage as you work, you will also be treating the deeper layer of muscles. As a guide, for most people you will be pressing one to one and a half inches deep into the muscle (depending of course on the size and strength of your client—for a very thin client you may be working at half an inch's depth). At all times obtain feedback from your client as to the depth that is appropriate for him or her.

If the cramps are usually experienced in the calves then you can complete the treatment with general massage work into the outer thighs and gluteus muscles; if the cramps are experienced in the thighs then carry on with this more detailed work further up the leg, focusing your attention on the mid and outer thigh where the problems usually occur. You can stroke up the full length of the thigh using the heel and palm of your hand, being careful to keep your fingers outward to avoid stroking the client's inner thigh, gradually getting deeper with each stroke but always within your client's tolerance.

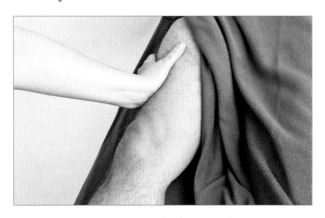

It is important to follow up this massage work with advice on stretching to help prevent the muscles shortening and therefore cramping. The two stretching exercises given earlier in this chapter can be supplemented with one that utilizes the bottom step of the stairs (below). The client, holding onto the banister or wall, should stand with the front of the foot on the stairs so that the ball of the foot is in contact with the stair.

The client can then allow the heel to drop over the edge of the step, and a deep stretch will be felt within the belly of the calf. The stretch should be held for 15–20 seconds, the heel lifted back up to counterstretch, and this repeated three or four times. This is a stretch that can be integrated into daily life as a single (not repeated) stretch every time the client goes upstairs. It takes seconds to do but has a very significant effect in helping to reduce cramps.

If the cramps do not improve or if the client has any concerns or a complex medical history, a visit to their GP should be encouraged. There are some medications for which cramps can be a side effect, including some diuretics and statins.

Dehydration is a major cause of cramp, as is an untreated underactive thyroid. Imbalances in body salts, such as a high or low sodium or potassium level, can lead to cramps, as can excessive alcohol and peripheral arterial disease, a narrowing of the arteries leading to poor circulation. If in doubt, ask your client to get checked out medically.

In athletes and amateur sports persons, not stretching after exercise can also be a cause and is a useful first line of questioning. A member of the local football team whose cooldown is going to the bar can often remedy their problem with stretches and water!

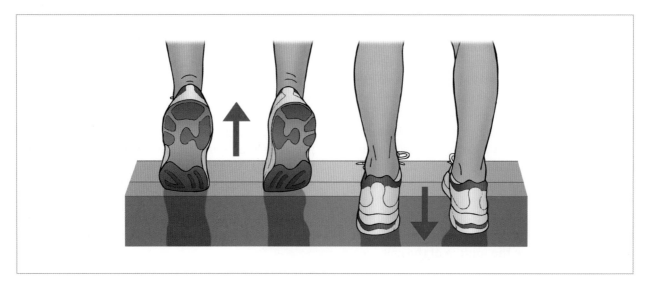

Down Syndrome

Background to the Condition

Down syndrome is a common genetic condition accounting for approximately 1 out of every 691 live births.[53] Most people have 23 pairs of chromosomes, giving a total of 46 chromosomes; someone with Down syndrome has an extra chromosome 21 (47 instead of 46) or one chromosome with an extra part of chromosome 21. There are three different forms of Down syndrome. Trisomy 21 comprises 95% of cases. This is due to an error in cell division called "nondisjunction," resulting in an embryo with three copies of chromosome 21 instead of the usual two. Prior to or at conception, a pair of 21st chromosomes in either the sperm or the egg fails to separate. As the embryo develops, the extra chromosome (or part chromosome) is replicated in every cell of the body.[54]

Mosaicism occurs when nondisjunction of chromosome 21 takes place in one—but not all—of the initial cell divisions after fertilization. When this occurs, there is a mixture of two types of cells, some containing the usual 46 chromosomes and others containing 47. Those cells with 47 chromosomes contain an extra chromosome 21. This accounts for 1% of cases.[55] In the remaining 4% of cases, Down syndrome is caused by translocation. In translocation, part of chromosome 21 breaks off during cell division and attaches to another chromosome, typically chromosome 14. While the total number of chromosomes in the cells remains 46, the presence of an extra part of chromosome 21 causes the characteristics of Down syndrome.[56]

While people with Down syndrome will share some common features, the condition varies greatly in its severity and impact.

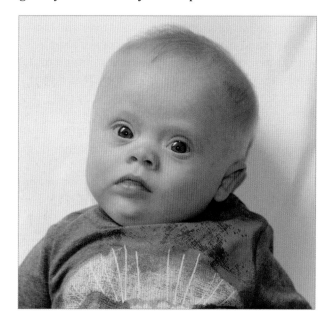

---

[53] http://www.specialolympics.org/Sections/Who_We_Are/Down_Syndrome.aspx

[54] https://www.ndss.org/Down-Syndrome/What-Is-Down-Syndrome/

[55] Ibid.

[56] Ibid.

The common physical characteristics of Down syndrome include: decreased or poor muscle tone; a short neck; excess skin at the back of the neck; flattened facial profile and nose; small head, ears, and mouth; upward-slanting eyes, often with a skin fold that comes out from the upper eyelid and covers the inner corner of the eye; a single crease across the palm of the hand; and a deep groove between the first and second toes.

In addition, cognitive impairment is common in people with Down syndrome and usually ranges from mild to moderate (this is only rarely severe), and may include: a short attention span, poor judgment, impulsive behavior, slow learning, and having delayed language and speech development. People with Down syndrome are also at increased risk for a range of other health conditions, including autism spectrum disorders, problems with hormones and glands, hearing loss, vision problems, and heart abnormalities.[57]

With good support and appropriate health care, life expectancy for someone with Down syndrome has increased massively over the last 25 years and is currently 60 plus; many people with Down syndrome will live independent, or semi-independent, and fulfilled lives. Massage at any stage of life will be good, as touch can be extra important to someone with Down syndrome, but there are also some specific therapeutic benefits, particularly in childhood.

Specific Contraindications

There are two specific areas to be very careful of; these are not contraindications, but where special care is needed. Apart from these two specific areas, each person needs to be treated simply as any other individual regarding health issues, which may or may not be associated with the Down syndrome, using the contraindications

and adaptations specific to that medical condition.

Some children with Down syndrome are hypersensitive to touch and do not like being touched, but this is an important part of life so gentle massage, done playfully with young children, can help to overcome this. However, avoid the mouth area; children with Down syndrome who are hypersensitive will particularly not like their mouth being touched,[58] so this area should be avoided during massage treatment.

The second factor to bear in mind with massage is that, for some people with Down syndrome, the upper part of the cervical spine under the base of the skull is different than for someone without Down syndrome. Muscles are weak and ligaments may be looser than they should be. Potentially, this can cause the vertebrae in the neck to press on the spinal cord, leading to an inability to coordinate muscle movement and weakness,[59] so it is important not to hyperextend the neck of someone with Down syndrome, nor to undertake any swift movements of the neck that could cause any compromise to the neck.

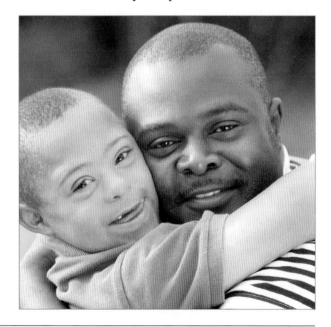

---

[57] http://www.specialolympics.org/Sections/Who_We_Are/Down_Syndrome.aspx

[58] http://www.cmdss.org/resources/therapies/speech-therapy/

[59] http://orthoinfo.aaos.org/topic.cfm?topic=A00045

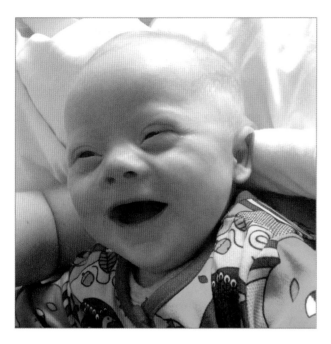

Massage Treatments

Hernandez-Reif et al., in the journal Early Child Development and Care, document a study in which 21 moderate-to-high functioning children with Down Syndrome, with an average age of two years and receiving early intervention (physical therapy, occupational therapy, and speech therapy) were randomly assigned to additionally receive two half-hour massage-therapy or reading sessions per week for two months. The children's functioning levels were assessed on the first and last day of the study. The study found that the children in the massage-therapy group had greater gains in fine and gross motor functioning and less severe limb hypotonicity when compared with the children in the reading/control group. These findings suggest adding massage therapy into an early intervention program may enhance motor functioning and increase muscle tone for children with Down syndrome.[60]

Massage can be introduced from birth and can be a great bonding experience for parent and child. Massage can also be introduced at any stage in life, both for children and for adults. Be gentle in your massage and, for older children and adults, offer a choice of massage oils for the client to choose. Start any massage with long strokes to warm up the muscle and be careful to avoid working close to joints, specifically the knees, elbows, and shoulders, where it might be easy to over extend joints. For the same reason avoid any strenuous or assisted stretches as part of the massage. Always work from the outside in, and don't neglect the client's hands, feet, and head; you can use the protocols in Chapters 2–4, just omitting any stretches.

There are two very specific techniques that can be utilized for clients with Down syndrome. With babies, there can be a problem with overfrequent discharge or tearing from the eyes due to tear duct abnormalities, this will be worse when the baby has a cold, and while this can need surgical intervention, massage can also be successful. The area to be worked is the tear sac, or lacrimal sac, region. This is in the area between the eye and the nose; be careful not to press onto the eye itself.

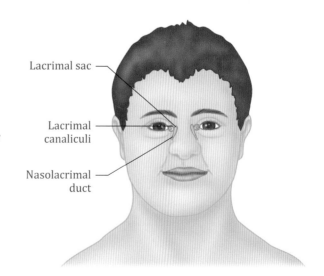

Lacrimal sac

Lacrimal canaliculi

Nasolacrimal duct

[60] http://www.tandfonline.com/doi/

Practice this on yourself before trying it on a client or your baby. Practically speaking, you need very short fingernails to do this and always wash your hands thoroughly before this treatment. Using your little finger, place the tip toward the inner corner of the eye and gently press against the nose, moving up and down the space close to the corner of the eye. Do this for around five to ten seconds, two or three times a day, every day. One in five babies will suffer from a problem with their tear ducts and this becomes more common in Down syndrome babies, but is something that usually resolves on its own by 12 months without the need for any surgical intervention; gentle massage can help in some cases so it's worth a try.

The second treatment that is worth giving, for a baby, child, or adult, is abdominal massage. With decreased muscle tonality, constipation can be a problem for those with Down syndrome, so gentle but frequent belly massage can help. This can either be carried out skin to skin if you are working with a young child or a close friend or family member, or done through clothes if that is more appropriate to your setting and therapeutic relationship.

For this abdominal massage you need to make circles around the belly, starting off with smaller circles around the belly button to help with the transit of digesting food through the small intestine and then in larger, wider circles around the belly to treat the large intestine and to assist with the flow and elimination of fecal matter.

You do not need to worry about knowing where one starts and the next begins, but always work clockwise around the belly so you do not disrupt the functioning of the ileocecal valve, which is the link between the two parts of the bowel, and so that you are encouraging rectal loading by increasing intra-abdominal pressure; this can produce rectal waves that stimulate bowel sensation,[61] helping the individual move their bowels.

After you have moved around the belly in gentle circles you can gently press on the belly as you circle; keep this as very gentle pressure with two or three fingers for babies, and this can be increased as necessary with older children or adults. You may find areas where the belly feels hard and that these soften as you gently press onto them; this is usually compressed fecal matter, and it's not unusual for clients to be quite gassy as you work the belly, so let them know that it's perfectly ok to pass wind as you work. Abdominal massage can work very quickly to relieve constipation so if a client has travelled a distance to you for a treatment this needs to be considered. This gentle form of abdominal massage can be effective and is very safe to do; some clients will also be able to self-administer it.

Massage for clients, friends, or family with Down syndrome can be a very loving part of life—and if you are working with a friend or family member you may well be able to teach the recipient to give you massage in return.

[61] http://www.nursingtimes.net/nursing-practice/clinical-zones/continence/does-abdominal-massage-relieve-constipation/5027718.article

Dupuytren's Contracture

Background to the Condition

Dupuytren's contracture is a condition that can cause the fingers to contract, sometimes meaning that the person loses normal functioning of the hands.

First, to explore some of the myths that surround Dupuytren's, this condition is not caused by overuse, operating machinery, or too much golf, nor is it a virus. Rather it is a thickening of the connective tissue below the skin—but on top of the tendons. In this way it is similar to scar tissue, and as it builds it pulls the fingers forward. Its exact cause is unknown but it is thought to have a genetic link, so runs in families. It is most common in the hands but can also occur in the knuckles, the soles of the feet, and, for some men, it can develop in the penis, causing a curvature.

Dupuytren's contracture is more common in men than women and is mainly a condition of middle age and onward. When women do get it they tend to present less severe symptoms. Men of northern European heritage seem to be at much greater risk than other groups. There appears to be an increased chance of men with Dupuytren's contracture also developing diabetes, but this is not yet fully understood.

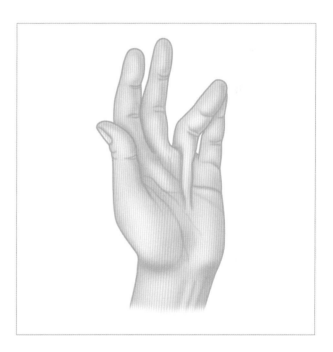

The condition is normally painless, but is very inconvenient as the affected fingers become progressively and permanently difficult, or impossible, to use. Surgery is often carried out to release the fingers, but with mixed results. Other specialists recommend injections or radiation treatment, but for some these cause unpleasant side effects.

Specific Contraindications

None.

Massage Treatments

Massage will not completely fix a hand that is already badly impacted by Dupuytren's contracture but it can make a positive difference, and the earlier the massage treatment starts, the better. In the first stages the condition can appear as nodules in the palm, most often (but not always) at the base of the ring finger or little finger. As the tissue thickens it causes a shortening of the palmar fascia, the fibrous tissue that lies under the skin of the palm. Releasing this contracture in the early stages will help the hand to remain more flexible.

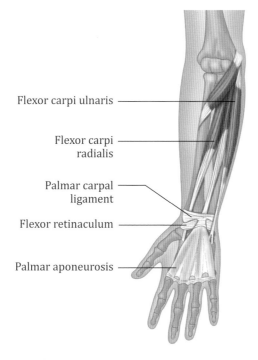

Flexor carpi ulnaris

Flexor carpi radialis

Palmar carpal ligament

Flexor retinaculum

Palmar aponeurosis

The protocol for massaging the hands is the same as that detailed in Chapter 2, and you should ensure you follow this in detail, not neglecting any part of the treatment. Massaging the hands in detail, and frequently, will be most effective, ideally working at least weekly to begin with.

The client also needs to commit to doing stretching exercises with the hands two or three times each day; pressing the hands together, palms and fingers touching, and then drawing the palms away so that the fingers stay connected. As the client is able to do this more easily, treatments can be drawn out to fortnightly, then every three weeks, aiming for a monthly maintenance

treatment—but with the stretching carrying on as part of the client's daily routine. A necessary part of that routine is the client stretching their hand to spread the fingers outward. Where the condition is more advanced, this initial stretching of curled-in fingers will need to be done manually, with the client pressing each finger backward with the thumb and holding the stretch for 20—30 seconds, or as much as is comfortable to do; this can be carried out at home by the client as part of his or her daily routine.

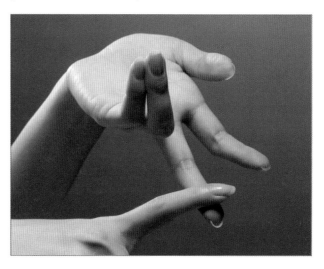

The stretching may feel uncomfortable but should not be too painful, if it is painful then just relax the stretch, and take your time to get to a fuller stretch. This exercise also needs to involve the wrist—with the wrist being stretched out by pulling the hand back, palm up so that the palm and forearm are stretched—again, this should always be done without causing pain by overstretching and without putting undue pressure on the joints.

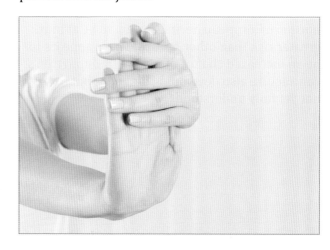

Aloe vera has long being used in natural medicine for burns and scars and there is growing evidence that it can help to break up old scar tissue. If you live in a climate where you can grow plentiful amounts then it can be used fresh from the plant; if not, then aloe vera in a 99% pure form is available from most good health food shops. You can opt to use the aloe vera in the place of massage oil, and your client can also apply it like a hand cream on a twice daily basis.

The combination of stretching and massage can help to alleviate the problems; this is particularly effective in the earlier stages but it can be of help at all stages. Adding in the aloe vera will hopefully assist in this healing process. You cannot promise your client that it will resolve the problem or provide a cure, but it should at least alleviate some of the discomfort and for some clients it will improve mobility, enable increased use of the hand, and prevent symptoms from worsening.

Eating Disorders

Background to the Condition

Eating disorders are complex, and a growing area of concern. In the United States alone, 20 million women and 10 million men suffer from a clinically significant eating disorder at some time in their life,[62] while in Australia it is estimated that over 1 million people have eating disorders.[63] As well as clinically diagnosed eating disorders, it is estimated that in the UK between 11 and 13 million people have psychological issues or problems connected with food that often leave them, in effect, on a permanent diet.[64]

There are different types of eating disorders. The three main types clinically diagnosed are: anorexia nervosa, where affected individuals will attempt to keep their weight as low as possible through starvation and/or exercise; bulimia, where weight is controlled by binge eating followed by vomiting or laxatives; and binge eating disorder, characterized by the need to overeat. Women are eight times more likely to develop anorexia than men and five times more likely to develop bulimia, whereas binge eating affects both sexes equally.[65] The fourth group of eating disorders is classed as "other specified feeding or eating disorders," and includes: atypical anorexia nervosa (where weight is not below normal), purging disorder (purging without binge eating), and night eating syndrome (excessive nighttime food consumption). Increasingly obesity is also being recognized as an eating disorder, with food often being used as a "prop" and for comfort, rather than any underlying issues being addressed.

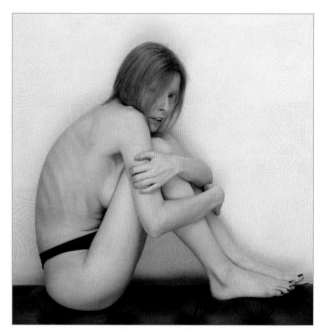

---

[62] http://www.nationaleatingdisorders.org/get-facts-eating-disorders

[63] http://www.eatingdisorders.org.au/key-research-a-statistics

[64] http://www.anorexiabulimiacare.org.uk/information-and-statistics-mediaqaswee

[65] http://www.nhs.uk/Conditions/Eating-disorders/Pages/Introduction.aspx

Eating disorders are serious emotional and physical problems that can have life-threatening consequences and have a huge impact on health, work, and relationships. Eating disorders come about from a number of physical, emotional, and social issues. Effective prevention is complex but there are a range of professional options to help, and early intervention gives a much better outcome, before behaviors have been strongly established.

Negative body image can be one of the first triggers of an eating disorder and one of the final and toughest stages of recovery.[66] However, eating disorders are not simply a problem with food and body image. Food can be used to regain a sense of control of feelings that can otherwise seem overwhelming, and to ease tension, anger, grief, and anxiety.

When people have an eating disorder they may be wary of massage; undressing or being uncovered on the table can be daunting for someone with a poor body image, but at the same time it can give an outlet for tension, anger, and anxiety.

Studies have also shown that women diagnosed with anorexia nervosa who were given massage therapy twice per week for five weeks reported lower stress and anxiety levels and had lower cortisol (stress) hormone levels following massage. Additionally over the five-week study they also reported decreases in body dissatisfaction on the Eating Disorder Inventory, and showed increased dopamine and norepinephrine levels.[67]

Careful management of the massage environment can support the client during the treatments, and help development of a confident client–practitioner relationship. If you are a friend or family member carrying out the massage, it is important not to comment on the client's body during treatment, or to use it as an opportunity to try to discuss their condition; instead make this a safe space where the person can be accepted and touched in a nonjudgmental and professional way.

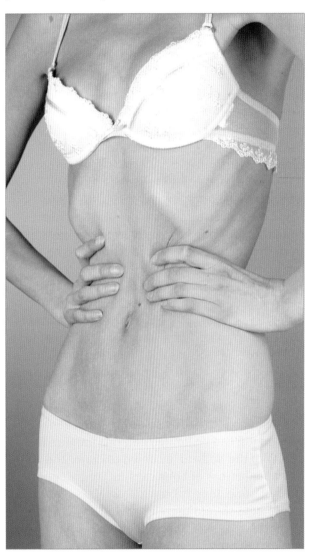

---

[66] http://www.nationaleatingdisorders.org/developing-and-maintaining-positive-body-image

[67] http://www.tandfonline.com/doi/abs/10.1080/106402601753454868#.UwPEgfl_vk0

Specific Contraindications

There are some specific contraindications and precautions for massage with clients with eating disorders, not least linked with some of the complications that can arise from eating disorders. Eating disorders can be associated with cardiovascular, gastrointestinal, endocrine, dermatological, hematological, skeletal, and central nervous system problems.[68] We will focus here on those that specifically impact on massage treatments.

Heart disorders are the most common medical causes of death in people with severe anorexia nervosa. The condition can lead to very slow heart rhythms, reduced blood flow, very low blood pressure, and damage to the heart muscles. It is vital to check with the client if there is a history of heart problems, fainting, or low blood pressure. If there are pre-existing heart conditions it is best to get clearance to massage from the client's medical practitioner, to be on the safe side. Electrolyte imbalance from a restricted diet can be dangerous to the heart's electrical impulses; otherwise be aware of the issues around low blood pressure, and ensure that on completion of the massage the client first rolls onto one side with the head supported on a pillow, then moves to a seated position, and only then to standing.

For women with eating disorders estrogen production can be limited and this impairs the ability of the body to lay down calcium, and osteopenia (loss of bone calcium) or osteoporosis (loss of bone density) can follow. Massage treatments should therefore avoid any cracking or manipulation of joints. The same applies for adolescent boys, as weight loss will result in a decrease in testosterone levels, which in turn will affect bone density.

Anemia is also common in those with eating disorders and this will make bruising from massage more likely. This does not mean that you cannot massage but you may need to build the depth very gradually over a number of treatments to avoid severe bruising. Using longer strokes rather than direct downward pressure will also help to limit bruising.

Eating disorders can cause bloating and constipation; you can use the techniques described in the chapter on constipation, but work gently as this area can be very tender and there can be a weakening in the rectal wall in people who have overused laxatives—this could potentially result in some fecal incontinence during massage if pressure is placed on the large intestine.

Hair loss, yellow skin, and poor healing of cuts are also frequent side effects of eating disorders as the body is missing the resources to heal itself. Avoid massaging over any broken skin and avoid the gentle hair pulling that would otherwise be a relaxing part of head and scalp massage.

Finally, for clients with bulimia, forced vomiting can cause erosion of and damage to the esophagus. If this is a problem then working with the client in a side position with a pillow under the head to raise and support it can be more comfortable.

A client who is morbidly obese may have problems lying on their back, side, or front as this may compromise their breathing; if this is the case you can adapt the massage so that the client can be seated. It can be tempting to think that for someone with a high body mass you have to work extra deeply to get through fat to muscle, but remember that working deeply will be painful and may cause medical complications so keep your pressure light to moderate. You can focus your treatments on the feet and lower legs, hands and arms, and head and neck, and progress to working on the back as you are able with client positioning and as you have released some of the initial tension by treating those areas first.

For all clients with an eating disorder be extra careful around your draping, so that the client always feels safe, supported, and dignified while on your table.

---

[68] http://www.aedweb.org/AM/Template.cfm?Section=Medical_Care_Standards&Template=/CM/ContentDisplay.cfm&ContentID=2413

Massage Treatments

There isn't one specific massage technique to be used for people with eating disorders. You can treat for any other problems or conditions they have using standard massage techniques, but bear in mind the issues discussed above.

Gentle massage for relaxation can also be helpful—this in itself can help improve body image, raise confidence, and improve mood. For people who do not have a good relationship with their body, touch may not be something they are comfortable with in everyday life, and massage can be part of a wider healing process. Healing therapeutic touch in massage is neither purely medical nor purely personal, so can be helpful in allowing the client to experience their body in a nonclinical, nonjudgmental way, and for some can be an integral part of a long healing journey.

While massage for people with eating disorders can be carried out by a friend or family member, being touched for massage by someone they know can be complex as the people involved may have what is referred to as a dual relationship.

A dual relationship means that you are trying to hold two roles: in this case as a friend or family member and the giver of therapeutic touch. For some people this can be too much; as the giver of the massage you may, for example, feel frustrated or even angry with the person with the eating disorder and this can come out in the treatment.

The person receiving the massage may have, even unacknowledged, issues that involve family members or friends and so may not feel able to fully relax or "let go" on the massage table. It is easy to unintentionally bring issues from the existing relationship into the massage and this can limit the effectiveness of the treatment; if this is a problem for either person it is best to engage the services of a professional to give the massage.

If anxiety is an issue, follow the protocol for anxiety massage; if headaches are a problem, follow the directions for massage for headache. You may need to adapt which part of your body you use—if someone is seriously underweight then you will not be able to use your forearm on their back, as your arm will be too big to avoid hitting ribs and spine. Work slowly and carefully and, as always, get continual feedback from the client as to the depth of your work. For people with very poor body image, touch can be incredibly powerful.

Emotional Issues and Post-Traumatic Stress Disorder

Background to the Condition

If you have not yet read the introductory chapter of this book it would be worth doing so now, as that gives some of the historic context for massage and how it has been used for millennia for a wide variety of conditions and problems. Some traditional massage systems were built on an understanding that problems were caused by spiritual influences, which the traditional healer would work to remove from the body. Other massage and healing practices work on the body's energy systems, and part of the aim of massage is to remove excess or stale energy from the body. Disease can be seen as an imbalance in the body's energetic system. Understanding the link between illness and emotional trauma is an integral part of massage for those working in this way. These beliefs come from understandings of the body and health that go back over 5000 years.

This began to change with the advent of Greek philosophy and, with that, what we now describe as modern medicine. Hippocrates stood out in a faith-based system to argue for a physically based medicine; this comment on epilepsy attributed to him is a good example of his position: "Men think epilepsy divine, merely because they do not understand it. We will one day understand what causes it, and then cease to call it divine. And so it is with everything in the universe."[69]

The end result of this was to change the practice of Western massage so that the focus was on the musculature and structures of the body. As our understanding of the body has grown, so too has this focus on the mechanics of massage to work with the systems of the body.

Sadly the two ways of thinking continue to divide and the massage world is still often split on a "scientific versus nonscientific" basis, and so massage becomes a political issue to be argued out and legislated both for and against. In a postmodern world, however, there is now room for both and for each to recognize the strengths and potential weaknesses of sticking rigidly to one system or belief.

Western versus Traditional Massage

When it comes to treating emotional issues, Eastern traditions have long focused on how the physical body will both hold and be impacted by emotional tension and trauma. Western traditions have more recently focused on the role of the vagus nerve and its possible role in emotional trauma, memory, and the parasympathetic nervous system; how to access this nerve is the focus of much study and also a certain level of debate. Rather than sticking

---

[69] http://www.eoht.info/page/Hippocratic+reductionism

rigidly to the argument from just one side or the other, we can simply see what works for us and our practice. How we understand the body changes with time, medical research and our philosophical approach, so we should perhaps worry less about clinging to our narratives of how and why things work as they do and allow our practice to develop on the basis of our own experience, ongoing training, insights and our client's results. So long as we "first, do no harm" then there is nothing to lose. Nothing here will promise that massage will instantly cure anxiety or post-traumatic stress disorder; if there was a one-cure-fits-all then it would be well documented and no doubt patented and sold. Nor, however, is it appropriate to say that massage cannot help with these issues; there should be no false promises but also no restrictions on what may or may not be achieved in helping to treat the individual person.

Can massage help people to overcome emotional issues or crises in their lives? Probably not for everyone, but it can for some people. Physical tension and mental/emotional tension share a common source in that they are both held in the body of the person experiencing that tension. Emotional tension can be felt as real physical pain; a tension headache, for example, is caused by tight muscles in the head, face, neck, and shoulders, but the reason for that tightness may be a stressful work environment, relationship breakdown, or any other stress or strain in the life of that person. Irritable bowel syndrome is at least made worse, if not caused, by stress, and the language of the more Eastern approaches to the body still finds its way into everyday Western language, so we talk about our stomach's churning or being in knots when the root cause may well be fear, grief, or anxiety.

Our bodies release complex hormones in response to fear (these are detailed more fully in the chapter that discusses anxiety), and they have a real and often detrimental effect on our health. Sometimes when faced with stressful situations there is the need to keep going for survival, and there is not the time to process the emotions and effect on our body, which can be stored in our muscles and whole body systems. A member of the armed services may witness and experience horrific situations but cannot stop and process that emotion on the field of war; a parent who loses a partner but has to keep going for the children or someone who just "keeps going" after a trauma may never get the chance to process what has happened, but this does not mean it does not have an impact on both body and mind.

For some this can lead to anxiety, depression, or anger and for others it will lead to post-traumatic stress disorder (PTSD). This is one aspect of how our bodies respond to stress. The Royal College of Psychiatrists (RCP) lists a number of events that can lead to PTSD; PTSD can start after any traumatic event. A traumatic event is one where you see that you are in danger, your life is threatened, or where you see other people dying or being injured. Typical traumatic events could be: a serious accident, military combat, violent personal assault, being taken hostage, terrorist attack, being a prisoner of war, natural or man-made disasters, or being diagnosed with a life-threatening illness.[70]

Just turning on the news suggests that these are risks for many people, worldwide, every day. The RCP argues that PTSD occurs as the events that take place undermine our sense that life is fair, that life is reasonably safe, and that we are secure. A traumatic experience makes it very clear that we can die at any time, therefore the symptoms of PTSD are part of a normal reaction to narrowly avoided death. The RCP goes on to describe the symptoms of PTSD as leaving people feeling grief-stricken, depressed, anxious, guilty, and angry. There are three main types of symptoms:

[70] http://www.rcpsych.ac.uk/healthadvice/problemsdisorders/posttraumaticstressdisorder.aspx

- Flashbacks and nightmares—this is where people find themselves reliving the event, again and again. This can be as a "flashback" in the day and/or as nightmares during sleep. Flashbacks can be so realistic that it feels as though they are living through the experience all over again. Not only will people see it in their mind, but they may also feel the emotions and physical sensations of what happened—fear, sweating, smells, sounds, and pain.

- Avoidance and numbing—it can be so upsetting to relive the experience over and over again that people will do anything possible to distract themselves. They will try to keep their mind busy by losing themselves in a hobby, working very hard, or spending time absorbed in crosswords or jigsaw puzzles. They will avoid places and people that remind them of the trauma, and will try not to talk about it. People may also deal with the pain of these feelings by trying to feel nothing at all—by becoming emotionally numb, communicating less and less with other people.

- Being "on guard"—people may find that they stay alert all the time, as if looking out for danger. Relaxation is impossible. This "hypervigilance" leads to anxiety and difficulty sleeping.

As the body is held at a heightened state, this may cause other physical symptoms, such as muscle aches and pains, diarrhea, irregular heartbeats, headaches, feelings of panic and fear, depression, and behaviors such as drinking too much alcohol and/or using drugs (including painkillers).[71]

Even if people do not develop full-blown PTSD they may develop some of the symptoms and may or may not seek help for this.

If we take a holistic approach to health and to massage, then massage can be an important part

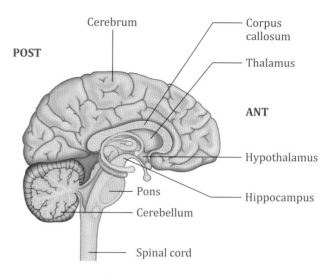

Mid-section through the brain

of treatment. Some people may need medication to help switch off the body's hyperalertness and allow relaxation to happen, but there is also an increasing awareness of the role that counseling, talking, relaxation, deep breathing, and treatments such as massage can bring to recovery. Not just in PTSD but also in other situations where the impact of an emotional event is affecting everyday life.

Massage can teach the body how to relax again and that it is safe to let go, even if just for a short period of time. Once someone feels safe relaxing for a short period of time, this relaxation can then be re-experienced until feeling more in control and more relaxed gradually starts to replace feeling anxious and alert. This can take many months; along with the emotional processing of coming to terms with what has happened, there is also a physical process going on. Adrenaline is a hormone the body produces when someone is under stress. Adrenaline "pumps up" the body to prepare it for action. When the stress disappears, the level of adrenaline should go back to normal. In PTSD, it may be that the vivid memories of the trauma keep the levels of adrenaline high. This will make a person tense, irritable, and unable to relax or sleep well.

---

[71] http://www.rcpsych.ac.uk/healthadvice/problemsdisorders/posttraumaticstressdisorder.aspx

The hippocampus is a part of the brain that processes memories. High levels of stress hormones, like adrenaline, can stop it from working properly—like "blowing a fuse." Flashbacks and nightmares continue because the memories of the trauma can't be processed. If the stress goes away, and the adrenaline levels get back to normal, the brain is able to repair the damage itself, like other natural healing processes in the body. The disturbing memories can then be processed and the flashbacks and nightmares will slowly disappear. Massage can provide a break in the body's flight or fight response, allowing the person to begin the de-escalation of symptoms.[72]

Specific Contraindications

While there are no specific medical contra-indications for this condition in isolation, treatment is best given in collaboration with the client's medical doctor so that the individual can access a range of treatments appropriate to his or her need to address what is a complex issue. Massage, combined with treatments that allow people to process the memories, can be very effective in aiding recovery.

Massage treatment is best given for the whole body, but also should also be given slowly. Extra care should be made to ensure the environment is comfortable and relaxing. If you are treating a friend or family member, choose a neutral space where the person will feel safe. If the client's PTSD has had an impact on your personal relationship with them—for example, if they are your partner or child—do consider the dual relationship that this gives for you treating them.

The person receiving the treatment needs to feel free to express anger or to cry and if there is a complex underlying relationship this may be difficult. Talk about this openly with the person to be treated, and without taking it as a judgment on your personal relationship; decide between you if you are the right person to give the treatment. Some clients may only feel safe with someone they know; for others, working with someone they do not have an existing relationship with may be easier. Judge each case on its own merits.

Along with making the room safe and comfortable, make sure it is warm—this allows the body to relax more. It will be worth investing in a portable massage table for this treatment, even if you are not working professionally, as this will allow you to work better and will help your client to relax as they will be able to rest their head in a face hole or cradle.

If you are living and working in a cold country, you can use an electric blanket to warm the massage table. Select some gentle music for the background, avoiding anything with too rhythmic a drum beat or any sudden noises. You could invite clients to choose their own music if they prefer. Keep the lights dimmed, unplug house phones, turn off cellphones, computers, TVs etc.—anything that will distract—and make sure that children are supervised by another adult so that you can work undisturbed and uninterrupted. Encourage the client to familiarise themselves with the room and its exit points before starting the treatment.

Allow at least two hours for each session and ideally work in a place where the client will not need to rush away at the end of the treatment.

---

[72] http://www.rcpsych.ac.uk/healthadvice/problemsdisorders/posttraumaticstressdisorder.aspx

Massage Treatments

You can follow the instructions included within these chapters to build a whole-body massage, but there are four other specific areas to consider for treating PTSD, depression, or other emotional issues: head massage, your communication, the client's breathing, and belly or abdominal massage.

Head massage is the "switch off" for anxiety and stress. Work on the head, face, and scalp allows the mind to switch off and the person to begin to relax. When treating someone who has any kind of emotional trauma, depression, or PTSD it is helpful to begin the treatment with gentle head, face, and scalp massage. After that you can move onto other areas of the body; work either upper or lower body first. If you are working upper body then, after the initial head work, start with the hands, moving up the arms and then into the shoulders, back, neck and chest as detailed in Chapters 2, 4, and 5.

If your client gets too distressed during a massage or cannot relax, keep returning to the head work; as your sessions progress and the client learns how to relax you may need to do this less, but don't worry if for the first few treatments you are constantly returning to massage the head. Finally, when you come to finish the massage ensure that you allow a good ten minutes at the end of the treatment to return to head massage to conclude your treatment.

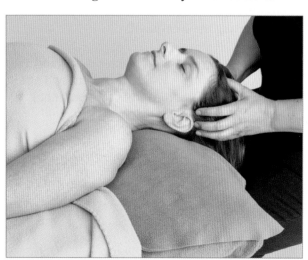

When working with clients who have PTSD it is important not to shock them during the treatment, so if you are moving from one area of the body to another, with soft speech, let them know that you are moving. Your communication should not be intrusive nor a constant chatter, so that the person can switch off, but it should be clear so that the person does not jump as you unexpectedly change the area you are working on. If move quickly or unexpectedly and make the client jump you will undo the work you are doing as the "flight or fight" reaction will be triggered by your unexpected touch.

Some clients will feel the need to talk during treatments; sometimes as you release tension they will want to talk about the stress or events that put that tension there—just allow them to talk, do not judge anything that is said, and always take your cue from your clients so that they know they can talk if they want to, but that they do not have to if they don't want to.

The client is not just passive during a massage treatment; you will be able to work more deeply and more effectively during a treatment if you work with the client's breath.

It can be worth spending a few minutes toward the start of the treatment establishing good breathing; if you watch babies and younger children breathe, they breathe from their bellies. As children get into adolescence and become more body conscious, this breath often gets more shallow as they start to hold their bellies in—a habit usually continued into adulthood. This results in chest breathing where breaths are shallow, often quicker, and not as efficient or effective. In massage you want to slow down and deepen the breathing.

It is worth making sure that your own breathing is deep and relaxed as it will be easier to teach this to your client if you have good breathing habits yourself.

Lying down, place one of your hands on your chest and the other on your belly so that it rests halfway between your belly button and your pubic bone—your breath should come from way down where the hand on your belly is. Try to relax and slow your breathing to the point where the hand on your belly rises and falls with each breath and the hand on your chest barely moves.

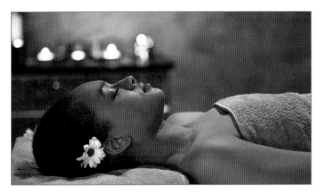

When you are massaging your client try to keep an eye on your own breathing so that you are always breathing deeply and relaxed—your client is likely to mirror your breathing patterns—and encourage your client to take these slow, deep breaths. This deep abdominal breathing alone can be very powerful in allowing the mind to regain control of thoughts and feelings and in calming down the flight or fight response. Use your client's breath to make the most of the massage; if you are going to use a particularly deep move, wait for you client's out breath before doing so—it will be less painful for your client, the tension will release more quickly, and you will automatically be working at a deeper level to clear tension, emotional as well as physical, as the deep breathing can also be a letting go of whatever has caused the tension to build up.

Finally, after you have worked all other areas of the body you can come to the belly or abdominal work. In many traditional understandings, the belly is where the soul or the life force of the person lives. In Western language this is reflected in expressions such as "my stomach was in knots," "my stomach sank," and "I had butterflies in my stomach," and working this region can not only help to release physical tension (and constipation) held in the bowels, but can also help to release deep-seated emotional tension.

If you are professionally trained and confident in your knowledge of human anatomy, then with your client's consent you can work more deeply into this area (if the client's general health allows you to do so). If you have not trained in abdominal massage or are working on a friend or family member then you can still work effectively on this area by working at a more surface level and working gently and with a light touch—it may just take more time to achieve the same results. Even if you are specifically trained, some clients just need to go slowly and lightly in this area so the slow and gentle approach will never be wasted.

Start by placing your hand on the client's belly with the palm of your hand positioned so that the ball of your thumb is flatly covering their belly button. Always work with your client draped; skin-to-skin contact in this area can be very confrontational and can feel invasive, so err on the side of caution.

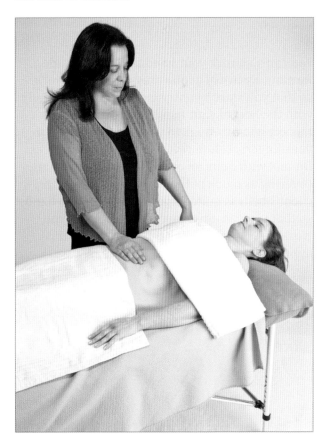

Just allow the client to breathe, encouraging that deeper breathing to take place. For some people just this alone will bring up emotion. Just allow that to happen. If someone wants to cry, just allow this to happen without any need to explain why; simply reassuring your client with "it's ok," "that's good, let it out" is enough. Don't be tempted to ask "are you ok?" or you are bringing the client back out of their relaxed state to a state where they have to think or engage in conversation, and this will interrupt the treatment. If you are being gentle and they are releasing, then it is ok, you don't need to ask.

Some clients can get angry at this stage and it's important to let them know that this is also ok—just ensure that the anger does not become directed at you. They may kick or thump the table and shout out, or similar; again, it is important not to pass judgment or try to explain anything. It's likely that they are processing quite complex situations so any comment you make might sound banal, but encouragement that what is happening is good is appropriate.

You can also rock your hand from side to side, forming a wave of gentle pressure as you work, so that you start by putting pressure on the belly with the heel of your hand, then transferring this pressure through to your palm and then to your fingers, before reversing the whole process. Do this with quite an open hand so that you are covering as much of the belly as you can. If the client's belly is quite large you can use two hands so that you can cross more of the belly as you work. Having completed this work, you can, if appropriate to your client, begin deeper work.

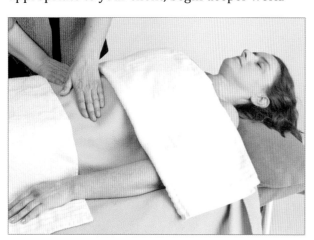

Always start either at the top right of the client's belly or at the bottom left, and the key thing to remember is that you need to work clockwise around the belly and work with the client's breath.

Start by working in a small circle around the outside of the belly button, one to two inches out depending on the size of your client (the bigger, the broader the circle). With the client's out breath gently press with the flat of your fingertips into the belly and hold for a few seconds—as the client begins to need to breathe always release your pressure. Only ever press into the belly as your clients breathe out and always release as they need to breathe in; they should never need to hold their breath.

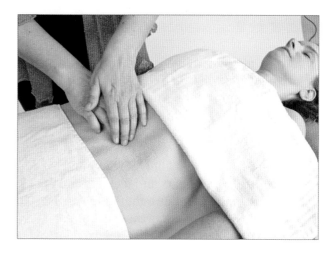

You are looking to sink in just a little—if you feel a strong pulse, pull back and readjust your hand position as you will be close to an artery. Simply work in a circle around the belly button, work slowly and avoid any jabbing movements—this is meant to be slow, rhythmic, and comforting. You may feel areas that do not easily yield to pressure; this may be something as simple as food/fecal matter in the bowel and it may move as you press onto it—just warn your client that there may be a bowel "clear out" post treatment. After you have worked in the circle close into the belly button, move outward and repeat the same thing in a bigger circle—this works the large intestine.

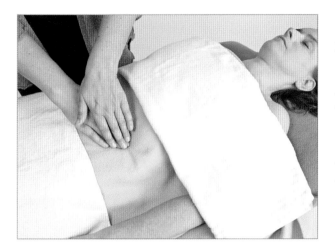

Again, always work clockwise and err on the side of caution with your pressure. This process should not be carried out on someone with Crohn's disease or ulcerative colitis, anyone who is pregnant, or someone who has had recent abdominal surgery. Never work higher than the ribs and avoid the pubic area, working on the area between the towels as shown in the photographs. Don't rush the treatment, and if your client cries, shouts, or has any other form of emotional release, just allow this to happen and be reassuring; wait for that wave of emotion to calm before moving onto another part of the belly.

Finish the treatment by returning to the head work to help ground and relax the client, and try to create a space for him or her to relax and come to after the treatment. There is no need to "dissect" the treatment afterward but if clients need to talk it is alright to allow them to lead the discussion so that the conversation is on their terms. Part of the reason that this treatment is best given in conjunction with other treatments is that they will then be able to access the other professional support to help them talk through their release appropriately with someone qualified and experienced to help. Massage can be a powerful tool as part of the healing process.

Fibromyalgia

Background to the Condition

Fibromyalgia is a very debilitating, and often misunderstood, condition. Because there is no single test for it, and there are no outward physical signs of the illness, it can be difficult to diagnose. A final diagnosis can only be made following analysis of the symptoms experienced and all other conditions being ruled out. Fibromyalgia is becoming more commonly known as fibromyalgia syndrome but has also been known in the past as unspecified rheumatism and muscular rheumatism. The growing body of medical opinion points to it being a disorder of the central nervous system; research is ongoing. It is a condition that affects many people, with estimates of seven million sufferers in the US alone and over one million in the UK.

The symptoms of fibromyalgia are many and varied but three of the central problems are chronic pain (and hypersensitivity to pain), chronic fatigue, and cognitive dysfunction.[73]

The chronic pain will usually be widespread; it may feel to sufferers as if they have just run a marathon or are coming down with flu, or it can instead be a sharp, intense arthritic pain. The pain can also be experienced as stabbing, shooting, or burning, for up to 24 hours a day, every day. This in itself is extremely debilitating, and if added to chronic fatigue to the extent where the limbs feel as if they are made of lead, and every movement takes immense amounts of energy, then a fuller picture comes together. "Brain fog" or "fibro fog" is common,[74] as cognitive function is impacted by the condition, with sufferers experiencing difficulty in concentrating and being easily distracted, and that can also lead to problems in decision making, memory, speaking properly, or even remembering which task the sufferer was halfway through.

Sleep disturbances are to be expected, which compounds the chronic fatigue. Medical research undertaken in the US has uncovered where exactly in the usual sleep patterns this disturbance occurs. There are "specific and distinctive abnormalities in the Stage 4 deep sleep"[75] of fibromyalgia patients. During sleep, individuals with fibromyalgia are constantly interrupted by bursts of awake-like brain activity, limiting the amount of time they spend in deep sleep." In practice this means that the fibromyalgia sufferer is not benefitting from the deeper, healing sleep that the rest of the population experience, making it difficult for the body to repair itself.

---

[73] http://www.fibroaction.org

[74] http://www.fmnetnews.com

[75] http://fmaware.org/site/PageServerb3b4.html?pagename=fibromyalgia_symptoms

Muscular tension, waking with stiff and sore muscles, digestive disorders, and recurrent headaches may all be experienced by the person with fibromyalgia. Many will also experience balance problems, which can result in painful falls; digestive disorders; and itchy and burning skin—all these making up the difficult package of fibromyalgia symptoms.

How, then, can massage help a person who may be experiencing both hyperalgesia—feeling more pain than would be usual from what would normally be a mildly painful event—and allodynia—feeling pain from a stimulus that would not usually be painful at all? In presenting the initial symptoms it seems that massage would be contraindicated; however, fibromyalgia self-help networks show that massage is the nondrug treatment of choice for the fibromyalgia patient.[76] There are, however, some very clear guidelines for safe and successful massage for people with this condition.

Specific Contraindications

The most important factor with any massage is to start treatment very gently. Even the lightest touch may be excruciatingly painful, so it is essential that you start very gently and perhaps build depth as sessions progress, and as you are able to receive feedback from your clients as to how their body has responded to the treatment.

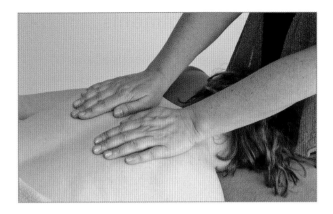

That said, it is also important to be "sure" in your touch; tentative or nervous contact may stimulate the skin too much and cause pain. Be gentle but confident.

It will be best to work in short sessions to begin with; this can be built upon as both practitioner and client learn how the fibromyalgia will respond to massage. Everyone will react differently so there is no one way to treat a client with fibromyalgia. If you are working in a friends-and-family context at home, even 10 minutes' work will help, while avoiding overstimulating the receiver. In a professional context it would be better to start with a 30 minute session and build on this over time. It would be rare to achieve a session length of over an hour but, again, see how your individual client responds.

---

[76] http://www.fmnetnews.com/fibro-basics/treatment/non-drug-therapies

Massage Treatments

One of the key elements to the successful treatment of fibromyalgia with massage is to ensure that you are releasing the fascia (example below). Without getting too complex, fascia is probably best described as "connective tissue"; it is made up of collagen fibers and it wraps and binds together muscles, bones, nerves, blood vessels, and organs. It provides a strong interconnection between muscles, ligaments, tendons, and bones, and the nervous and blood systems that supply them.

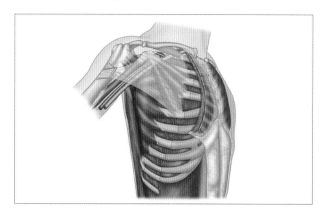

Fascia covers the whole body, from head to toe; the combined fascia and muscles together being known as the myofascial system. There are three types of fascia: superficial fascia, primarily to do with the skin; deep fascia, the fascia that encases the muscles, bones, nerves, and blood vessels; and finally visceral fascia, which is mainly connected with the internal organs. Massage will primarily work on the first two types of fascia, although some specialist massage will begin to impact on the final category. It is the superficial and deep fascia that we are focusing on working with now.

When fascia stops moving properly then both the fascia and the underlying muscle can get "stuck." Reasons for the fascia ceasing to move can be numerous; it could be as simple as a lifestyle that does not involve much movement or stretching. It could be due to chronic dehydration, or that an injury causes pain so, instead of keeping mobile, the patient keeps still to protect the injured area.

The starting point for massage for someone with fibromyalgia is to begin to release the fascia. It does not matter at this stage whether you work from the center of the body outward or the outside of the body inward, or if you start with the upper body or lower body. Fascia lies in all directions across and through the entire body so you can't go wrong no matter where you start or which direction you work in; the priority is that you work all of the main areas. It can feel good for the client if you start working outward from the spine but this is a guide, not a rule. The areas around the shoulders, neck, and down the full length of the spine can be very tight, as can the fascia around the ribs. The rib area will most likely be very tender so work gently and slowly. The treatment can be broken down into smaller sessions so that it is more bearable for the client. You will need to work across the whole body in this way (excluding all intimate areas).

To encourage the fascia to release there are two useful techniques that can be used simply and effectively. The first is to roll the skin—practice this move on yourself first so that you are confident using it on your client. Pick up the skin between your fingers and simply roll it so that you are moving across the area you are working on. You don't need to work in any particular direction and it's better if you change direction; unless the client has very dry skin, avoid using oil as it will be difficult to grasp the skin once oiled.

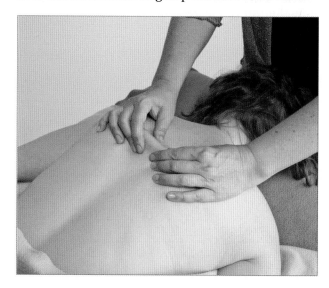

Next, using your thumbs, place your thumb tips together on the client's skin and, without releasing your grip, slide your thumbs so that the tip of the nail and the first knuckle are parallel as shown in the paragraphs below.

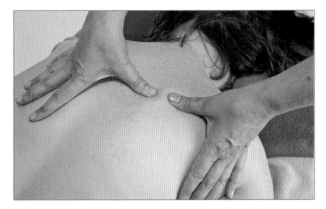

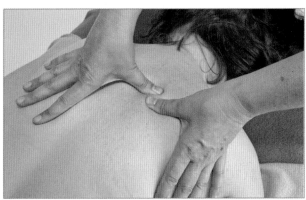

You are eventually aiming to work across the whole of the body in this way but you may need to break this down into shorter treatments, working on different areas at different times, so that you do not overwhelm your client.

Once you have worked the superficial fascia your next objective is to begin to release the deeper fascia, and you can do this through your massage. Take extra care not to work too deeply or too quickly for the client, and for this it is best to work outward in. Remember that the fascia covers all of the body so working the hands, feet, and head is really important, and this should be the starting point for your massage.

There is no one set way to work, so be flexible to meet the needs of your client. You could opt to treat the whole body in one treatment at a surface level through the rolling and gentle twisting and to leave any deeper massage work to a later date. Alternatively you could treat the whole upper body with both the surface and deeper work and then return to the lower-body work at a later date. There are positives and drawbacks for both of these approaches; fascia is a very integrated structure and in an ideal world you would treat the whole body at both the surface and deep level in one treatment— but that could be two to three hours' work and would likely be far too much for most people with fibromyalgia, so a compromise needs to be reached; how you reach that compromise is flexible and can be tailored to meet the needs of individual clients and their wishes.

You can start with the head, the hands, or the feet and follow the protocols in Chapters 2–4 at the start of this book for all of those treatments. Make sure you complete the head and hands treatments before moving onto the upper back, and if the client suffers from pain in the lower back you should also treat the feet and legs before the back work. You can then follow the protocols for other conditions to suit the client's needs; if your client has tension headaches, follow the instructions for that treatment, having completed the initial work detailed above; likewise if your client has plantar fasciitis follow that treatment protocol but integrate the work above too.

Foot Drop

Background to the Condition

Foot drop is one of the most common mobility problems following a stroke. Foot drop (also called dropped foot or drop foot) is the inability to lift the foot and toes properly when walking.[77] It can lead to trips and falls, and a loss of confidence when walking. Someone with foot drop will find it difficult, if not impossible, to control their foot and to turn the foot and ankle upward (known as dorsiflexion). As the person walks the foot will flop rather than be able to be placed, with little or no strength or control of the foot.

A foot drop is a symptom of something else going on in the body. This could be anything from lead poisoning to spondylolisthesis, a spinal cord injury; herniated disk; tumor; multiple sclerosis; Parkinson's disease; Lyme disease; or a whole host of other illnesses or injuries that can weaken the central or peripheral nervous systems. Occasionally drop foot can occur simply owing to the foot lift being hampered by tight or overactive calf muscles due to spasticity.[78]

Specific Contraindications

As a dropped foot is a symptom of another condition it is vital to get immediate medical attention if these symptoms start suddenly or develop as a new condition.

Any massage treatment should be carried out in partnership with the client's medical team once the underlying cause can be identified and addressed.

Massage Treatments

There are a number of treatments available, most of which are long-term. In some cases normal functioning can return with time and treatment—for others the focus will be on managing symptoms. There are surgical treatments available for some clients, including bone fusion and implants that artificially fire the nerves to stimulate the foot to lift as the heel lifts from the floor. These are not suitable for everyone, nor are they necessary for everyone, and there is no harm done in trying other treatments before looking at surgical options.

---

[77] http://www.dropfoot.co.uk/uploads/media/_33031-Manual_Mobile_200_Re.pdf

[78] Ibid.

As the client loses, or has lost, control of the foot, to avoid tripping up as the foot fails to rise off the floor as the heel is lifted, the temptation is to swing the hip out in order to lift the foot. Massage for foot drop should therefore work from the feet right up to the hips. If necessary also working the upper back, as the leg swing, although coming from the hips, may originate in the muscles of the back and shoulder. Even if only one foot is affected by the foot drop, still work both legs as the other leg is likely to be overworking to compensate for the lack of control and strength in the other foot.

Start by massaging the feet and, provided the client's medical team has no objections, the massage can also include some gentle stretches. With the client lying faceup, take the foot in both hands so that your thumbs are on the sole of the foot. Starting in the center, and with a little oil to lubricate the skin, stroke upward and outward across the sole of the foot with your thumbs, working toward the toes. You can repeat this eight to ten times, and after the first four or five warm-up strokes you can begin to work a little more deeply with each stroke, but always within the client's tolerance. After applying a little oil, use your fingers across the top of the foot to warm up the upper side of the foot, stroking in either direction up and down the foot and being careful not to massage across the metatarsal bones. Work each toe in turn, gently rolling them between your fingers, avoiding putting any pressure on the nail bed or the knuckles.

Next turn your attention to the sides of the feet. You can place the foot between your hands so that you have a hand on each side of the foot and gently roll the foot between your hands. This can be a very relaxing technique but it also helps to release the fascia of the foot and introduce gentle movement into the muscles and connective tissue of the ankle. A nice stretch at this point in the massage is to hold the heel of the foot in one hand, so that you are securely cupping it, and use the other hand to, in turn, place pressure on the sole of the foot, pushing the foot upward, and then on the top of the foot, pushing the foot downward. This is a gentle stretch and can be repeated five or six times. Next, keeping one hand

underneath the heel, bend the foot inward and find the groove that lies between the heel and the outer side of the ankle bone; place your thumb at this point and gently rotate the ankle left and right, keeping your thumb in place.

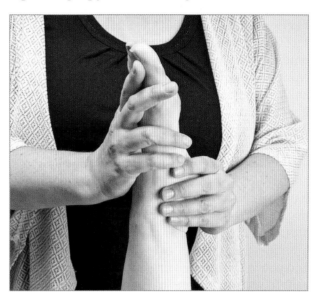

Moving upward into the lower leg, it is important not to neglect the muscles that run alongside the shin bone (shown below). The tibialis anterior is the muscle responsible for pulling the foot up as the leg moves and it is this muscle that positions the foot so that the heel will come down first when walking or running.

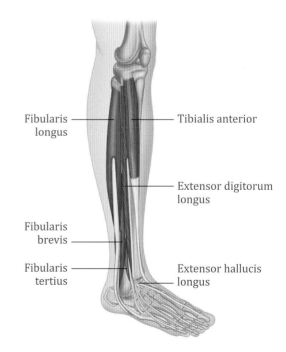

Fibularis longus — Tibialis anterior

Extensor digitorum longus

Fibularis brevis —

Fibularis tertius —

Extensor hallucis longus

Any lesions in the nerve roots that come from spinal problems between the L5 and S1 vertebrae (the lumbar and sacral vertebrae at the bottom of the spine) are likely to cause problems with the tibialis anterior and can lead to foot drop. Massaging this and the surrounding muscles will help keep blood flow healthy and assist in the recovery process. Being careful to avoid pressing onto the shin bone and using a little massage oil, work upward from the big toe, crossing at the ankle to the outer leg, and continue to massage upward until just below the knee, following the line of the muscle.

Avoid pressing onto the joints, but you will be able to work very close to the ankle bones and it is important to do so, in order that you are massaging the whole muscle and not ignoring its attachments. Don't restrict yourself to this one muscle—the whole muscle group needs massage and you will also need to work on the back of the calf. To save your client having to keep rolling over, you can, however, finish working the front of the leg first by working above the knee, paying particular attention to the outer leg. Use massage oil to lubricate the skin and use long strokes upward from just over the knee to the top of the leg. Placing a rolled-up towel under the knee to support it will ensure that you do not place any strain on the knee joint.

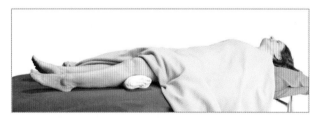

Work in long, slow strokes, always upward toward the heart and being careful to avoid pressing directly onto the IT band (iliotibial band). This will be tender to touch and the area will bruise easily; it can be worked carefully but not specifically for this condition. You can use either the flat of your hand or the side of your arm for this upper-thigh work; begin by working slowly and superficially and, as you have warmed up the area, you can then increase your depth.

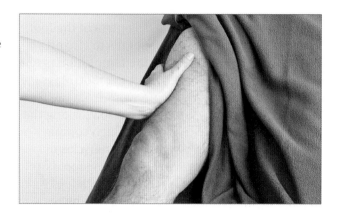

You should feel the muscle start to soften under your touch; if it is resistant, try placing three or four fingers onto the belly of the outer thigh muscle and shaking the muscle, before returning to the long strokes. Once you have worked both legs in a similar way you can then ask your client to turn over to lie facedown, and place a rolled-up towel underneath the ankles to support the feet (this is especially important for the foot affected by the foot drop).

Using long strokes to warm up the muscles, work up the calf muscles on both the inside and outside but increasing your depth more on the outside as you work. Use massage oil to allow you to slide over the skin without dragging it; you will need more oil if the client has hairy legs. The inner calf can bruise very easily and needs much lighter work. Once you have warmed up the muscles, you can use your thumbs to work more deeply up the outer calf, first with a stroke of the thumb moving up the leg a couple of inches at a time, and then following up with the other thumb.

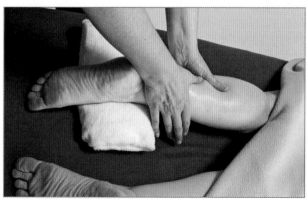

This should allow you to cover the whole outer calf in depth in three to five minutes; repeat on the other leg. Avoid massaging the area behind the knee as this is easily damaged. Working just on the outer thigh, repeat the same moves that you did on the front of the thigh, stopping just before you reach the top of the leg. Ensure that you drape your client fully so that the towel covers their underwear and inner thigh area—they are much more likely to relax and allow you to massage more if they feel secure on the table.

If your client has had a stroke, you will need to use your discretion with this next part of the treatment. You must judge whether they are ready for this more complex movement and whether they have enough control over their balance to be able to get into this position. If not, you can simply omit it. Having worked both legs, ask your client to lie on his or her side. The head should be supported with a pillow or cushion, the bottom leg (as lying on the table) should be straight, and the upper one bent upward. Both arms should be in front of the client in a comfortable position. Place your hand on the top of the upper leg with your fingers pointing upward so that your middle finger continues straight up from the top of the leg; you are effectively following the femur in a straight line.

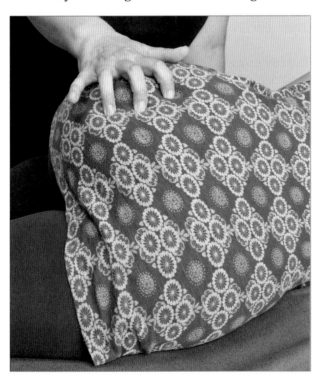

Before you get to the hard bone of the sacrum there should be a soft area between the palm of your hand and the top of your fingers—if the person was standing upright this would be the side of the buttocks. If you gently press into this area you will find usually three areas that are more tender than the rest of the area and more resistant to touch, these are the areas that you now need to work. If you are an experienced and qualified practitioner you can use your elbow here; if you are working to help a friend or family member use the flat of your knuckles, or if they are strong enough, your thumbs.

Ask your client to take a deep breath and on the out breath press down into this area; you should be pressing straight down into the side of the buttocks. Your client should feel this as a "good pain"; that is, they can tell you are on the right spot so it's tender, but it does not make them want to pull away. Hold this point for 30–40 seconds until the client feels that the tension has released; this may feel as though you have released your pressure, even though you have not. Repeat this move an inch or so up from your first point, and then an inch or so below that original starting point, and repeat on the other side.

This massage will help to strengthen the area and, along with the client's physiotherapy rehabilitation and other medical treatments, help to restore movement where that is medically possible (depending on the original cause), while at the same time it will help to loosen tension that may have built up in the other muscles, which may be working extra hard, or in an unusual way, because of the foot drop. Don't underestimate the importance of what you are doing; keeping the rest of the body moving and supple when there is one problem area can be a great boost to muscle health generally, and help to manage the aches and pains that come from unusual or additional muscle usage.

Frozen Shoulder

Background to the Condition

A frozen shoulder, or adhesive capsulitis, is a very painful condition that will limit the amount of movement in the shoulder, sometimes meaning it can barely be moved at all.

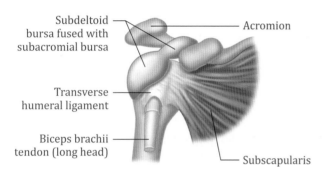

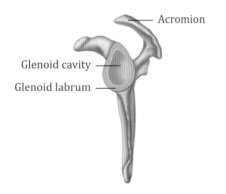

The shoulder is a ball and socket joint. The end of the upper arm bone (humerus) sits in the socket of the shoulder blade (scapula). The shoulder capsule is fully stretched when you raise your arm above your head, and hangs down as a small pouch when your arm is lowered. In frozen shoulder, bands of scar tissue form inside the shoulder capsule, causing it to thicken, swell, and tighten.[79] This means there is less space for your upper arm bone in the joint, which limits movements. This makes the joint, which usually has more mobility than any other in the body, severely restricted in its movement. Left untreated the condition will usually fix itself, but it can take around two years (some report seven years) and within that time the muscle will lose strength and flexibility; early treatment is therefore recommended.

The reasons why someone might get a frozen shoulder are not fully understood but recent injury, diabetes, thyroid problems, heart disease, Parkinson's disease, long periods of immobility, and Dupuytren's contracture are thought to increase the likelihood of a frozen shoulder. However, sometimes there is no apparent reason and it's not uncommon for clients to report that they just "woke up that way." It is twice as common in women than in men and most likely to affect those in the 40–60 age range.

---

[79] http://www.nhs.uk/Conditions/Frozen-shoulder/Pages/Causes.aspx

There are three phases to the progress of a frozen shoulder. Phase one is the acute or "freezing," painful, phase; typically this lasts between two and nine months. The first symptom is usually pain followed by stiffness and limitation in movement. The pain is typically worse at night and when the client lies on the side of the body that is affected. Phase two, the subacute, is the frozen, stiff, or adhesive phase. This typically lasts between four and twelve months. The pain gradually eases but the stiffness and limitation in movement remain and can even get worse. All movements of the shoulder are affected. However, the movement most severely affected is usually rotation of the arm outward. The muscles around the shoulder may shrink and waste as they are not used. Phase three, the chronic phase, is the "thawing" or recovery phase. This typically lasts between one and three years. The pain and stiffness gradually go and movement gradually returns to normal, or near normal.[80]

How serious the symptoms are will vary from person to person but they can interfere with everyday life, even dressing or brushing hair, and depending on the client's job it can also interfere significantly with work.

As any athlete who has taken a couple of months off training will testify, a muscle needs to be used to retain its strength and flexibility. The natural thing to want to do with a frozen shoulder is to not use it—simply because using it causes pain, sometimes very intense pain—but in order to restore the muscle to its full function quickly and effectively, the muscle needs to be used.

A frozen shoulder is normally diagnosed from a review of the symptoms but an X ray or scan may be needed if the diagnosis is unclear. Traditional treatment can include painkillers, anti-inflammatory painkillers, shoulder exercises, steroid injections, and, in the worst cases, surgery.

Specific Contraindications

If a client presents with a frozen shoulder and there has been a significant trauma to the shoulder in a recent accident or a sporting injury then medical help should be sought for an X ray or scan to check that there has been no structural damage to the shoulder before any treatment takes place. If this has already been checked or if there has been no trauma to the joint then massage treatment can be very effective, ideally with some stretches and exercises for the client to carry out at home between treatments. According to the American Academy of Orthopaedic Surgeons, "More than 90% of patients improve with relatively simple treatments to control pain and restore motion."[81]

Massage Treatments

It can be tempting simply to massage the shoulder, but massage on a frozen shoulder needs to include massage on both the hands and the head. Someone with a frozen shoulder will often also complain of pain in the rotator cuff at the front of the shoulder (these are the muscles that stabilize the shoulder—rotator cuff injuries being a common complaint from baseball players and drummers). Following the muscle tension from this area leads back to the front outer part of the thumb, so be sure to work the hands in detail and as deeply as is comfortable for the client, to release the tension. There are detailed instructions for hand massage in Chapter 2; do ensure that you work the hand in detail with particular focus on the thumb, and then work up the arm as you follow the tension through the palmaris longus, flexor carpi radialis, brachioradialis, and pronator teres—you do not need to worry too much about which muscle you are working on so long as you work the whole of the front of the forearm as it comes up from the thumb.

---

[80] http://www.patient.co.uk/health/frozen-shoulder

[81] http://www.frozenshoulder.com/frozen-shoulder-diagnosis. php?gclid=COXHmdnC7b0CFSfmwgoduH8AhQ

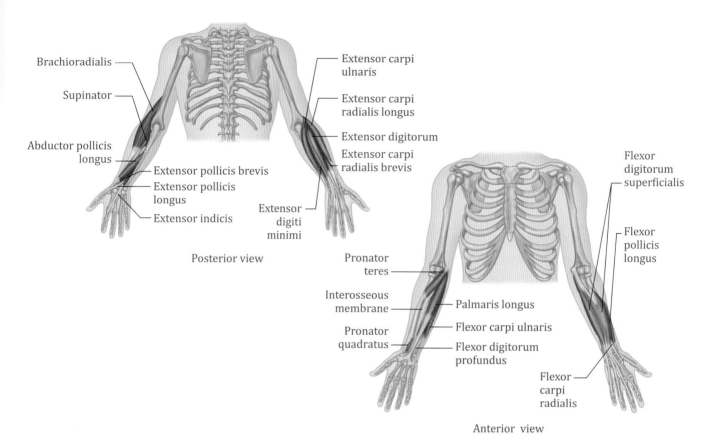

Brachioradialis

Supinator

Abductor pollicis
longus

Extensor pollicis brevis

Extensor pollicis
longus

Extensor indicis

Extensor carpi
ulnaris

Extensor carpi
radialis longus

Extensor digitorum

Extensor carpi
radialis brevis

Extensor
digiti
minimi

Posterior view

Pronator
teres

Interosseous
membrane

Pronator
quadratus

Palmaris longus

Flexor carpi ulnaris

Flexor digitorum
profundus

Flexor
digitorum
superficialis

Flexor
pollicis
longus

Flexor
carpi
radialis

Anterior view

Using a little massage oil and the flat of your thumb to stroke up the muscles, gradually increasing your depth as you repeat this stroke can be a very effective way to work. For some clients this work alone will give an immediate improvement in shoulder movement and a decrease in pain. Follow this work up the arm into the biceps, but working more gently as this can be a tender area to work.

It may be more comfortable for your client to remain seated for the hand and arm part of the massage. When the client is lying down for other parts of the massage, be careful to support the shoulder; you may need to place a rolled-up towel under the shoulder, particularly for female clients, so that the shoulder is not left pointing down (the larger breasted the client, the more shoulder support that will be needed). With the client lying faceup make sure you support the arm fully as you work on it, perhaps resting it on a towel on your knee as you work so that, again, there is no pulling on the shoulder itself. Do not allow the arm to fall down the side of the table as this will put pressure on the joint.

After you have worked from the hands and up the arms you can then do some head massage, following the instructions in Chapter 4, but you then need to approach the neck and top of the shoulders very carefully. This work is important as it will gently start to release any tension held in the neck, which may be contributing to tightness in the shoulder.

After this, working with your client facedown (or seated facing forward against the back of a chair if you do not have a massage table with a face hole), use a little massage oil and begin to warm up the back of the neck, top of the back, and across the top of the shoulders, avoiding the shoulder joint. Use sweeping motions moving out from the edge of the spine down across the top of the shoulders and then moving from the center out and down toward the shoulder blades; work both sides at once, being careful not to apply any pressure on the spine itself.

As you work you will find tender spots and some areas that feel firmer than others—these are the areas where the muscle tension is held. Don't be tempted to ignore these areas because they're tender; instead, once you have spent three or four minutes with the sweeping and warming up motions, bring your attention to these tender and resistant areas and give them extra attention, but work slowly and gently so that you release them gradually.

There are two key ways that you can do this safely and effectively. The first is to find the individual tender or tight spot and, only working these one at a time, simply press onto that point in the muscle and hold your static pressure there until you feel the muscle soften and release under your pressure. You can use your finger or thumb but, in order to protect yourself, place another finger or your other thumb on top of the first one to give it some added support—this will help to ensure you don't cause damage to yourself while you are trying to help someone else. You may need to hold this pressure for one or two minutes. Move slowly around all of the tight and tender spots around the back of the neck, top of the shoulders, and upper back. The other technique is to gently shake the muscle; again, find that tight and tender spot and, using your first two fingers, apply moderate pressure so that you are not simply moving the skin and then move quickly back and forth across the muscle. You should work the across the run of the muscle. Most of the muscles in the neck run up and down the body so moving across them left to right and back should be effective.

Continue the shaking for up to a minute before moving onto the next tight area. Don't worry if the skin on the area appears a little red—this simply happens as you encourage blood flow to the area and it is a positive part of the treatment. After you have worked all of the tender and tight areas, finish this part of the treatment by repeating the earlier long stroking movements downward, moving with the flow of the muscle.

If your client is lying down, ask him or her to move to lie faceup and cradle the client's head in your hands so that your fingers rest underneath the curve of the base of the skull; this is likely to be a tender area. (Note: do not use this particular move for a client with Down syndrome.) Gently curl your fingers upward and hold that upward pressure, encouraging your client to rest the head back in your hands. Heads are heavy so your hands should feel weighed down by the pressure of the client's head.

Hold this position for around one minute and then slowly and gently rock your client's head in your hands, the range of motion for the rock is no more than half an inch in each direction, and work very slowly with this move. Release the client's head and then repeat this whole part of the treatment, but this time raising the client's head no more than half an inch higher than you did the first time. This allows the whole area very gently and naturally to stretch, but without putting any pressure on the neck. When you have finished this move, gently place the client's head back down—do not let it drop back.

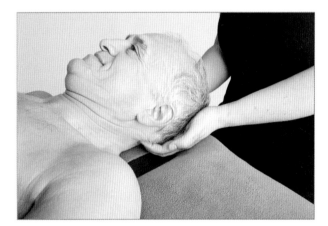

Only after all of this work do you come to touch the shoulder itself; do so carefully, you may be breaking down scar adhesions, which can be very painful for your client, but you also want to work at a depth that does not then mean that the body will form new scar tissue. It is better to have a few more sessions working slowly than to try to fix everything in one session. In the acute stage you will only be able to work very lightly over the shoulder joint itself; do not press into the shoulder or apply any great pressure—as the area is inflamed this can cause more problems. For direct work on the actual shoulder, on the front or the back of the body, simply use light strokes in phase one and move in gentle, small circles in phases two and three. Do not rush a treatment—it is better to work slowly and effectively than to risk causing more pain or injury.

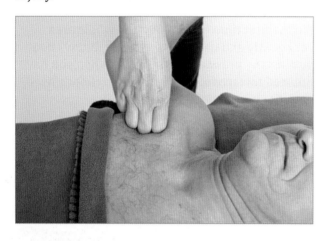

As the frozen shoulder moves into phase two, along with this gentle massage work you can also ask your clients to do some stretches between massage sessions to keep the joint mobile and the muscles working. You can go a little more deeply with your massage but keeping focused on the hand, arms, head, and neck as this will be of great benefit in releasing the shoulder without risking any damage to it.

You can also now begin to massage the muscles that come from the front of the body into the shoulder, specifically the deltoids and pectoralis major; these can be very tender muscles so work gently and slowly.

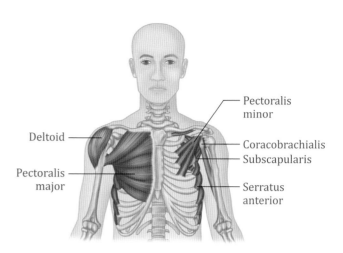

Deltoid

Pectoralis major

Pectoralis minor

Coracobrachialis

Subscapularis

Serratus anterior

With the client's shoulder supported by the massage table and using the flat of your knuckles as shown in the picture below, work across the pectoralis major by pressing and then holding your hand still for 30–60 seconds; release to move around the chest so that you work the whole of this area.

Be careful when working with women clients that you do not press onto breast tissue, and avoid pressing onto the collar bone. Having done this, use the flat of one finger to work with this same press and release technique, moving down the deltoid muscle from just below the collar bone to the top of the arm—don't slide down the muscle but release your pressure between each press.

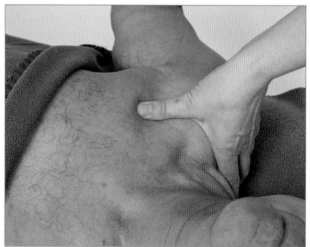

With regard to stretches: working with a physiotherapist where appropriate and with the client seated, ask the client to roll the shoulders gently down and backward, then move the shoulder in small circles (working up to larger circles as the joint gains mobility), and then to repeat this in the other direction, moving the shoulder upward and forward. Each can be repeated ten times (start with five if this is difficult).

In phase three, more exercises can be introduced and you can also begin to increase the depth of the massage into the shoulder, still working the same areas as above. Still act with caution and get constant feedback from your client; the depth of massage at this stage should mean that your client can feel that you are working there but should not be experiencing pain from what you are doing—if there is pain during a treatment then pull back on your depth.

With your client seated, ask him or her to put one arm out in front of them with the fingers pointing upward and the palm forward. Then ask your client to hold the fingers of the outstretched arm with the other hand, gently pulling the fingers back. The client will feel the stretch through the arm and into the shoulder. Releasing that, then ask the client to turn the hand so that the fingers point to the floor, using the other hand to, again, gently pull the fingers toward the body. Hold each side for a maximum of 20 seconds.

Shoulder blade squeezes can be done anytime, anywhere. Ask your clients to imagine that there is a tennis ball between their shoulder blades and they are trying to squeeze the ball. Hold the squeeze for five seconds and release; repeat 10 times.

There are a lot more exercises available: some should be done under the supervision of a physiotherapist, all are aimed at *gently* mobilizing the shoulder, and the phases may pass more quickly with this combined approach. Your massage work, combined with these, can get the shoulder moving again and your client should see a much shorter recovery time, a reduction in pain, and an increase in mobility.

Gynecological Issues

Background to the Conditions

There are a large number of gynecological problems encountered by women and an equally large array of both conventional and alternative treatments on offer to treat them. There are massage treatments that can help with painful or scanty periods and some women have found massage has helped with issues around fertility.

Massage can be helpful for some women with endometriosis, particularly to help with the pain of adhesions. But for all of these, and other, issues it would be remiss to promise "cures" for what can be complex physical and emotional issues that can reach right to the core of how a woman might feel about herself. So while this chapter will look at how massage can help with some gynecological issues, there will be no promises about what that massage can and cannot do.

These massage techniques can, however, be tried either through a professional practitioner or in the comfort of your home with the massage carried out by a friend or family member.

This section is divided into three main topics, looking at problem periods, endometriosis, and polycystic ovaries. We will also touch lightly on unexplained infertility. There will be a significant focus on acupressure points as this can give a targeted treatment, in addition to looking at the benefits of abdominal massage.

Specific Contraindications

None of these techniques should be used on anyone who is pregnant or who has given birth within the last three months. If clients are experiencing heavy bleeding or are on blood-thinning medication you should seek the approval of their medical practitioner before treatment.

Massage Treatments

Drawing on traditional Chinese medicine (TCM) and acupuncture techniques, there are some acupressure points that can be used as part of massage to give a general treatment for problematic periods. They can be included in a general massage or given as a stand-alone treatment. Pregnancy should be ruled out before commencing any treatment or massage for gynecological issues.

Problem periods may come in a variety of forms: amenorrhea (absent periods), dysmenorrhea (painful periods), or menorrhagia (heavy periods).

Problem Periods: Amenorrhea

There can be a number of reasons why periods are absent. Young women under the age of 16 may just be late developing and, once they do start, will have normal cycles—this is known as primary amenorrhea. When it occurs in later life it can be due to a number of reasons, including menopause (early or normal onset).

Hypothalamic amenorrhea is an absence of periods usually due to extreme weight loss, excessive exercise, stress, or some long-term conditions. Polycystic ovaries can lead to amenorrhea, as can hyperprolactinemia—when a person has abnormally high levels of the hormone prolactin. This can be a side effect of medication, but if periods stop suddenly a medical practitioner should be consulted to assess the underlying reason.

Some thyroid treatments will interfere with the menstrual cycle; premature ovarian failure will lead to amenorrhea, as, of course, will pregnancy.

TCM works on the understanding that the body's energy (qi, or ch'i) runs through the body along meridians, and problems occur when energy is blocked and becomes stagnant or where there is too much or too little energy. Accessing these points through acupuncture (using needles) or acupressure (using fingers, thumbs, or specialist acupressure tools) allows this system to restore its flow.

The meridians have names, and the points on them numbers and names—these are referred to here and are shown in the diagrams below. The acupressure point K 3 (kidney 3), located below SP 6 (spleen 6) on the inside of the ankle and used in conjunction with SP 6 and SP 8 (spleen 8 on the inside lower leg), can initiate the menstrual cycle.

TCM could attribute scanty menstruation to a number of different causes, representing both deficiencies and stagnation in the body's energy system, but these three points are common to most treatments. You can apply static pressure to the point simply by pressing into that point with your thumb; this may be tender when you first apply pressure but this tenderness should ease as the point is stimulated.

Problem Periods: Dysmenorrhea

Painful periods (dysmenorrhea) can usually be treated at home; there are numerous over-the-counter medications and traditional/home remedies that are in use around the world every day. Period pain happens when the muscular wall of the womb contracts; this is normally very mild. As the period progresses the womb contracts more and the lining is shed, causing normal menstrual bleeding. When these contractions take place, the blood vessels in the womb are compressed and the womb is starved of oxygen. When part of the body is without oxygen the body produces pain. It's not known why some women have more pain than others but the pain can be very debilitating for a number of days each month.

In a small number of cases there are underlying problems that need investigating; these include: endometriosis, fibroids, pelvic inflammatory disease, and adenomyosis (where the tissue that normally lines the womb starts to grow within the muscular wall of the womb), or pain can be triggered by an intrauterine device.

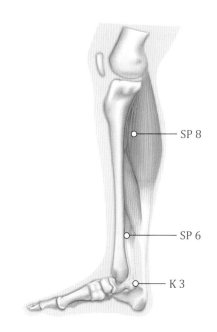

There are two very useful points in acupressure that are supported by research to show their pain-relieving qualities for period pain. LI 4, a point on the large intestine meridian, is a good point for pain relief for any part of the body. In a study in Taiwan this point alone was used for six months to effectively treat women with painful periods.[82]

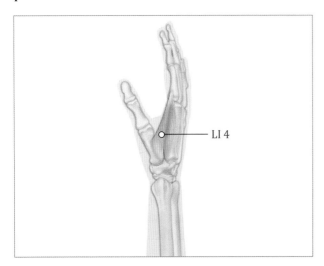

LI 4

In another study, the point SP 6 (on the spleen meridian) was found using the width of three fingers above the ankle bone on the inside of the ankles. Pressure was applied with the thumb at SP 6 for six seconds and then released for two seconds, and this repeated during two five-minute cycles on each leg. The women were asked to rate their pain and anxiety levels using four questionnaires before and immediately following treatment at both sessions. Pain and anxiety scores improved significantly more after the initial session in the women who received acupressure than in those who rested; pain, but not anxiety, was significantly reduced after self-administered therapy.[83]

Problem Periods: Menorrhagia

Heavy periods, or menorrhagia, is when a woman loses an excessive amount of blood during consecutive periods. Heavy blood loss is normal for some women and does not necessarily mean that there is anything wrong, but it can be very debilitating. The average amount of blood lost during a period is 30–40 ml (two to three tablespoons), with nine out of ten women losing less than 80 ml. Therefore, heavy menstrual bleeding is considered to be 60–80 ml or more in each cycle.[84] Underlying causes to rule out include: uterine fibroids, polycystic ovary syndrome, problems with intrauterine contraceptive devices, and anticoagulant medication.

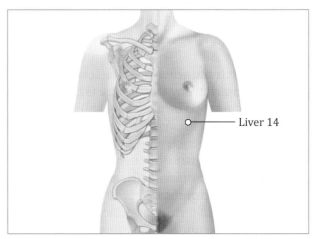

Liver 14

To self-treat for heavy bleeding you can use the point Liver 14; this is located below the breast where the bra wire sits.

This tender point is located between the ribs in a little nook closer to the sternum or hard part of the breast plate. If this is a tender point then it likely that the liver could use a little boost. Hold the point with firm pressure for up to five minutes until the pain subsides. The point should soften and will not be as sensitive. Liver 3 is located on the foot between the first and third toe, up into the fleshy part of the foot about

[82] http://www.massagemag.com/acupressure-found-beneficial-for-menstrual-problems-7456/

[83] http://www.bastyrcenter.org/content/view/363/

[84] http://www.nhs.uk/conditions/periods-heavy/Pages/Introduction.aspx

two inches up from the web. It is usually very sensitive. This is one of the most powerful points in the body as well as being the source point of the liver. It must be avoided during pregnancy. [85]

Abdominal massage can also assist with these three issues and you can follow the instructions from the chapter on emotional issues, on page 108, for this massage. Abdominal massage can bring on a period outside of the regular pattern; when this happens, it is usually shorter than a normal period and may contain small clots or darker blood. This is a clearing out of the area and is nothing to be concerned about; it should stop in two or three days and hopefully periods will be lighter and less painful afterward.

It is also important for menstrual problems to massage the sacrum. The uterosacral ligaments connect the uterus to the sacrum so don't miss this important area. The sacrum is a flat area of bone at the base of the spine; it is a very strong bone that supports the weight of the upper body as it is spread across the pelvis and into the legs. The sacrum forms from five individual vertebrae that begin to join together during late adolescence and early adulthood to form a single bone by around the age of 30. It is one of the few bones that it is possible to massage directly onto.

You can do this using the flat of your hand, the heel of your palm, or the flat of two or three fingers held together. Simply make small circles around the whole of the area, stopping as you get to the intergluteal cleft; on most clients you should be able to feel the edges of the sacrum. Circle over the whole area slowly three or four times—this may be tender at first but the tenderness should drop as the tension in the area relaxes. This area is particularly good for treating period pains.

Endometriosis

Endometriosis gets its name from the word *endometrium*, the tissue that lines the uterus or womb. Endometriosis occurs when this tissue grows outside of the uterus on other organs or structures in the body. Most often, endometriosis is found on the ovaries, fallopian tubes, in the tissues that hold the uterus in place, on the outer surface of the uterus, and on the lining of the pelvic cavity. It can also grow in the vagina, cervix, vulva, bowel, bladder, or rectum, and there are some rare cases where it has been found in other parts of the body, such as the lungs, brain, and skin.[86] It can also lead to very painful menstrual cramps, pain in the lower back and pelvis, pain during or after sex, abdominal pain, exhaustion, stomach upsets, and infertility.

Traditional treatments for endometriosis are hormonal and surgical. A study by the *Iranian Journal of Nursing and Midwifery Research* found in clinical trials that massage for women with endometriosis significantly helped to reduce their pain.[87] Abdominal massage, as detailed on page may also help to increase blood flow to the area and can, for some women, help to regulate periods—something that can be very welcome with the heavy and prolonged bleeding associated with endometriosis. This is a condition that can have a profound effect on a woman's life, so gentle, supportive whole-body massage can also bring a very welcome and healing touch.

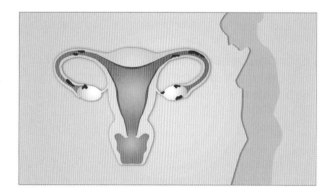

[85] http://www.self-helphealth.com/topics/acupressure_woman.html

[86] http://www.womenshealth.gov/publications/our-publications/fact-sheet/endometriosis.html#a

[87] http://www.ncbi.nlm.nih.gov/pmc/articles/PMC3093183/

Polycystic Ovary Syndrome

Polycystic ovaries, more correctly termed polycystic ovary syndrome (PCOS), is a hormonal disorder among women of reproductive age. The name of the condition comes from the appearance of the ovaries in most, but not all, women with the disorder, where the ovaries appear enlarged and contain numerous small cysts located along the outer edge (polycystic appearance).[88]

The exact cause of PCOS is unknown but excessive insulin, low-grade inflammation, genetics, and being exposed to too much male hormone in the womb may all be implicated. Common symptoms include infrequent or long menstrual periods, excess hair growth due to elevated levels of male hormones (androgens), acne, and obesity. The Australian Natural Therapy Pages website suggests that massage can help with PCOS by encouraging good circulation in the area, stimulating the release of natural endorphins and neurotransmitters such as serotonin to improve the mood and decrease the effects of stress; lowering the levels of adrenaline, noradrenaline, and cortisol—all associated with the "fight or flight" response—that cause feelings of stress; and helping to normalize sex hormone levels that are often unstable throughout PCOS.[89] By decreasing stress, massage also helps to increase immunity.

Massage for PCOS can be general massage, and upper-body massage is very effective in lowering stress levels; however, don't ignore the lower body as gentle abdominal massage with the flat of the hand is helpful for gynecological issues, and this should ideally follow from lower-body massage to free the tension from its source.

Unexplained Infertility

The most controversial part of massage for gynecological issues is probably that surrounding the treatment of unexplained infertility. There have been numerous promises made by some practitioners. Act with caution here—massage may help someone overcome unexplained fertility, but it also may not. This is not to say that massage cannot help, for some women it can and it does, but it is unethical to promise a "cure" for something that may be causing couples a great deal of distress. Sometimes the stress of potential infertility can itself be enough to cause fertility problems, and massage to relax will not cause any problems; the instructions in the chapter on massage and anxiety can be followed.

Abdominal massage may help to increase blood supply and decrease pain, which can also help. Acupuncture and TCM have much to contribute and some people find these effective; it's worth a try but within clear ethical boundaries around promises or even hints at what can and cannot be guaranteed.

---

[88] http://www.mayoclinic.org/diseases-conditions/pcos/basics/definition/con-20028841

[89] http://www.naturaltherapypages.com.au/article/PCOS_and_Massage

Irritable Bowel Syndrome

Background to the Condition

Irritable bowel syndrome (IBS) is a common condition of the digestive system whose full cause is unknown. Inspection of the gut through scanning, surgery, or under the microscope shows no abnormalities, but the condition gives rise to stomach cramps, bloating, diarrhea, and constipation. IBS is the most common gut problem worldwide, with an estimated 20% of the population of the US experiencing symptoms,[90] 13% in Canada, 12% in the UK, and 6.9% in Australia. Full and reliable statistics are not available for the whole world and diagnosis varies from place to place.[91] IBS can affect anyone at any age, but it commonly first develops in young adults and teenagers. IBS is twice as common in women as in men.[92]

The pain experienced in the stomach can be mild to severe and will often vary from time to time with each individual. The area of the stomach where the pain is felt will also move around, and IBS usually happens in bouts that can last for very varied lengths of time—this changes from individual to individual and for each individual between different bouts. The pain usually eases with passing stools and someone with IBS will usually experience a lot of gastric gas. In IBS the gut appears to be overactive in specific areas; it is not yet fully understood why this overactivity of the nerves or muscles of the gut occurs, although stress, anxiety, and emotional upset appear to play a role. About half of people with IBS can relate the start of symptoms to a stressful event in their life and symptoms tend to become worse during times of stress or anxiety.[93] Food intolerances may play a part, and some cases of IBS follow gastroenteritis or traveller's diarrhea, while other cases appear to be linked to antibiotic use.

Some medications are used to treat IBS but increasing soluble fiber can help; eating regular meals, increasing the intake of probiotics, and trying to decrease sources of stress and anxiety are all things that the person with IBS can do that help ease their symptoms. Massage can also be a positive aspect to treatment, including self-massage of the abdomen.

Specific Contraindications

- Do not use this treatment on anyone who is pregnant.

- Do not use this treatment if the IBS has not been medically diagnosed so that other, more complex, conditions have been ruled out.

---

[90] https://www.floridahospital.com/irritable-bowel-syndrome-ibs/statistics

[91] http://www.worldgastroenterology.org/assets/downloads/en/pdf/guidelines/20_irritable_bowel_syndrome.pdf

[92] http://www.patient.co.uk/health/irritable-bowel-syndrome-leaflet

[93] http://www.patient.co.uk/health/irritable-bowel-syndrome-leaflet

- Do not use this treatment on someone who has Crohn's disease or a leaky gut.

- Do not use this treatment on anyone who has had recent abdominal or gynecological surgery.

- If clients have blood in their stools, do not massage; refer to their medical practitioner.

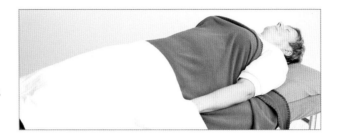

Massage Treatments

For guidance of how to give an abdominal massage to someone else please follow the detailed instructions given in the chapter on Constipation. It is also possible to self-administer this treatment.

Before doing any detailed work simply circling clockwise around the belly can give some people release by relieving bloating. This can be done on a self-care and as-needed basis. If you are at home, find a warm and comfortable place to lie down and warm some high quality massage oil in your hands. Place the flat of your hand to the bottom right of your belly button and stroke around your belly button clockwise in small circles; you can rock your hand as your work to vary the gentle pressure as you move around the inner belly, working on the small intestine.

Finish in the same place as you started, at the bottom right of the belly, this time lower down and further out so that you are resting your hand just above the inside of your right hip bone. If you are big bellied, you can use two hands to ensure you cover the whole of your belly. Use your hands to stroke upward toward the bottom of your right rib, across to the bottom your left rib, down toward the left hip, and then back across to the right. You are aiming simply to move your hands in a large circle around your belly, gently rocking your hand as you move so that you are softly stimulating the bowel.

As IBS tends not to strike at very convenient times, you can also do the same moves discretely through clothes at work as and when you get the chance. Some people find that it does help relieve trapped wind, so try to do this in a place where

releasing gas is not a problem so that you don't end up confounding the problem by deliberately holding on to gas.

You can also treat someone else with this same massage; be careful that you are always working clockwise on the client. If you are treating someone else with IBS you should do this work through a towel or blanket for privacy. Do not work higher than the bottom of the ribcage and do not go too low—placing an additional towel across the hip bones will give you a guide of how low to work, as shown in the photograph. If you are a parent working with your child you can do this gentle treatment as part of your nighttime routine.

For some people this will be enough and all that can be tolerated; if you or your client is able to take deeper work then follow the detailed directions given in the chapter dealing with constipation.

As IBS is also made worse by stress, massage that releases stress can also be effective for general wellbeing and in helping to reduce some symptoms. Massage work to relax the shoulders, neck, and head is very effective in treating stress and tension. With your client faceup, start by massaging the head following the directions in Chapter 4.

There is evidence to suggest that many people fear their IBS is actually cancer, and discussing this can help to alleviate IBS symptoms by addressing some of the underlying health fears.[94] If your clients are at all concerned about their symptoms, if symptoms change over time, or if there is blood in stools then they should speak to their medical practitioner.

[94] http://www.worldgastroenterology.org/assets/downloads/en/pdf/guidelines/20_irritable_bowel_syndrome.pdf

Lumbar Spondylosis

Background to the Condition

Lumbar spondylosis is a term used to describe lumbar osteoarthritis, disc degeneration, and degenerative disc disease. What they have in common is that they are all degenerative lumbar spinal problems. Lower-back pain affects approximately 60–85% of adults at some point in their lives.

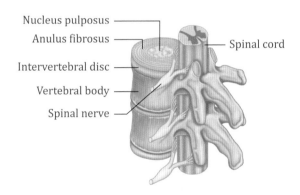

Nucleus pulposus
Anulus fibrosus
Intervertebral disc
Vertebral body
Spinal nerve
Spinal cord

Chronic low back pain, defined as pain symptoms persisting beyond three months, affects an estimated 15–45% of the population.[95] The impact of this on the physical and economic wealth of individuals and a country are considerable.

Lumbar spondylosis is a degenerative disorder that may cause loss of normal spinal structure and function. Although aging is the primary cause, where and how this happens is very individual. The intervertebral discs and facet joints are affected and changes occur as an individual ages.[96] "Normal wear and tear" is an expression many people will hear from the medical world when diagnosed with this problem. Understanding how the spine works is useful in understanding what goes wrong in lumbar spondylosis.

The spine is our body's central support structure. It keeps us upright and connects different parts of the skeleton to each other, such as the head, chest, pelvis, shoulders, arms, and legs. Although the spine is made up of a chain of bones, it is flexible owing to elastic ligaments and spinal discs.[97]

These discs between each vertebrae normally work like shock absorbers. They protect the spine against the daily pull of gravity. They also protect the spine during strenuous activities that put strong force on the spine, such as jumping, running, and lifting. The lumbar spine is supported by ligaments and muscles.

[95] http://www.ncbi.nlm.nih.gov/pmc/articles/PMC2697338/

[96] http://www.healthcentral.com/chronic-pain/c/17554/24809/lumbar/

[97] http://www.ncbi.nlm.nih.gov/pubmedhealth/PMH0005179/

The ligaments, which connect bones together, are arranged in layers and run in multiple directions. Thick ligaments connect the bones of the lumbar spine to the sacrum (the bone below L5) and pelvis. Between the vertebrae of each spinal segment are two *facet joints*.

The facet joints are located on the back of the spinal column. There are two facet joints between each pair of vertebrae, one on each side of the spine. A facet joint is made of small, bony knobs that line up along the back of the spine. Where these knobs meet, they form a joint that connects the two vertebrae. The alignment of the facet joints of the lumbar spine allows freedom of movement as you bend forward and backward.[98]

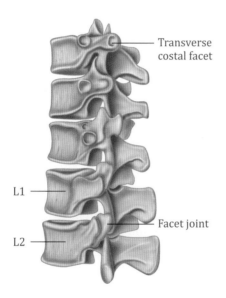

Transverse costal facet

L1

Facet joint

L2

Lumbar spondylosis occurs when the degeneration in the disc and facet joints allow the vertebrae to move more than they should. Spondylosis changes the weight-bearing relationship between the disc and facet joints. Normally the disc will handle the majority of the load and the facets "guide" movement. As the disc degenerates (wears, loses water content and thins) the facets bear more weight. The facet joints thicken (facet hypertrophy) and the bony end plates of the vertebrae above and below the disc can thicken and develop spurs (syndesmophytes).

Eventually, the support from the facet joints becomes ineffective.[99] This causes disc and facet joint pain, but also narrowing of the central canal of the spine and the lateral canals where the nerves exit, causing numbness, tingling, weakness and often considerable pain. The World Health Organization estimate that in the industrialised world 60–70% of the population will suffer from back pain at some point in their lives[100] and it is the leading cause of activity limitation and work absence throughout much of the world—imposing a high economic burden on individuals, families, communities, industry, and governments.[101]

Pain from lumbar spondylosis is usually worse when the person is standing, walking, or bending backward, and it can be eased by resting or bending the spine forward. There may be spasms in the lower-back muscles and the hamstring muscles may be tight. Diagnosis is usually through a physical examination, X-rays, CT scans and MRI.

In addition to degenerative spondylosis, about 6% of the population has a pre-existing problem. Other than obvious trauma and fracture, not much is known about how this happens but it probably occurs around adolescence.

Another term used in describing lower-back problems is spondylolisthesis. Spondylosis and spondylolisthesis are often related. Spondylosis refers to the deterioration of the vertebrae described above, while spondylolisthesis if often the result of this and describes a misalignment of the vertebrae in the spine, where a vertebra might 'slip', either moving into the spinal canal or over the top of the vertebra below.[102]

---

[98] http://www.methodistorthopedics.com/lumbar-spondylolisthesis

[99] http://www.methodistorthopedics.com/lumbar-spondylolisthesisIbid.

[100] http://www.who.int/medicines/areas/priority_medicines/Ch6_24LBP.pdf

[101] Ibid.

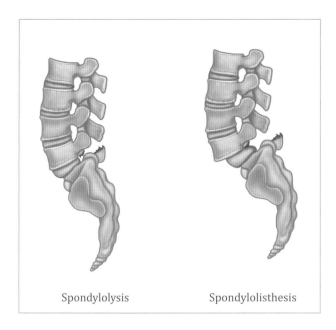

Spondylolysis   Spondylolisthesis

This is different to a slipped disc—also known as a prolapsed or herniated disc—which occurs when one of the discs that sit between the vertebrae is damaged and presses on the nerves. While spondylosis and a slipped disc can overlap, spondylosis is degenerative and more likely to occur as age increases; slipped discs are more likely to happen to those between 35 and 55. After 60 years of age, the water content of the disc is reduced, and slipped discs are less likely.

If the nerves at the very bottom of the spinal cord become compressed it can lead to complications, the symptoms of which include: numbness in the groin, paralysis of one or both legs, rectal pain, loss of bowel or bladder control, or pain in the inside of the thighs.[103]

If any of these complications arise then the client should seek medical advice to prevent longer-term nerve damage, and surgery to release the nerve and prevent further damage may be necessary—this would be assessed by a spinal specialist.

The treatment protocol usually involves rest, particularly rest from sporting activities, and in addition may include some of the following treatments: epidural steroid injections, chiropractic treatment or acupuncture, physiotherapy, strengthening exercises and in a small minority of cases, surgery.

Specific Contraindications

If the problems arise following an accident or injury the client should be checked by a medical practitioner prior to massage treatment.
If the client is experiencing numbness, tingling, slowed reflexes, muscle weakness in the legs, or bladder or bowel problems, they should get medical clearance prior to receiving massage to rule out any other causes.

Massage Treatments

If there are no complications, massage may help to alleviate pain and can be done gently, safely, and effectively. If the person has a history of slipped discs then do not work on the muscles immediately beside the spine; instead concentrate on the feet, legs, sacral, and upper-back work, using only superficial massage over the muscles surrounding lumbar spine. The body is very good at protecting the spine; at the first sign of any danger to the spine the muscles react to protect it. Even after this perceived danger passes, the muscles can take a while to relax and muscular tension can cause significant pain.

[102] http://www.rushortho.com/spondylolisthesis.cfm

[103] http://www.methodistorthopedics.com/lumbar-spondylolisthesis

This massage should be carried out with the client facedown; work for no more than 45 minutes so that the muscles of the lower and middle back do not stiffen up. Place a pillow or cushion underneath the ankles to provide support to the legs and to prevent further pressure on the spine. Begin by working the feet as detailed in Chapter 3. Then, holding the foot securely, gently stretch from the base of the toes up towards the front of the body; only stretch within the client's comfort zone, holding each stretch for 20–30 seconds, and repeat with the other foot—this completes the foot treatment and begins to stretch out the Achilles tendon in the calf.

Next you need to massage up the back of the legs, focusing on the calves and thighs. You should only apply light pressure to the inner calf as this can easily bruise, and avoid massaging close to the groin to protect your client's dignity. Start with the calves.

You can use your thumb or the flat of your palm to massage the outer calf muscles, focusing specifically on the soleus and gastrocnemius muscles as shown in the diagram. To begin with focus on the gastrocnemius lateral head on the outside of the leg and when you have massaged this well you can also work the gastrocnemius medial head.

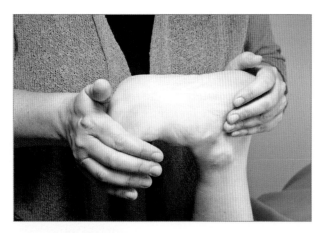

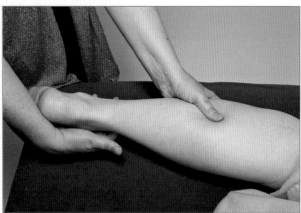

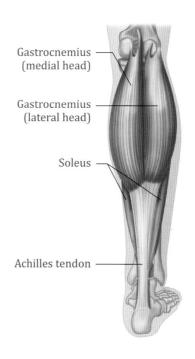

Gastrocnemius (medial head)

Gastrocnemius (lateral head)

Soleus

Achilles tendon

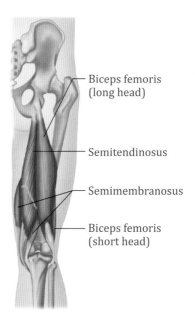

Biceps femoris (long head)

Semitendinosus

Semimembranosus

Biceps femoris (short head)

Posterior view

Use long strokes to begin with and if there is a particularly tender spot you can either shake the muscle at that point using two fingers or you can use your thumb to apply moderate static pressure to that point. After either of these techniques have been used you should repeat the long strokes over the whole of the muscle, being careful to lift away from the calf before you reach the back of the knee.

Move up to above the knee to massage the thigh. You will see from the diagram that there are a number of muscles in the upper thigh; do not worry too much about the names of the muscles but aim to massage the whole of the back of the thigh, while avoiding the inner thigh.

You can use the flat of your hand or the flat of your arm to warm up the muscles using long strokes and gentle pressure; having done that you can work a little deeper, always within your client's tolerance, using the same strokes but at a greater depth. You can also knead the muscles with the palm of your hand, holding the pressure on areas that are resistant to touch.

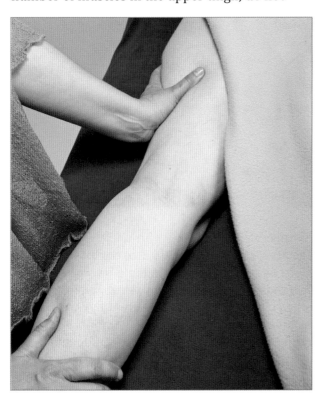
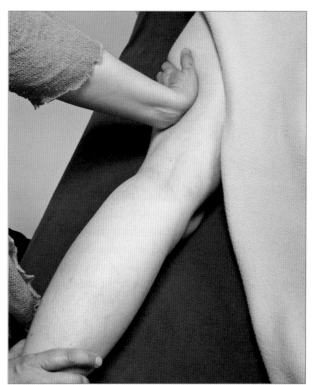

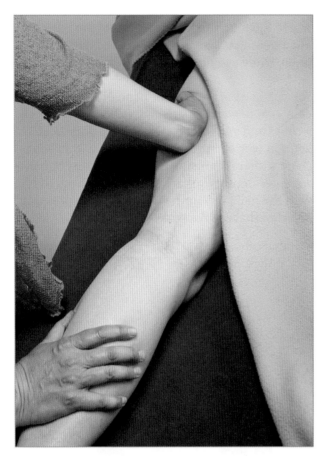
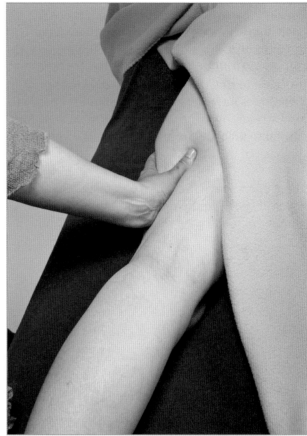

Having worked the feet and legs you can then gently work the sacrum. The sacrum is a flat area of bone at the base of the spine; the sacrum is a very strong bone that supports the weight of the upper body as it is spread across the pelvis and into the legs.

The sacrum is formed from five individual vertebrae which begin to join together during late adolescence and early adulthood to form a single bone by around the age of thirty; it is one of the few bones that it is possible to massage directly onto.

You can do this using the flat of your hand, the heel of your palm or the flat of two or three fingers held together. It is very important when treating this problem to work gently so that you do not pull or put any strain on the spine itself.

Simply make small circles around the whole of the area, stopping as you get to the intergluteal cleft; on most clients you should be able to feel the edges of the sacrum. Move with these small circles over the whole area slowly three or four times; this may be tender at first but the tenderness should wane as the tension in the area relaxes.

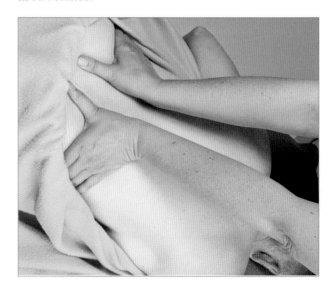

You can now work the main area of the lower back but do so very gently, be careful not to put any pressure onto the spine itself so take great care not to touch the spine. Use lots of massage oil so that you can glide across the back. Placing your thumbs either side of the spine gently roll your thumbs away from the back until you reach the edge of the hips; repeat this four or five times.

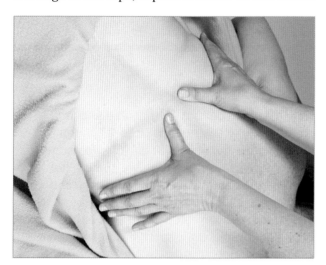

As your client's pain levels decrease and they are able to stay on the massage table longer you can also include more general back massage, as detailed in Chapter 5, always being careful not to put any downwards or sideways pressure onto the spine itself.

Stretching the hamstrings is something that your client can do between treatments––if they are a sports person they will already have their own ways to do this, if not then the simplest way is, while seated, for your client to stretch their leg out straight and curl the toes up towards the front of the body, repeating this movement on both sides.

The massage for this condition is aimed at relaxing the muscles, relieving pain, and assisting the body in recovery. As a bonus, massage encourages the body to produce endorphins, which are the natural pain relievers for the body, so massage should have both short- and longer-term positive effects.

Menopause

Background to the Condition

The menopause starts with the perimenopause, when a woman's estrogen levels decrease, and then develops into the full menopause when ovulation and monthly periods stop. The average age for a woman to go through the menopause in Western society is 52 but it can happen from 30 onward; below 45 would be classed as an early menopause. The fall in estrogen not only prevents ovulation but also causes a number of other symptoms including hot flushes, night sweats, mood swings, and vaginal dryness.

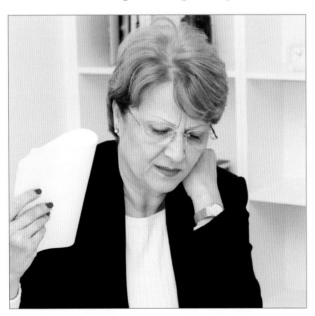

How a woman deals with the menopause emotionally will vary: for some it signals a loss of youth and an end to any possible new pregnancies; for others it's a welcome relief from periods and worries about contraception. If there are children, they are often close to adulthood, and new careers and adventures may become possible. October 18 has been named as World Menopause Day by the World Health Organization and International Menopause Society; this is designed to raise the profile of the menopause, making it a more visible public health issue, and easier for women to discuss.

The physical changes that take place during the menopause are not restricted to hormonal ones—there is a knock-on effect into the rest of the body, and decreases in bone mass density, muscle mass, and strength have been reported.[104] Estrogen is partly responsible for maintaining muscle tone and contributes to skin collagen, so both muscle and skin can suffer during and after the menopause. Osteoporosis can impact on bones and teeth; joint and muscle aches and pains are common symptoms during menopause.[105]

---

[104] http://www.ncbi.nlm.nih.gov/pubmed/19949277

[105] https://www.menopause.org.au/consumers/information-sheets/33-menopause-and-body-changes

These are major hormonal and metabolic shifts that occur during menopause, and the body needs adequate rest,[106] maintenance, and a good dose of TLC. Massage during this time can be both relaxing and therapeutic. Simply receiving a positive loving touch at a time when your body seems to be doing strange things is nurturing and supportive. Having body work that helps to resolve aches and pains and stretch out the muscles is a positive treatment that women can add to their self-care routine at this time of change.

Specific Contraindications

There are no specific contraindications for massage during the menopause. If the client has any specific medical conditions the contraindications for those conditions should be followed.

Massage Treatments

Whilst there is no particular recommended massage, you can work with any of the treatments in this book to help alleviate the problems encountered by the individual woman. There are some specific acupressure points for use in the menopause and there are certain aromatherapy oils that can help relieve symptoms and these can be used on a "try and see which works best" basis.

There is evidence to suggest that acupressure can be effective in treating hot flushes, and also any anxiety and depression related to menopause.[107]

Acupressure and acupuncture work on an understanding of the energy flow within the body; qi (ch'i) or energy—qi flows along meridians, the invisible pathways in the body. Good health depends on the smooth and free flow of qi along these meridians and for this to happen the body and mind need to be in harmony. When hormonal changes occur at menopause this can create an imbalance and so acupressure and acupuncture work to restore harmony. The symbol of yin and yang below is used to demonstrate this balance. Yin and yang are balanced opposites and everything in the universe consists of both elements.

Yin originally meant the shady side of a slope. It is associated with such qualities as cold, rest, responsiveness, passivity, darkness, interiority, downwardness, inwardness, decrease, and femininity. Yang, by contrast, originally referred to the sunny side of a slope. It implies brightness, and is associated with qualities such as heat, stimulation, movement, activity, excitement, vigor, light, exteriority, upwardness, outwardness, increase, and masculinity.[108] Where there is in a blockage in qi flow or where the energy is deficient, this area is treated to bring about a balance.

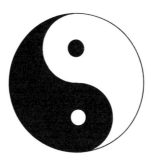

---

[106] A Stengler and M Stengler, *Your Menopause, Your Menotype.* New York, NY: Avery, 2002, pp. 51-52.

[107] http://www.acupuncture.org.uk/a-to-z-of-conditions/public-review-papers/menopause-and-acupuncture-the-evidence-for-effectiveness.html

[108] http://www.dailyom.com/library/000/000/000000268.html

There are five key areas that should be treated for the menopausal woman: (CON 4) conception vessel 4, (L1 11) large intestine 11, (K3) kidney 3, and (SP6, SP9) spleen 6 and 9.

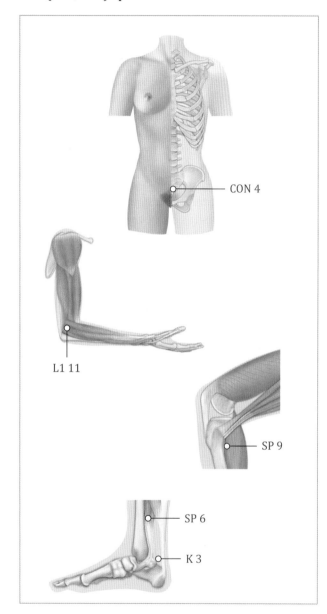

Point 4 on the conception vessel meridian is on the midline of the abdomen about three-fifths of the way between the belly button and the top edge of the pubic bone. In traditional treatments this point is for exhaustion, weakness, chronic fatigue or diseases, and menstrual and sexual issues. In acupressure there are three different ways to treat this spot; a steady pressure with a fingertip or knuckle (or even a rubber-tipped

pencil) is "tonifying." Hold this steady pressure for up to two minutes; a clockwise circling motion can be used to move blocked energy and to calm excessive energy use the flat palm of the hand to stroke the area.

Large intestine 11 (known as "the pool at the bend") is used to treat hot flushes and is on the outer arm at the side of the elbow. If you bend your forearm bringing your hand toward your neck, LI 11 is located halfway up width of the arm at the end of the crease at the elbow. To reduce hot flushes circle anticlockwise on this area.

Spleen 6 is used for reducing hot flushes, anxiety, and other gynecological issues. This is located by asking the client to place the hand flat with the little finger across the middle of the ankle bone on the inside of the leg on a line with the second knuckles. SP 6 is where the index finger rests, in a direct line from the inner ankle bone. This point is also good for treating insomnia and dizziness.

It can be a very tender point so work gently and gradually increase the pressure with each treatment. If it is simply too painful to treat with direct pressure, begin by holding your flat hand over the point to begin with.

Kidney 3 (the "great steam point") is an effective point to work for an energy boost and for detoxification along with treating backache, headache, dizziness, and insomnia. This point is found on the inside of the foot, halfway between the Achilles tendon and the side of the ankle bone.

Spleen 9 helps with fatigue, lack of energy, abdominal bleeding, and pain in the genitals. It is located below the inside of the knee, just off the bone where the tibia begins to curve. This point can be very tender; if it too tender to press straight into gradually increase your depth as tolerance increases.

All of these points can be used either as a separate treatment, as part of a general massage treatment, or by the individual menopausal woman for self-treatment.

Aromatherapy oils can also be used to support the menopausal woman, these should be blended into a base oil—do not use them neat on the skin as they are too powerful, and do not ingest them. You can use them in base bubble baths and lotions. A base oil is the oil into which you put drops of essential oils, grape-seed is one of the most natural and low-allergen oils and is suitable for use on most people. It is available to buy online or at health food shops and some supermarkets. Try to use an organic base oil where possible.

Different essential oils have distinct properties; there are three main groups of oils to use. Firstly essential oils that affect estrogen and balance the hormones; these include cypress, geranium, lavender, neroli, rose, and clary sage. Next, essential oils that will help to ease hot flushes; these include clary sage, grapefruit, lemon, lime, and peppermint. Finally essential oils that are good for emotional ups and downs include chamomile, cedarwood, jasmine, and neroli. You can blend any of these oils together—be guided by your preferences or those of your client.

Essential oils should be bought by their botanical names to ensure you are buying a pure oil and not a chemical-based copied oil; some are fairly cheap (for example lavender and citrus oils), whereas neroli is a very expensive oil—you do get what you pay for with essential oils so it is worth the investment. As you are only using a tiny bit of oil at any time they should last you a long time.

Blending essential oils is both a science and an art but you can also just experiment at home and blend according to needs, mood, and preference. The starting point is to know the blending ratio of the oil—this is the number of drops that you need to use in a base oil or lotion and some of these are given in the table.

The table gives the oils' botanical names and whether they are top, middle, or base notes. Top notes are the lightest fragrances; these will be the first thing that you smell and tend to be uplifting, energizing oils. Middle notes are warm, soft, and subtle fragrances that will linger for longer than the top notes. These oils are good for metabolism, balancing, and relaxing the mind. The base notes are the deep and often heady smells; these will linger long after the other fragrances have faded and are the most relaxing and sedating aromas.

Name	Botanical Name	Note
Cedarwood	*Cedrus atlantica*	Base
Chamomile	*Anthemis nobilis*	Middle
Chinese grapefruit	*Citrus grandis*	Top
Clary sage	*Salvia sclarea*	Top–middle
Cypress	*Cupressus sempervirens*	Base
Geranium	*Pelargonium odoratissimum*	Middle
Jasmine	*Jasminum grandiflorum*	Base
Lavender	*Lavandula angustifolia (officinalis)*	Middle
Lemon	*Citrus limonum*	Top
Lime	*Citrus aurantifolia*	Top
Neroli	*Citrus aurantium amara*	Middle
Peppermint	*Mentha piperita*	Top
Rose	*Rosa damascena*	Base

To simplify, initially blend on the basis that you should have a 3:2:1 ratio—three drops of top notes to two middle notes to one base note. In a 20 ml base you can have 12 drops in total, so you can either have a lighter blend of 3:2:1 or a stronger blend of 6:4:2. This is, however, a generalization: if your client really needs a lift you could, for example, opt for 10 drops of top notes alone in the base oil, but avoid using just base notes as these on their own can induce a headache in some people.

You will need to experiment; most people will end up throwing a few blends away (remember that oil should not be flushed into sewage systems), and what is a beautiful blend to one person may be the worst smell ever to someone else. Some blends do have "synergy"; that is, their combined effect is more powerful than the individual aromas, so feel free to experiment and enjoy combining oils. All of the oils given in the table are useful during the menopause so you will not go wrong with any of them.

Do remember to store essential oils out of the reach of children and animals; essential oils should be kept in a dark box away from strong light and heat. If you are in any doubt about how to blend you can always ask an aromatherapist to blend the oils for you, or you can look out for preblended oils with these essential oils added.

You can also put a few drops of essential oil into your bath; just be careful as the oil can make the bath a little slippery—alternatively use a foot bath or sprinkle the oil onto a tissue or bed linens (but away from where it might come into contact with your eyes).

While different oils have their own contra-indications, as a general rule you should not use these oils if you or your client is pregnant or breastfeeding, or has blood pressure problems or epilepsy, unless under the guidance of a trained aromatherapist. Many of the citrus oils can make the skin photosensitive so avoid direct sunlight after their use. There are also some good books on the topic of aromatherapy that will give much greater detail than is possible here—but have fun as you experiment with these great natural resources.

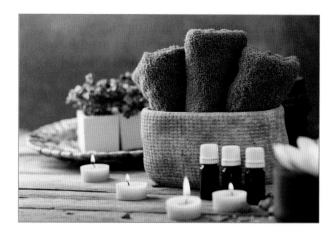

Multiple Sclerosis

Background to the Condition

Multiple sclerosis (MS) is a disease affecting the nerves in the brain and spinal cord, causing problems with muscle movement, balance, and vision.[109] Each nerve in the brain or spinal cord is surrounded by a layer of myelin, which is made up of lipids and proteins; its job is to protect the nerve and help transmit the electrical signals from the brain to the rest of the body. In MS, the myelin becomes damaged.

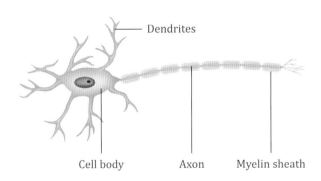

Dendrites

Cell body   Axon   Myelin sheath

The most common symptoms of MS are fatigue; numbness of various parts of the body; problems with walking, balance, and coordination; bladder and/or bowel dysfunction; problems with vision, dizziness, and vertigo; sexual dysfunction; pain; cognitive dysfunction; emotional changes and depression; and spasticity (particularly in the legs).[110] MS is an autoimmune condition in that the individual's immune system mistakes the myelin for a foreign substance and attacks it. This results in messages travelling along the nerves becoming slower, distorted, or completely lost.

While the cause of MS is still unknown, there are some clues emerging as to what could be the trigger. It is not a genetic disease although there could be a genetic predisposition that may make someone more likely to develop MS. Geography is a factor; MS is almost unheard of in countries near the equator and much research is ongoing to see if this could be a bacterial issue,[111] or if it is to do with a lack of sunshine that interferes with vitamin D levels and immunity.[112]

Another recent theory is that the development of MS could be linked to blood flow and the narrowing of veins inside the brain and spinal cord. It is thought that the blood supply to the brain and spine has trouble returning to the heart, which could lead to a buildup of tiny iron deposits inside nerve tissue, which may damage the nerves and/or trigger an autoimmune response.[113]

---

[109] http://www.nhs.uk/Conditions/Multiple-sclerosis/Pages/Introduction.aspx

[110] http://www.nationalmssociety.org/about-multiple-sclerosis/what-we-know-about-ms/symptoms/index.aspx

[111] http://www.nationalmssociety.org/about-multiple-sclerosis/what-we-know-about-ms/what-causes-ms/index.aspx

[112] http://www.nhs.uk/Conditions/Multiple-sclerosis/Pages/Causes.aspx

[113] http://patientmemoirs.com/condition/912-multiple-sclerosis/details

The research into the cause and therefore future possible treatments of MS is ongoing. As yet there is no cure for MS but there are a number of treatments available to help manage the symptoms. Massage can be an important tool in helping to manage some of these symptoms.

Medical practice divides MS into four different types.

• Relapsing remitting MS (RRMS) is the most common form of multiple sclerosis, accounting for around 85% of initial diagnoses. This form of MS is marked by flare-ups of symptoms followed by periods of remission when symptoms improve or disappear, with periods of remission potentially lasting for many years.

• Some patients with RRMS go on to develop secondary progressive (SPMS), where the disease course continues to worsen with or without periods of remission or leveling-off of the severity of symptoms.

• Primary progressive MS (PPMS) accounts for around 10% of initial diagnoses; here, symptoms worsen gradually from the very beginning with no relapses or remissions, although there may be occasional plateaus.

• Finally and most rarely, in less than 5% of diagnoses is progressive relapsing MS; this is progressive from the start, with intermittent flare-ups of worsening symptoms along the way and no periods of remission.[114]

While there have been few clinical trials as to the effect of massage on physical symptoms, there is evidence to show that massage has a positive overall effect on people with MS. In a study where patients received a 45-minute massage twice weekly for five weeks, it was shown that the massage group had lower anxiety and a less depressed mood immediately following the

massage sessions and, by the end of the study, they had improved self-esteem, better body image and image of disease progression, and enhanced social functional status.[115]

While the evidence from clinical studies is lacking, there is good anecdotal evidence to say that massage will also help to relieve the symptoms of MS, specifically the muscle spasms and tremors. On the basis of "first, do no harm," there is nothing to be lost in the individual trying massage to relieve symptoms, to reduce pain, and increase sleep.

Specific Contraindications

Bone density: There are some contraindications for massage which need to be taken into account for people with MS. For reasons yet not fully understood, people with MS can have a lower bone density than the general population, and this can lead to osteoporosis. While this does not rule out massage per se, care needs to be taken not to manipulate bones during massage and any pressure on the sacrum and hips should only be light.

Avoid assisted stretches: It is important to avoid stretching the limbs of someone with MS to avoid any sympathetic nerve firing that might cause muscles to spasm. It is absolutely fine for the client to stretch, and yoga has been helpful for many people with MS; during massage you are avoiding stretching that is not within the client's control.

Heat and vibration: Avoid using any heated pads or mechanical vibration massage as this can cause the nerves to fire. Be very careful when your client moves position on the bed, and particularly when getting up after a treatment, as vertigo can be a problem for people with MS. Some treatments for MS involve self-injecting,

[114] http://www.nytimes.com/health/guides/disease/multiple-sclerosis/print.html

[115] M Hernandez-Reif, Multiple sclerosis patients benefit from massage therapy. *Journal of Bodywork and Movement Therapies*, 1998, 2, 168-174.

so take care not to massage over recent injection sites. If you spot an area that is red or inflamed on an area of the body that is not directly visible to the client, make him or her aware of it so that medical attention can be sought if necessary.

As the symptoms of MS can vary for each individual, and also over time, it is important to start each treatment with a consultation. Ask where pain or stiffness is being felt and how this is affecting everyday life; this will allow you to target the treatment to the client's current concerns.

Massage Treatments

This is a suggested protocol for a full treatment; if this is too long for you or your client you can break it up into an upper body and a lower body treatment, but, if you can, do try to make time for a full regular treatment.

As you repeat the massage your client will be able to say which aspects seem the most useful, and you can then use those techniques between full treatments. It is important that a client with MS should feel very secure on the table; massage could be done with the client clothed and, if you both agree on skin-to-skin contact, ensure that you have blankets or sheets for draping rather than smaller towels, which could become dislodged during tremors or muscle jerking. This will help the client to feel safe and secure, which in turn helps with relaxation. It is also useful to have spare blankets or a light duvet to hand, as someone with MS may also feel cold on the massage table.

As with a number of other conditions it is important to work the fingers and toes in detail, so begin any treatment with the hand and foot massage detailed in Chapters 2 and 3.

As you move to the larger muscles of the arms and legs you are aiming to apply medium pressure to help release any spasticity or tightness in the muscle and to help calm tremors.

Tremors in MS clients can be a daily battle—and a nightly challenge that can result in disturbed nights and a severe lack of sleep. Tremors can be present during a massage as much as they can be at any other time. If tremors occur, don't back off entirely, just place a hand on the affected limb(s) and apply gentle pressure—remember you are not trying to restrain your client at all, you are simply reminding the muscle that it can relax. If the tremors are particularly bad your client may also start to panic at the lack of control; if this happens, focus with your client on deep, slow breathing to help relax and quell any anxiety, and you can do some gentle head massage. A spoken meditation that focuses on the breath can be very helpful for some clients; talk your client through calmly and gently.

Begin the leg work with long, gentle strokes up the leg, working from foot to hip and avoiding the knee and the area behind the knee. Fluid retention can be an issue with MS and this stroking (effleurage) massage helps to stimulate lymphatic flow. Always work upward toward the heart and use a good quality naturally based massage oil to lubricate the skin, unless you are working through clothes. It is important to work both sides of the body as tightness in one muscle will have an effect on the opposite side of the body. Starting with the client facedown will mean less moving around on the table, as you can do this work straight after the work on the hands and feet.

Avoid massaging into the groin when working on the leg, coming off the leg halfway between the knee and the groin. Use the flat of your hand for these long strokes and work with your hands following each other, moving upward all the time.

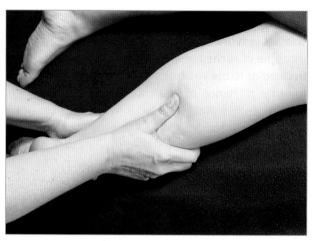

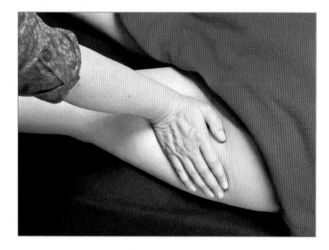

Repeat on both legs and ask your client to adjust position to face upward, so that you can repeat this work on the front of the body. You will need to return to the legs at a later stage to do much deeper work.

With the client still faceup, move to the head and neck. There is a detailed protocol for head massage in Chapter 4, and this should be followed.

Having completed the head massage, you should now continue by following the back massage protocol in Chapter 5, taking care that when you need to move a limb, you ask clients to move it themselves rather than moving it for them.

Once you have completed the work on the back of the body you can return to the legs for deeper work. Having already completed the full foot massage you can move to the ankles. Begin by warming up the calf, paying particular attention to the outer calf. Starting just above the ankle use your thumb or the flat of your hand to knead and gently stretch the outer calf; you are not aiming to stretch any joints, just the actual muscle.

You may feel "knotty" or resistant areas in the outer calf and these are the areas that your client will report as being tender. When you reach such a spot put medium pressure on and hold for 30 seconds to two minutes; you should feel a change in the muscle as it relaxes and your client should report the tenderness diminishing. When this happens, release the pressure and move further up the muscle.

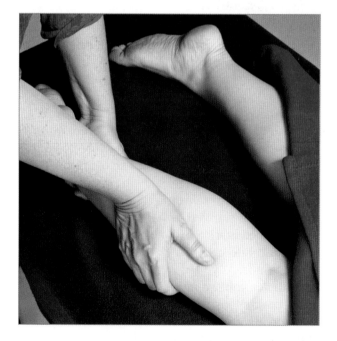

Moving up the leg and avoiding the knee, repeat this same work up the outer thigh, stopping a couple of inches below the client's bottom. Instead of using your thumb on the thigh, use the flat of your hand. When you have finished the back of both legs ask your client to turn faceup so that you can then work the outer front of the legs.

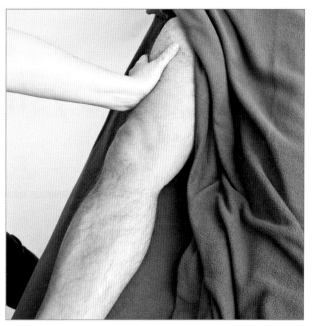

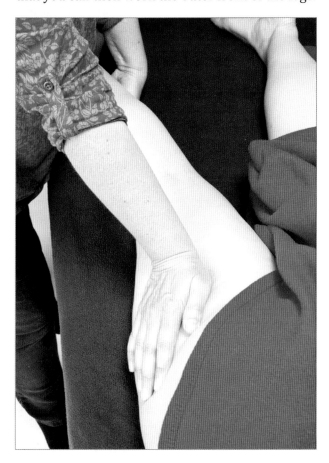

It can be incredibly relaxing to finish the treatment with some gentle head and scalp work, and then allow your client a good 10–15 minutes to relax before starting to get up. Ask clients to raise themselves slowly, first moving onto their side, then to a seated and, finally, if appropriate, to a standing position. Be ready to support them if necessary. Treatment will be most effective if carried out weekly. As this is a whole-body treatment it will take one to two hours, but you can always split the treatment into upper and lower body if time is a limiting factor.

On the lower legs you need to work the area to the outside of the shin bone; this is usually small enough to be worked with a thumb, or the heel of your hand side-on if you need a break from using your thumbs. As you move to the outer upper thigh, place your hand with the fingers pointing outward so that you do not end up sliding your hand up the inner thigh as you work. Focus your work along the center and outer quarter of the upper thigh, using the flat of your hand in long and gentle to moderate strokes.

Muscular Dystrophy

Background to the Condition

Muscular dystrophy is a genetic disorder that causes muscle weakness and wastage. The term muscular dystrophy (MD) is an umbrella term for a number of muscle-wasting conditions that vary in severity from very mild to severe. The Muscular Dystrophy Campaign lists over 60 different muscle-wasting conditions covered by their campaign,[116] and for which they provide support.

Different types of MD will affect different muscles. Most MD is progressive, meaning that the condition gets worse with time; there is currently no cure for MD although there is some promising early research work around the possibility of gene repair. There are, however, a range of treatments designed to help manage symptoms.

MD is a genetic disorder that may or may not be inherited. A parent of a sufferer may be a carrier for the condition but never develop symptoms, and sometimes the problem will be a genetic mutation that occurred in that individual's genes in the early stages of development and there will be no family history. A person's genes are the "control center" of each cell in the body, including muscle cells, and these genes control the proteins made by the muscle cell—the proteins that are needed for muscle fibers to work properly.

These are the genes that are affected in people with MD, where either the protein is lacking, or is a "faulty" protein that does not work well. This leads to damaged muscle fibers and to muscle weakness. Depending on the exact type of faulty gene and faulty protein, different types of muscle weakness result. This is why there are different types of MD.[117]

Some forms of MD limit life expectancy and have a severe impact on the person's mobility; others may have little impact on everyday life. While many cases of MD become apparent in childhood or adolescence, others may not become evident until much later in life, even into old age. When the muscles of the heart and lungs are affected the condition can become life threatening, so for anyone with MD there should be a complex medical support system in place to monitor and help to manage symptoms and their side effects.

---

[116] http://www.muscular-dystrophy.org/

[117] http://www.patient.co.uk/health/muscular-dystrophies-an-overview

The NHS in the UK list the most common varieties of MD as:[118]

- *Duchenne muscular dystrophy*: one of the most common and severe forms, it usually affects boys in early childhood, and men with the condition will usually only live into their twenties or thirties.

- *Myotonic dystrophy*: a type of MD that can develop at any age; life expectancy is not always affected, but people with a severe form may have shortened lives.

- *Facioscapulohumeral muscular dystrophy*: a type of MD that can develop in childhood or adulthood; it progresses slowly and is not usually life threatening.

- *Becker muscular dystrophy*: closely related to Duchenne MD, but it develops later in childhood and is less severe; the effect on life expectancy is less than with other forms.

- *Limb-girdle muscular dystrophy*: a group of conditions that usually develop in late childhood or early adulthood; some variants can progress quickly and be life threatening, whereas others only develop slowly.

- *Oculopharyngeal muscular dystrophy*: a type of MD that usually does not develop until a person is 50–60 years old and does not tend to affect life expectancy.

- *Emery–Dreifuss muscular dystrophy*: a type of MD that develops in childhood or early adulthood; most people with this condition live until at least middle age.

A diagnosis of MD is likely to be a shock for both the person with the condition and his or her family, and the best-practice medical approach will be a package of care bringing together treatments and support tailored to the individual needs of the person with MD. Massage can be an integral part of that package of care, and while some will seek professional massage treatment, there is also much that can be achieved at home from friends and family massaging.

It is an important starting point to understand a little of what is happening to the muscles affected by MD; there are four main features to be aware of. The first is muscle wastage, where the muscles become thin and weaker. Secondly muscle hypertrophy can take place; this is where the muscles are bulkier than usual but, despite this size, the muscles do not work well. The person with MD may experience aches and/or pains in the muscles and, finally, there may be contractures—this is when the movement of joints is reduced or restricted because of the tightness of the muscles. Muscle weakness or impaired childhood muscle development in itself does not give a diagnosis of MD; there may be many other causes for these and it is important that muscle weakness is investigated properly by appropriate medical professionals.

Specific Contraindications

There are no specific contraindications to massaging someone with MD, but if the heart is affected then checks need to be made with the supervising medical practitioner and the massage will need to be slower and more gentle than that which might otherwise be given. Depending on the individual client you may need to either massage in a chair or take extra care that the client does not roll off the massage table when turning over, as movement could be difficult. Allow the client plenty of time to get on and off the table, and ensure that changing position is not rushed as, if the client's lung capacity is impacted by the MD, this in itself could be exhausting.

---

[118] http://www.nhs.uk/conditions/Muscular-dystrophy/Pages/Introduction.aspx

Finally, if lung capacity is an issue, ensure that you have pillows or cushions so that the client's head can be raised, which will help make breathing easier, or use a massage table that can be lifted at one end so that when working with the client faceup, you can raise the table so as not to compromise the breathing.

Massage Treatments

Your aim in the massage is to try to gently stretch out the muscle and, where possible, to introduce movement to the muscle—this in turn will help alleviate muscle pain. While there is little high-quality research available, there is evidence emerging that massage therapy blunts muscle pain by the same biological mechanisms as most pain medications.[119]

It is worth keeping in mind that, depending on the stage of the MD, the muscles might be small and very tight, feeling almost solid to the touch; however, this does not mean that you need to work more deeply than usual.

As ever, gauge your depth by the level the client wants to go to and how the muscles respond. If a muscle only needs gentle pressure to relax and soften, then only use gentle pressure. What you are aiming to do in the massage is release any residual tension in the muscle to allow the muscle to relax. While you cannot alter the degree of muscle wastage, you can introduce movement and increase the blood flow to the muscles, which can help to counter muscle weakness.

Hypertrophy refers to an increase in the size of muscle fibers, not an increase in the number of muscle fibers, so while in some instances a client may appear to have enlarged muscles, these will not be extra strong muscles and the same weakness will exist in these muscles as in the muscles that are smaller due to muscle wastage.

Do not mistake size for strength and be tempted to work too deeply; this could be very painful and counterproductive. As you release the tension held in the muscle and allow the muscle to relax that will help to address the muscular aches and/or pains in the muscles.

Massage can also help to address problems where contractures have taken place, ideally to a stage where, depending on the client and the severity and duration of the problem, more movement within the joint may be possible. A contracture is a shortening of the muscle or other soft tissue that causes a joint to be in a fixed flexed position.[120] This can be permanent or temporary; if the person with MD is treated from an early stage and treated very regularly, then it may be possible to slow the development and severity of the contracture.

It is possible to massage any area of the body of the person with MD but always start at the extremities of the limb that you are working on, and work the limbs before the back, hips, or chest.

As this is a full-body massage you can choose to start by following the instructions for massaging the hands and arms, head, or feet, based on the client's choice. These massages are detailed in Chapters 2, 3, and 4. Ideally you need to work all of these areas, and it does not matter which you start with.

After you have massaged all of these areas you can also work on the back, following the directions given in Chapter 5, but begin this with warming up the area and doing some basic fascial-release work. Fascia lies in all directions across the entire body so you can't go wrong no matter where you start or which direction you work with—the priority is that you work all of the main areas.

[119] http://www.sciencedaily.com/releases/2012/02/120201173226.htm

[120] Susan G. Salvo, *Mosby's Mosby's Pathology for Massage Therapists*. Mosby, 2008:, p. 137.

When you are working on the back it can feel pleasant for the client if you start by working outward from the spine, but this is a guide, not a rule. The areas around the shoulders and neck and down the full length of the spine can be very tight, as can the fascia around the ribs. The rib area will most likely be very tender so work gently and slowly, especially if your client is underweight. If this area is too ticklish for your client don't worry too much about this, as you will still get a good release from working the main part of the back and the area around the ribs can be omitted.

To encourage the fascia to release there are two useful techniques that can be used simply and effectively. The first is to roll the skin; practice this move on yourself first so that you are confident using it on your client. Pick up the skin between your fingers and simply roll it so that you are moving across the area you are working on.

You don't need to work in any particular direction and it is better if you change direction; unless the client has very dry skin, avoid using oil as it will be difficult to grasp the skin once oiled.

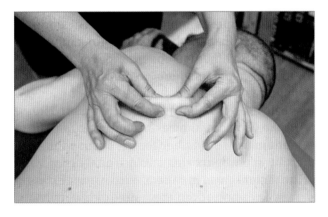

Next, using your thumbs, place your thumb tips together on the client's skin and, without releasing your grip, slide your thumbs so that the tip of the nail and the first knuckle are parallel.

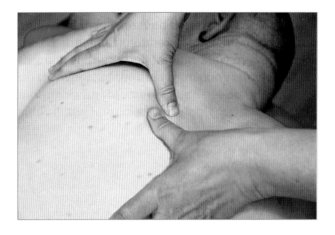

After this initial work use a little massage oil and gently glide over the skin, always working upward toward the heart. So if you are working on a leg, work from ankle to knee and then from knee to the top of the thigh, and if you are working on an arm, first work from wrist to elbow and then elbow to shoulder.

After you have glided up the muscle three or four times you can repeat this movement, slowly adding depth by increasing the pressure you put on with your hand; you may become aware of areas that feel tight and less mobile and these are the areas that you then need to pay specific attention to. You can use your hand to gently knead the muscle, applying the heel of your hand to move across and into the muscle, as though you were trying to roll the muscle under your palm.

Finally, for each area, as you work it stretch the muscle out with long strokes. If you are working from wrist to elbow, hold one thumb at the base of the wrist and use the other to gently glide to the top of the arm, stopping just short of the elbow, to stretch the whole of that muscle. You can repeat this on any muscle on the arms or legs.

One additional massage technique for MD clients is to try to help release the diaphragm. The diaphragm is a large, flat, dome-shaped muscle that sits under the lungs and above the digestive organs. The diaphragm contracts downward as we breathe in, drawing air into the lungs. As air is released from the lungs the diaphragm relaxes. As a result, the diaphragm, which is a huge muscle, is rarely fully contracted and relaxed. Without proper deep breathing, the rib cage can become more rigid, constricting the diaphragm, and the diaphragm becomes tight.[121] This massage can be self-administered or can be provided by someone else.

With the client lying on their back (or lie on your back if you are self-administering this part of the treatment) and with the head and shoulders raised with a pillow if needed, focus on taking as deep a breath as is possible; this should be slow breathing rather than shallow, quick breaths.

The aim of this part of the massage is to help the diaphragm relax to allow deeper breathing to take place. As the person breathes out for the fourth or fifth time, with your hand palm up, curl the tips of your fingers very gently underneath the ribcage at one side (it is usual to start on the left side but this is not critical); make sure that your fingers stay right underneath the rib cage so that you are not poking fingers into vital organs.

Gently tease out tension in this area, moving your fingers very minimally (up to around an eighth of an inch or so) underneath the rib cage. This should not cause any pain. If your client experiences any pain you should stop immediately. You can also practice this on yourself so that you know how it feels and how you need to position your fingers.

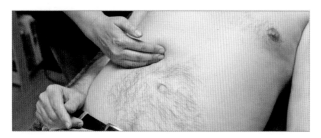

Turning your fingers around so that you are palm down, with the next out breath tease your fingers underneath the ribcage so that your fingers are flat and the fingertips are just underneath the lower ribs; do this one side at a time and work slowly and gently. With the in breath the ribs will raise upward naturally, and it is now that you need to gently pull downward, this helps to create space between the diaphragm and the stomach and will allow the diaphragm to relax.

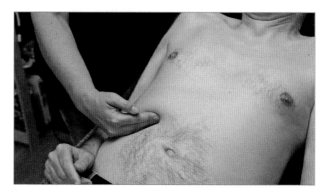

Repeat this slowly all along both sides of the rib cage at the top of the abdomen. This is a great technique for self-massage as the client is in control of the depth and pace of the treatment, which can feel better for the client.

Any of these massage techniques can be carried out safely for the MD client and it is also fine to split the treatments into blocks, spread across the week.

Working together you and your client should be able to evaluate the best frequency to gain maximum effect. Massage for the client with MD can safely be carried out by a qualified practitioner—who may be able to work a little more deeply where appropriate—or by a friend or family member, and the massage can improve the individual's quality of life.

[121] http://lifespa.com/cool-your-digestion-self-massage-technique/

Parkinson's Disease

Background to the Condition

Parkinson's disease (Parkinson's) is a progressive neurological condition and is remarkably common, with 1 person in every 500 developing Parkinson's.[122]

Most people who develop Parkinson's are over 50 but it can affect younger people, with 1 in 20 people being diagnosed under the age of 40. There is no cure and it is a progressive illness. The physical root of Parkinson's is not having enough dopamine owing to nerve cell degeneration in the brain. Without dopamine movements become slower, so it takes longer to do things and the typical symptoms of tremor and rigidity become more visible. At an early stage Parkinson's often causes tiredness and weakness. It may also include poor hand coordination, problems with handwriting, and tremor (shaking) in the arm.

In a study by Hernandez-Reif et al.,[123] a small group of 16 Parkinson's sufferers received 30-minute massage therapy or progressive muscle relaxation sessions twice a week for five weeks, both the physicians assessing the participants and the participants themselves reported an improvement in daily living activities by the end of the study, including having more effective and less disturbed sleep. Massage will not be a cure for Parkinson's but it can give symptomatic relief. The tremors and rigidity that come with the disease are linked in with muscle tension and tightness, and with that comes muscle pain, sometimes very severe.

Specific Contraindications

There are some key pointers in massaging someone with Parkinson's that need to be taken into consideration. Getting on and off a massage table may be a problem for people with Parkinson's as they may not be in full control of their bodily movements. As an introductory massage it would be worth considering an initial treatment on the client's hands, arms, and shoulders with the client seated. This will reduce anxiety for clients who may be new to massage and will allow them to approach subsequent treatments in a more relaxed manner. Always, whether it is the first or a subsequent treatment, and if the client is confident to be on the table, take care to assist your client on and off to minimize the risk of falls. You can work with the client clothed to avoid any draping issues, or the client could bring a friend or partner to assist them with dressing and undressing and getting on and off the table.

---

[122] source http://www.parkinsons.org.uk

[123] Parkinson's disease symptoms are differentially affected by massage therapy vs. progressive muscle relaxation: a pilot study, M Hernandez-Reif et al., *Journal of Bodywork and Movement Therapies*, 2002, 6: 177–182.

Make sure you get a full list of the client's medications. Antidepressant use is higher than in the general population, and you should work in conjunction with the client's medical practitioner if you are at all unsure of the prescribed medications and their interactions with massage.

Hypotension (low blood pressure) is characteristic of Parkinson's, so changing positions and getting up from the table after a massage must be supported and done slowly, as there is a risk your client may pass out. Take your time and never rush clients or allow them to "jump up" after their massage.

Make sure you work inward to release the area where tension in the muscle and fascia is held. So hands before arms, feet before legs, and head before neck—gradually working your way inward on the body.

Loss of sensation can be a part of Parkinson's symptoms so be careful to work very gently where there is reduced feeling so that you do not accidently apply too much pressure. Working in longer and slower movements will make the treatment more tolerable for the client. Work gently for at least the first few treatments so that you can gauge with clients the amount of recovery time they need to allow them to process the massage, and the effects of it on their body, and at all times get feedback from clients as to whether your pressure is right for them.

Finally, don't be nervous about treating someone with Parkinson's; it is a condition that can respond well to massage, and as practitioners or friends and family members offering massage, we have much that we can offer to our clients. Just be gentle; you are working at all times to slowly release the tension running through the muscles, always working inward toward the heart and with the precautions mentioned above.

Massage Treatments

Begin the treatment by following the detailed instructions in Chapter 2 on hand massage, making sure you spend a good 15–20 minutes on each hand. The hands are often the key to releasing lots of arm, shoulder, upper-back, and neck tension. Trying to control hand tremors can result in a great deal of tension through the arms and shoulders, so working the hands will help to relieve this tension and the consequent pain, making this is a particularly useful treatment for someone with Parkinson's.

Your recipient will gain even more benefit from the massage if you also continue up the lower arms. Making sure the client's arm is supported, gently move the wrist through its normal range of movement; do not force any movement that is not free and natural and work slowly, rotating the hand three or four times in each direction. This gentle stretch can help to release the tension held further up the arm.

With the client's arm flat and supported against a firm surface, turn the arm so that the thumb is turned outward with the hand resting on the side with the little finger.

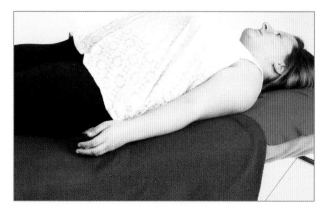

Gently grip the arm so that your palm can knead the large muscle in the forearm that leads up from the thumb and so that your fingers can knead the opposite side of the arm.

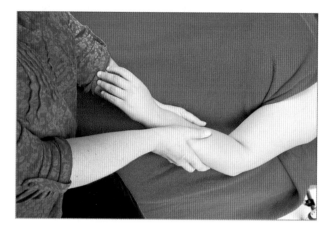

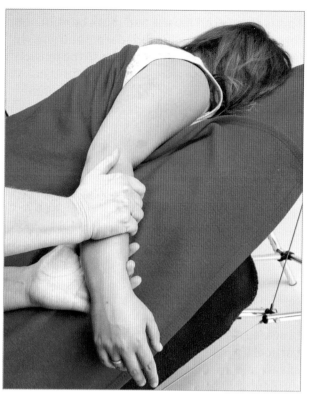

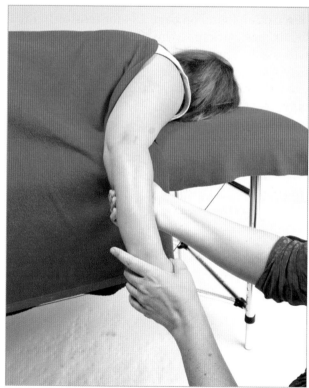

Next, using oil or cream, use deep strokes up from the thumb from just above the wrist to just below the elbow.

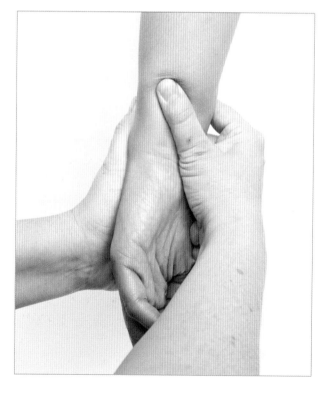

Work from just above the wrist to just below the elbow, repeating the whole sequence four or five times. Lay the arm palm down and adjust your grip so that your palm now works the outer part of the forearm and your fingers can knead the muscle coming up from the side of the little finger and ring finger.

This is a powerful muscle and it can be tight and sore, so work gradually more deeply and you will feel the muscle soften as you release the tension from it. You can use your own thumb for this or your own palm, depending on the size of the person's forearm that you are massaging and how strong or fragile he or she is.

The outer part of the lower arm needs a little less work. Running up the center of the radius and ulna bones is the muscle that is primarily responsible for extending the arm and you can work this with your thumb and fingertip, either pressing and releasing the muscle as you move inch by inch up the center of the arm, or using oil or cream and sliding up the muscle. Be careful not to exert too much pressure as this can be a sensitive area and, in elderly clients, can bruise easily; always err on the side of caution, particularly when you begin treatments with new clients and are unsure how they will respond to the depth.

The benefits of hand and lower-arm massage should be felt immediately by the person with Parkinson's but they will also be cumulative, so don't be disappointed if you do not see immediate great results in terms of the massage assisting with the tremors. Any lessening of the tremor symptoms will be welcome; remember you are alleviating not curing the tremors so the treatment will need to be repeated. This massage could be carried out daily but once or twice a week should be enough to make an impact. You may be able to lengthen the time between treatments as the muscles relax, depending on how advanced and symptomatic the Parkinson's is for that particular person.

While the hands are the key area to massage, the client may also benefit from wider massage. Treating the head and neck can be both relaxing and pain relieving and you can follow the protocol in Chapter 4 for head treatment, and if you want to extend this further use the detailed description found on page 234 for tension headaches. Back massage and foot massage work will also be appropriate (Chapters 3 and 5) and may be both beneficial and relaxing for your client. Provided you always work to a depth that is correct for the individual, work systematically and slowly and your massage should be a positive experience and be beneficial for your client.

Peripheral Neuropathy

Background to the Condition

Peripheral neuropathy refers to damage to the peripheral nervous system. The peripheral nervous system is all parts of the nervous system that are outside of the brain and spinal cord (the central nervous system) and includes the motor nerves, used by the brain to control muscles.

As well as the muscles, the peripheral nervous system also controls the automatic nerves whose job it is to regulate the automatic functions of the body, including blood pressure, sweating, and bladder function, along with the sensory nerves that pass sensations, including pain signals, to the brain. Peripheral neuropathy often affects the hands, feet, and lower legs; the longer a nerve is, the more vulnerable it is to injury.[124]

It is vital that treatment for peripheral neuropathy is carried out in conjunction with other appropriate medical treatment through the client's doctor or specialist.

Anyone presenting with numbness and tingling in the feet and hands; consistent burning, stabbing, or shooting pains; loss of coordination in affected body parts, including loss of bladder control; or muscle weakness or wastage needs to be directed to a medical practitioner for diagnosis and treatment.

Peripheral neuropathy usually occurs as a result of diabetes, as a result of high blood glucose levels damaging the small blood vessels that supply the nerves, preventing essential nutrients reaching the nerves. The nerve fibers are then damaged or disappear.[125] Peripheral neuropathy can also be the result of chemotherapy and some anticancer drugs, long-term alcohol addiction, AIDS, vitamin B12 deficiency, exposure to some heavy metals, and shingles. According to the US-based National Institute of Neurological Disorders and Stroke, more than 100 types of peripheral neuropathy have been identified, each with its own characteristic set of symptoms, pattern of development, and prognosis.[126]

Specific Contraindications

If symptoms are newly developed, clients should consult their medical practitioner to discover the underlying cause of the problem.

Particularly for clients with diabetes, it is important for the affected limbs to be closely monitored to check for problems as the condition can lead to diabetic ulcers that, if left untreated, can lead to gangrene, which may require amputation. With this in mind, an important part of the massage treatment is to observe and monitor any changes to those areas, particularly

---

[124] http://www.macmillan.org.uk/Cancerinformation/ Livingwithandaftercancer/Symptomssideeffects/Othersymptomssideeffects/ Peripheralneuropathy.aspx

[125] http://www.diabetes.org.uk/Guide-to-diabetes/Complications/Nerves_ Neuropathy/

[126] http://www.ninds.nih.gov/disorders/peripheralneuropathy/ peripheralneuropathy.htm

if it is the feet that are impacted as these can be more difficult for some clients to check themselves, and to refer clients back to their medical practitioner if changes are noticed. Do not massage over broken skin.

Massage Treatments

The starting point for discussing massage and peripheral neuropathy is that it is a long-term commitment to treatment. Treatments need to be frequent and over a lengthy period to be effective. Massage can, however, be carried out at home by a friend or family member, making it a very accessible treatment. Massage will not cure peripheral neuropathy but it can assist in maintaining the health of the affected area.

Begin the treatment by looking at the feet; reduced sensation in the feet from the condition may mean that the client is not aware of cuts or blisters, which can go on to become ulcers.

A person with peripheral neuropathy is also more prone to athlete's foot and fungal nail infections. If these are a problem consider wearing disposable gloves to give a treatment as they can be highly contagious conditions. It can be more pleasant for the practitioner or giver of the massage to begin the treatment by washing the feet in warm soapy water; do not soak the feet but do ensure you dry them thoroughly afterward.

Clients should contact their medical practitioner if any of the following problems occur: changes in skin color or temperature; swelling in the foot or ankle; pain in the legs; open sores on the feet that are slow to heal or are draining; ingrowing toenails or toenails infected with fungus; corns or calluses; dry cracks in the skin, especially around the heel; or an unusual and/or persistent foot odor.[127] Some clients / friends and family members may not notice some of these conditions for themselves depending on their general health so if you as a massage practitioner spot any of these issues, gently let your client know and encourage them to see their doctor.

Begin to warm up the foot with gentle strokes upward toward the leg. Even gentle touch may be painful, but your aim is to increase the circulation in the foot so deeper than just surface work will be necessary, and build this slowly so that your client can tolerate the treatment.

To begin with use feather-light strokes, and you can use this part of the treatment to moisturize the legs with a good-quality pure massage oil; use a natural oil such as grape-seed or coconut oil that will nourish the skin as well as providing lubrication for your treatment.

Start at the toes, stroke up the sole, side, and top of the feet, around the ankles, and up the leg to the knee on all sides. After you have covered the whole feet and lower legs, go back to the toes and work all of these same areas but stroking a little more deeply. Use the palm and heel of your hand to apply moderate pressure to the feet, supporting the opposite side of the foot with the other hand. Use small kneading movements on the feet to apply this pressure, starting at the toes and working all the way around the foot moving just an inch or so at a time; be careful as you knead the top of the foot not to put too much pressure onto the delicate bones. As you move up the leg use longer strokes, so that you are kneading upward four to five inches at a time.

Taking the foot in both hands with your fingers on the sole, gently squeeze the foot, working from the toes to the heel. Get feedback from your client as to how hard to squeeze—this can be an unexpectedly pleasant move for the receiver and you may be able to work more deeply than you think.

---

127 http://www.medicinenet.com/diabetes_foot_problems_pictures_slideshow/article.htm

Working each toe individually, hold the toe between your thumb and two or three fingers. Start at the tip and simply roll the toe between your fingers; you will need to move your hand position to be able to work the whole of the toe, to ensure that you work both the bottom and top of each toe, gradually moving from tip to base of the toe. Work each toe in turn on both feet. With the same thumb and fingers, you now need to work up the outside of each foot; place your fingers on the under outside edge at the toes and your thumb opposite so that you can just feel the edge of the bones of the foot—but you will be pressing away from and not onto the bones.

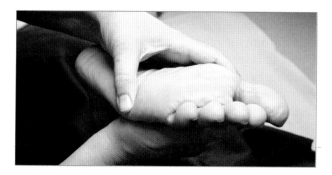

Roll the fleshy part of the outside of the foot between your thumb and fingers, gradually working upward from toes to heel; repeat on the other foot.

Next, working on the top of the foot and using just the tip of one finger, place it between the little and next toes; feel for the groove between the toes and, making sure you have a little oil to lubricate the skin, gently glide up the groove between the metatarsal bones. You should be able to feel the groove until you are approximately halfway up the front of the foot. Move along a toe and repeat, continuing until you have worked the front of both feet.

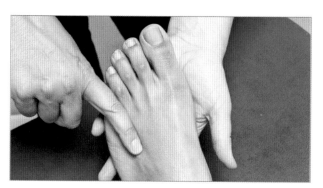

The last deep move is to form a fist with one hand, with the thumb tucked in, and use the knuckles to work the sole of the foot.

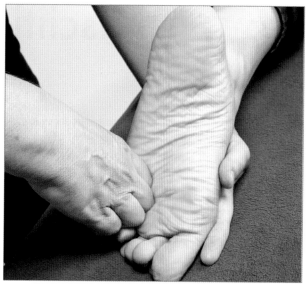

Start where the toes join the foot and draw semicircles with your knuckles, working in lines across the foot, working backward to the heel and ensuring that you also cover the sides of the foot. Do not work the top of the foot with your knuckles. This move may be painful to begin with so only work to your client's tolerance but aim to build depth with subsequent treatments, remembering that the aim is to improve the circulation of the foot. If this is too hard on your hands you can get clients to do this move themselves by rolling a tennis ball under the foot while they are seated. Clients should wear socks for this and do it for only three to four minutes per foot to avoid blisters.

The final part of the treatment is to return to the long strokes that you started with, from toe to just below the knee. If able, your client should sit with the feet raised on a small footstool for the next 20–30 minutes.

Peripheral neuropathy can also be experienced in the hands; to treat this you can follow the hand massage protocol in Chapter 2 but work extra gently, especially along the fingers and on the back on the hand. Using a little massage oil or cream on the back of the hand will prevent you dragging the client's skin while you work.

Plantar Fasciitis

Background to the Condition

Plantar fasciitis is a painful foot condition that can be very debilitating and often strikes people who are fit and active; it used to be called "policeman's heel" as it was an occupational hazard for police officers walking the beat. The plantar fascia is a strong band of tissue that stretches from the heel to the middle foot bones. It supports the longitudinal arch and acts as a shock absorber for the foot.

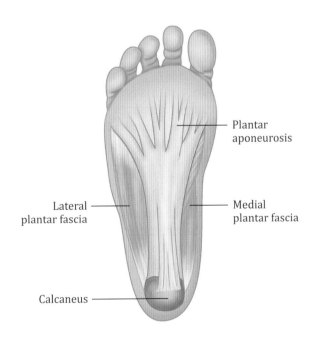

Lateral plantar fascia

Plantar aponeurosis

Medial plantar fascia

Calcaneus

Someone with plantar fasciitis (PF) has developed microtears and subsequent inflammation in the plantar fascia, and even placing the foot flat on the floor can cause excruciating pain. It is a condition that can develop slowly or appear seemingly instantly. The pain is usually worse first thing in the morning or after resting. This is because of the microtears starting to heal and then being torn apart by using the foot, so each day, or every time someone starts moving having rested, the tears are retorn, causing pain.

There are a number of causes: an increase in usual activity (e.g. runners increasing their training regime for a race), introducing new activities, a change in the surface usually trained on, obesity, poor running technique, wearing shoes with inadequate heel protection, and, in some cases, tightness of the Achilles tendon. It can affect one or both feet. The location of the pain will usually be in the main pad of the heel and it will often be tender just to touch.

As a massage practitioner it is ideal to work alongside a professional podiatrist. While there are off-the-shelf orthotics and they can be bought cheaply online, a podiatrist will be able to assess the extent of the PF and prescribe orthotics that are appropriate to that specific client's needs. These orthotics are supports that fit inside the shoe and are usually worn for a minimum of 12 months. Bare-foot walking should be avoided and supportive shoes worn at all times. PF will usually self-resolve but this usually takes between 6 and 18 months and it can be both a painful and a frustrating time.

Specific Contraindications

- Massage is safe in the treatment of PF but you should always avoid any pressure directly onto the client's heel.

- Avoid work into the side of the Achilles tendon if your client is pregnant.

- Do not use this massage if your client has a deep vein thrombosis.

- Do not massage over any varicose veins if present in the leg.

Massage Treatments

Massage can help alleviate the symptoms of PF and if someone comes to you with this condition then there are a few things that can help. It is important to begin any massage session for PF with gentle stretching first to ensure the release begins prior to applying any pressure. Gentle stretching can be key in the treatment of plantar fasciitis; in one study, 83% of clients involved in stretching programs were successfully treated, and 29% of clients in the study cited stretching as the treatment that had helped the most compared with any other treatment.[127]

The aim of the stretch is to increase the flexibility of the calf muscles, the Achilles tendon, and the plantar fascia. Arthritis Research UK recommend a simple stretch for the Achilles tendon: The Achilles tendon comes from the muscles at the back of the thigh and calf muscles. Along with the client repeating these exercises at home twice a day, they should be performed at the start of a massage treatment. The exercises need to be performed first with the knee straight and then with the knee bent in order to stretch both parts of the Achilles tendon. Do the following wall push-ups or stretches twice a day:

- Face the wall, put both hands on the wall at shoulder height, and stagger the feet (one foot in front of the other). The front foot should be approximately 12 inches from the wall. With the front knee bent and the back knee straight, lean into the stretch (i.e. toward the wall) until a tightening is felt in the calf of the back leg, and then ease off.

- Repeat 10 times.

- Now repeat this exercise but bring the back foot forward a little so that the back knee is slightly bent.

- Repeat 10 times.[128]

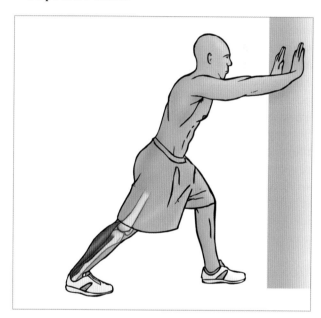

The second stretch is aimed specifically at the Achilles tendon and the plantar fascia; it can be done either with the client holding a handrail and standing on the bottom step of the stairs or on a large, thick textbook. The client should stand with the foot on either the stair or the book and, allowing the heel to hang down, will instantly feel the stretch as body weight and gravity stretch the area. This stretch should be held for 30–40 seconds and then the client should step back off

---

[127] http://www.aafp.org/afp/2001/0201/p467.html

[128] Plantar fasciitis exercises, Arthritis Research UK, 2004. Available to download as PDF at: http://www.arthritisresearchuk.org/%20 infoandexercisesheetsfile

the step or book to neutralize the stretch, and repeat this five or six times. If working on a step, both feet can be stretched at the same time; using the book work one foot at a time. These exercises should be repeated twice a day at home.

The final stretch is most effective when using cold treatment at the same time. A small bottle of water in the freezer would be ideal, but make sure your client either keeps his or her socks on or provide a towel to go between the bottle and the client's foot, as direct skin contact with the frozen bottle must be avoided.

With the client seated, the bottle should be rolled back and forth under the foot, across the whole foot in all directions for two to three minutes, ensuring that the whole foot is used, including into the arch. The coldness of the bottle will help as pain relief on the plantar fascia so should come as a welcome relief.

This dynamic stretch also starts to gently massage the area and is ideal as a bridge between the stretches and the massage. This should be repeated twice daily at home; if the client is at work and cannot access an iced bottle then a tennis ball will do, but the added benefit of the icing will be lost. With the stretches complete, you can now begin the main massage treatment.

Your aim in the massage is to release any tension that is holding the area tight. Although conventional medicine has for many years pointed to the ligaments as being the main support for the foot arch, the evidence is growing that the muscles of the foot also play a critical role;[129] as all parts of the foot are interconnected, massage will work on all of the foot structures so it is important to massage the whole foot.

Begin working by releasing tension in the toes—following this up into the foot will help alleviate any tightness that is pulling into the plantar fascia.

To massage the foot, follow the detailed instructions in Chapter 3, but when you are following the instructions to massage down the side of the foot, avoid the side of the heel, and as you are massaging down the arch of the foot, stop just short of the heel or at the point in the arch where the client reports any plantar fasciitis pain.

You now need to work into the Achilles tendon. The Achilles tendon is a tough band of fibrous tissue that connects the calf muscles to the heel bone. The gastrocnemius and soleus muscles (calf muscles) unite into one band of tissue, which becomes the Achilles tendon at the lower end of the calf. This will be a tender area and it is important to encourage your client to breathe deeply, to work slowly and within your client's tolerance, but warn your client that this may initially be painful.

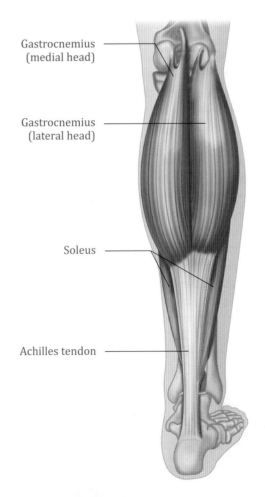

Gastrocnemius (medial head)

Gastrocnemius (lateral head)

Soleus

Achilles tendon

---

[129] http://www.futurity.org/muscles-just-ligaments-support-foots-arch/

You are working the area to the back of the heel, not the heel pad but the area below the ankle on the very bottom on the back of the foot. Starting just below the ankle, squeeze the back of the heel with short movements, holding for just two to three seconds at a time. As you work upward you will find that your fingers come closer together, this is as you follow the Achilles upward; be careful not to pinch the actual Achilles—you are working the muscle and fascia that surrounds it, so squeeze rather than pinch. You should omit this part of the treatment if your client is pregnant.

If you have been working until now with your client seated until, you will need to move him or her to a facedown position. If you are working with a friend or family member at home you could use a bed or even the floor for this next part of the work, provided the client has no neck problems, using a pillow for support of the neck and head with the client's head turned to one side.

As the Achilles is integral to the calf, you now need to focus on releasing the back of the leg. Be careful to warm the calf muscles up first using both hands and starting with gentle movements, only moving deeper into the calf as the muscles warm and begin to release; otherwise it will be painful and muscles may start to cramp.

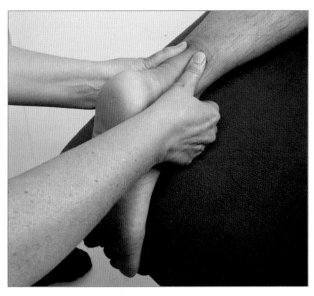
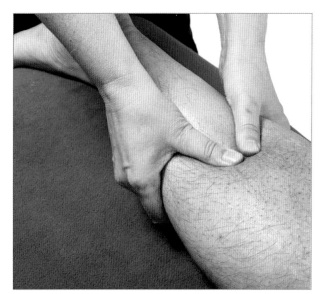
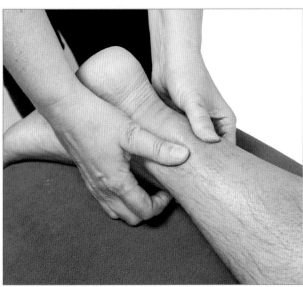
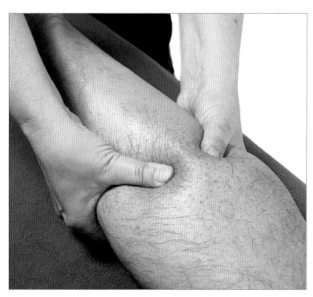

You can do this by kneading the muscles and using long strokes up the leg, focusing particularly on the outside of the leg. The inner calf can bruise very easily so be more careful and gentle when massaging this area. Stretching the foot as part of the treatment will also help, gently bringing the foot upward as if pushing the toes toward the face, while keeping the foot flat and supported with your hand. Hold for five to ten seconds and slowly release, repeating this stretch three or four times.

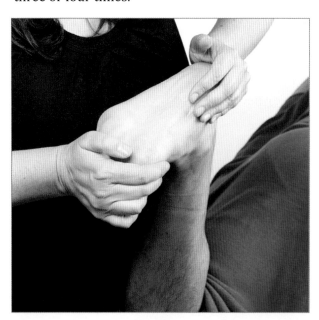

Once you have warmed up the area you can begin to work more deeply; hold the leg with your thumbs at the center just above the heel and stroke upward and outward, using your thumbs to work more deeply into the Achilles as you go. You will need to repeat this move three or four times as you work up the calf to ensure you cover the whole area. Work slowly as this area is inclined to cramp if you work too deeply or too quickly. Finally, shake the calf muscle using your fingers—this will help to resettle the muscle after the deeper massage.

Repeat the whole treatment on the other leg. Ideally you would carry out this treatment twice a week for the first month and then weekly as the problem starts to resolve until the pain has fully subsided and the plantar fascia has healed. This treatment can be carried out as a preventative massage—ideally once a month, or more if the client is starting a new fitness or training regime.

Rest is important for the treatment of PF, as are correct shoes and orthotics, so work holistically with a team of practitioners to give your client the best chance of a quicker recovery.

Pregnancy

Background to the Condition

Massage and touch have been an important part of both pregnancy and labor for women the world over, throughout the ages, but more recently a fear has become attached to massage during pregnancy. The starting point for this chapter is that pregnancy is not an illness—if the pregnancy is progressing with no problems and the mother is healthy then massage should be safe and beneficial at a time when the mother-to-be is experiencing stresses and strains on her body and emotions that may leave her nervous and stressed, with sore feet and an aching back from carrying the baby, and shoulders tender and pulled forward in an attempt to carry enlarged breasts. What better time could there be to have a massage?

Mainstream medical opinion is also coming to this conclusion. The Royal College of Midwives in the UK comments that midwives know massage has much more to offer than the feel-good factor, and can make a big difference to women on their way through pregnancy and labor—and really help them form strong relationships with their babies afterward.[130] It produced a booklet examining peer-reviewed studies, concluding that the benefits of massage in pregnancy include: a general reduction in stress and anxiety, pain relief during pregnancy and labor, and helping newborns to stay warm, to feed, and (in preterm) gain weight.[131]

There is still some controversy as to whether massage should be carried out during the first trimester. The NHS in the UK advises avoiding abdominal massage during the first three months of pregnancy,[132] whereas a number of spas will not allow any massage during pregnancy. This, however, is more to do with a fear of litigation than any evidence of a risk of harm; many women who have regular massages will have had massage in the very early stages of pregnancy without knowing they were pregnant and have come to no harm. If you or your client wants to wait until the pregnancy has reached the second trimester then that's fine; providing you massage using the protocol for pregnancy then this is a better option than allowing a problem area of pain or muscular tension, and the mother-to-be taking painkillers.

Pregnancy can be a tumultuous time. The woman's body is changing, additional hormones are circulating, and some angst about the ability to cope is normal. It is both an exciting and a challenging journey.

---

[130] http://www.rcm.org.uk/college/about/alliance/johnsons-baby/magicoftouch/

[131] RCM Alliance Programme, Revealing the Evidence Behind the Magic of Touch, http://www.rcm.org.uk/college/about/alliance/johnsons-baby/

[132] http://www.nhs.uk/chq/Pages/957.aspx?CategoryID=54&SubCategoryID=129

Specific Contraindications

The one caveat to any suggestions in this section is that this is for a normal, healthy pregnancy. If the mother-to-be has a history of miscarriages then massage should only be by written consent of her midwife or medical practitioner; if she is experiencing any bleeding or abdominal pain then medical advice must be taken immediately.

Pregnancy isn't always straight forward and the mother-to-be may also have a number of other pre-existing conditions for which she is already receiving treatment. It is important to adapt these treatments to account for the pregnancy. Pregnancy massage should be gentler—less deep and less vigorous than other massages. An hour is usually a sufficient length for a treatment for a pregnant woman; if you need longer or if your client tires after half an hour, just divide your treatment into two or three shorter sessions. There are also some specific factors to take into account.

There are some areas that should not be massaged during pregnancy. Unless you are specifically training in pregnancy massage you should not massage the abdomen at any stage of the pregnancy. This does not prevent the woman from gently massaging oil onto the belly to help prevent stretch marks.

In traditional Chinese medicine there are a number of "elimination points" that should be avoided during pregnancy, along with the following points:

- The first key point is L1 4 (large intestine 4), the "great eliminator" point on the large intestine meridian; this is in the area between the thumb and first finger and that area should be avoided altogether.

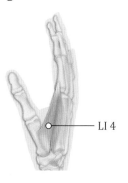

- SP 6 is on the spleen meridian—this is three (of the client's) finger widths above the ankle bone on the inside of the calf. All inner calf and inner thigh work should be avoided during pregnancy.

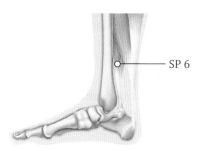

- The bladder meridian point BL 60 is on the outside back of the ankle, between the ankle bone and the strong Achilles tendon that runs up from the heel into the calf. This area should be avoided. Avoid all work around the heel to be on the safe side.

- Kidney 6 (K 6) is on the inner ankle one hand's width above the protruding ankle bone—it is a point used to treat a number of gynecological issues and should therefore always be avoided in pregnancy.

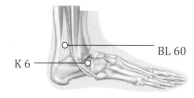

- Stomach 36 (ST 36) on the outside upper shin just below the knee is to be avoided as it is believed to induce labor.

There are other points that are less of an issue but should still be avoided unless you are specifically trained in pregnancy acupressure:

- Kidney meridian point (K 1) should be avoided—this is on the sole of the foot between the second and third metatarsal bones, and is found around one-third of the way between base of the second toe and the heel. Avoid direct pressure here.

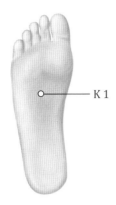

- Spleen 10 (SP 10) is on the inside of the thigh just above the knee—as all inner thigh work is contraindicated in pregnancy massage, this area should not be worked at all.

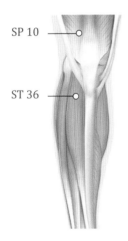

Shin, anterior view

- Liver meridian point 3 (Liv 3) is between the first and second tarsal bones on top of the foot, about an inch above the gap between the toes—you should avoid putting any direct pressure on here.

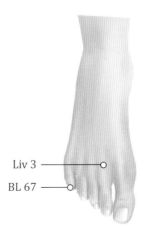

- Bladder 67 (BL 67) is on the upper edge of the little toe next to the nail.

It's important to remember that just casually rubbing or touching these areas is not going to do any harm, it's deep and prolonged work into these areas that should be avoided. All of these points are contraindications during the normal term of pregnancy, but there may come a point if the woman is past 40 weeks and there is no sign of the baby that these points could be used to encourage the body to move into labor. They can also be used during labor if things start to plateau, or if the gaps between contractions start to lengthen rather than shorten.

As pregnancy is not an illness, with these contraindications in mind, you can carry out massage as needed for a pregnant woman. There are also some specific treatments that can help with some of the effects of pregnancy.

Pregnancy massage should be given with the woman in the side position only; she should not be lying on her back or front as that can affect negatively the baby. Have two or three pillows available—one for under the head to support the neck, one to be placed between the knees to support the hips, and one to tuck under the bump so that the stomach and baby are not pulled down to one side. Have large, fleecy blankets, sheets, or sarongs for draping so that the client is not having to keep adjusting smaller towels during the treatment—this should help to give a sense of relaxation and safety. Complete as much of the massage as you can with the woman on her left side; you will eventually need to ask her to turn and lie on the right and this should not be a problem for most women with a normal pregnancy for a short period of time. If your client has been told not to lie on her right side by her doctor or midwife for a specific personal health reason, adapt the massage by having the client seated for the treatment.

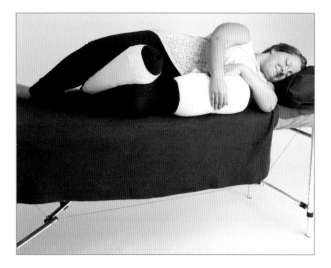

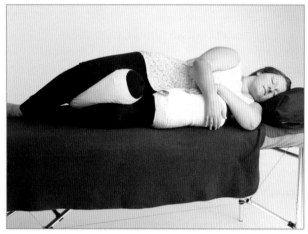

Massage Treatments

Most massage treatments given in this book for whichever condition is being treated will still be appropriate during pregnancy, with the exception of any abdominal massage. If the mother-to-be is suffering from headaches then you can treat for tension headaches following the directions in that chapter; if she has fibromyalgia, Down syndrome or dropped wrist, just treat as appropriate to that condition using the precautions above to avoid any specifically contraindicated areas. You may need to adapt your treatment to the client being on her side, but there are always ways to do this, and you may simply need to be creative about where you stand, sit, or kneel to work in relation to the client on her side.

If the woman has very swollen legs, using oil to moisturize the skin (which is likely to be dry with the swelling), use long strokes up the feet from toe to heel and then from heel to knee, finally from knee up the outside of the leg toward the buttock. Remember not to massage the inner leg and to avoid pressing onto the back of any joint. Use long, gentle strokes gliding over the skin to encourage lymphatic flow, to allow the body to clear the excess fluid.

Be careful of which oils you use—many aromatherapy oils are contraindicated in pregnancy. The molecules in essential oils are small enough to pass through the placenta, so avoid preblended oils unless they are specifically blended for pregnancy. Pure grape seed is a good light oil and if you are qualified in blending oils you can add other appropriate oils; chamomile is always a good option as this is not only safe for the mother and baby, it can also help to ease the churning stomach of morning sickness. It is also one of the few oils that you can use, appropriately blended, on newborns.

As pregnancy progresses many, if not most, women will suffer from lower-back pain. Along with the extra weight of carrying the baby, the uterosacral ligaments also come under stress. The uterosacral ligaments attach the cervix to the sacrum, the flat bony structure at the bottom of the spine. Backache in late pregnancy may be due to the stress of the weight of the uterus on the uterosacral ligaments attached to the spine.[133] Massaging this area with slow circles with the heel or your hand or three fingers together can give great relief, can be carried out through clothes, and can also be carried out as part of the woman's care during labor by the midwife or

---

[133] http://www.childbirthconnection.org/article.asp?ck=10244

support partner. To give a more complete back treatment you can also follow the instructions in Chapter 5 on back massage, with the client in the side position.

Hip work during pregnancy can be very effective and welcome, and it is important to keep the hips flexible ready for labor. Hip work in pregnancy is a little different from hip work at other times, and you will need to adapt the techniques given elsewhere in this book. Your client should already be lying in the side position with pillows under the knee to support the bent leg and to prevent any pressure onto their pregnancy bump—just check that this padding is sufficient before moving to do the hip work and add more if necessary. The bent leg should be kept at hip level.

Place your open hand at the head of the femur of the raised and bent leg; you will feel this at the very top of the leg—place your palm on the top of the head of the femur and spread your fingers outward. The area under your fingers is the area you are going to work.

This should feel soft to the touch but there may be tender and tight areas within it. If you are a friend or family member giving a treatment, use the flat of your knuckles for the next move; if you are a trained professional you can use your elbow. Try to feel the more resistant areas by applying gentle pressure—these will also be the more tender spots. There are usually three points that need release on each side. Ask your client to take a slow, deep abdominal breath and, on their out breath, press slowly and deeply into the muscle. At the same time as you press in you need to support the knee so that the leg is not being pressed into the belly.

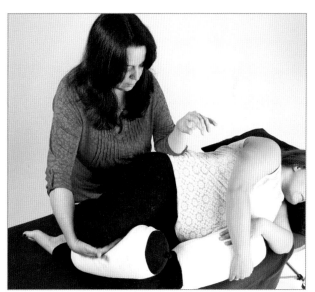

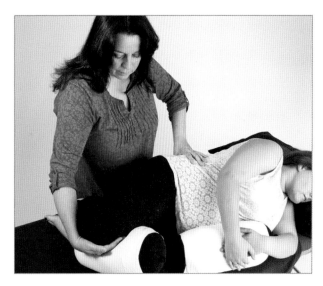

Ask your client to let you know when this starts to become painful and stop at that point (or professionally working to the maximum depth your client is happy to work to); hold the pressure without moving or otherwise changing depth or position. There should not be any pain in the back, so if this is reported stop immediately. After 30–60 seconds you will feel the muscle under your hand or elbow relax and your client will report that it no longer hurts. Slowly release the pressure and feel further down and repeat so that you have treated all three points. Carefully assist your client to turn over and repeat on the other side, being extra careful with your draping as your client turns over.

Massage on the hands as detailed in Chapter 2, avoiding the fleshy part at the base of the thumb, following up into the shoulders can also help to alleviate the extra stress placed on the shoulders and neck that enlarged breasts put onto them.

Head massage can be a great relaxer when sleeping is difficult. Massage by one partner to the other can be a great bonding experience during a time when life is changing and can allow the partner to be involved more actively in the pregnancy.

Raynaud's Syndrome

Background to the Condition

Raynaud's syndrome, also known as Raynaud's phenomenon, Raynaud's disease, or simply Raynaud's, is a condition that affects the blood supply to the extremities of the body. The areas most frequently affected are the fingers and toes, but occasionally the earlobes, nose, nipples, or tongue can be affected. It is a common condition, more so in cold climates as cold is one of the prime triggers of an attack.

The fingers are the most commonly affected area, with an additional 40% of sufferers also experiencing symptoms in the toes.[134] For ease, we will refer to fingers in this chapter but the same information and treatments apply to the toes. Raynaud's is a common problem, with up to 20% of the population affected in countries with colder climates. It affects more women than men and has a high hereditary factor, with the onset of symptoms usually coming before the age of 30.

Raynaud's is most commonly triggered by cold temperatures but it can also be triggered by anxiety or stress. During an attack the digital arteries that supply the blood vessels in the fingers contract and blood flow is severely restricted. At first the fingers go white and will feel very cool or cold to the touch. Then the fingers will go a blue as the oxygen from the blood in the narrowed blood vessels is quickly used. Finally the fingers go bright red as the blood vessels reopen and the blood flow returns—at this stage the fingers may also throb, tingle, burn, or feel numb. Attacks may last from a few minutes to several hours; for many people this is a mild and minor irritation that doesn't have a significant impact on life, for others the symptoms will be more severe and there may need to lifestyle changes—for example, not working outdoors—to manage the condition. There are medications available that can help,[135] and these should be discussed by the sufferer with their health care practitioner.

There are two forms of Raynaud's and the treatment given will depend on the form. More than 90% of sufferers have primary Raynaud's.[136] The cause of primary Raynaud's is not known—it is not a symptom or part of another illness and symptoms completely disappear after each bout. Massage is very safe for people with primary Raynaud's and self-massage can be applied when a bout occurs.

Secondary Raynaud's occurs as a result of another condition or as a result of medication or injury. Most cases of secondary Raynaud's are associated with autoimmune conditions, such as scleroderma (a condition that causes thickening and hardening of the skin), rheumatoid arthritis,

[134] http://www.nhlbi.nih.gov/health/health-topics/topics/raynaud/

[135] http://www.raynauds.org.uk/raynauds/treatments

[136] http://www.patient.co.uk/health/raynauds-phenomenon

Sjögren's syndrome (a condition where the immune system attacks the body's sweat and tear glands), lupus, or multiple sclerosis. Some forms of cancer may also cause Raynaud's, but secondary Raynaud's does not always mean a severe underlying illness, as it can also be caused as a side effect of migraine medications, beta blockers, some decongestants, the contraceptive pill, or hormone replacement therapy.

When the Raynaud's is secondary there will be other symptoms and onset is often much later in life; while primary Raynaud's almost always affects all the fingers, secondary Raynaud's symptoms may start with just one or two fingers. Secondary Raynaud's always needs medical investigation so that the underlying cause can be diagnosed and treatment given.

Specific Contraindications

If the underlying cause of the condition has already been diagnosed then massage treatment can be given, using the precautions given for the underlying condition.

In rare cases there can be complications with secondary Raynaud's with ulceration, infections, or in extreme cases gangrene. If there are any signs of damage, infection, or dead tissue (brown/black tissue that is shrinking) then immediate medical help should be sought and any massage would be very strongly contraindicated. Always warm your own hands first before treating someone with Raynaud's as applying cold hands will make the client's condition worse.

Massage Treatments

The starting point for massaging someone with Raynaud's is to make sure that your own hands are warm—for some people, being touched by cold hands would be enough to trigger an attack—and make sure that you prewarm any massage oil that you might be using. Massage can be applied gently during an attack or more deeply between attacks.

Begin massaging the hand at the fingers; curling your hand into a loose fist, support the finger against the palm of your hand and use your fingers to massage—this will allow you to massage the whole finger at once.

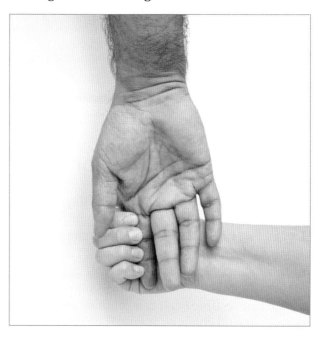

Starting at the end of the finger, press with your fingers in a wave down the client's finger. By doing this you are applying and then releasing pressure at the end of the finger, then a little further down, then further down still, finishing as you get to the palm of the hand. Work your way all around the finger, always working from the tip of the finger into where the finger joins the palm.

Keep moving your hand position so that you massage right around the client's finger. When you have worked your way down all around one finger, move on to the next. The same technique can be applied to thumbs. Depending on the length of the client's toes, you can either use the same technique or, alternatively, use your thumb to press down on the toe, working in a straight line from toe tip to where the toe joins the foot, and, again, work all the way down and around the toe so that there is no part of the toe or finger that you haven't touched. Be care with fingers and toes not to press directly onto, or onto the side of, the nail bed as this will be painful for the recipient.

Next work from where the fingers join the hand upward toward the wrist—you are looking to be gently squeezing over the whole of the palm. Supporting the other person's hand in your hand, use the length of your thumb to press across the whole width of the palm—press just for a second, release, and move your thumb higher up the palm and press again. If the other person's hand is much bigger than yours, work on half a palm at a time; when you have worked from the finger base to the wrist on one half, go back and start again at the finger base of the other half. Do this four or five times and repeat on the other hand.

The same techniques can be applied to the foot, working from the toe base to the heel. Be careful with both hands and feet that you are squeezing only with your thumb and are not putting pressure on the bones at the back of the hand or top of the foot.

and roll the soft flesh at the side of the hand or foot—this loosens up any tension within this area and will feel wonderful to the recipient.

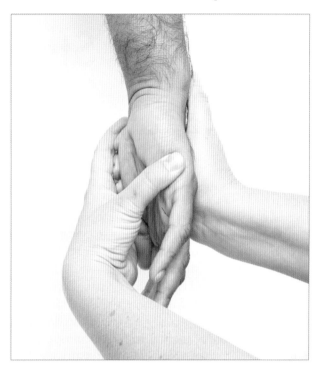

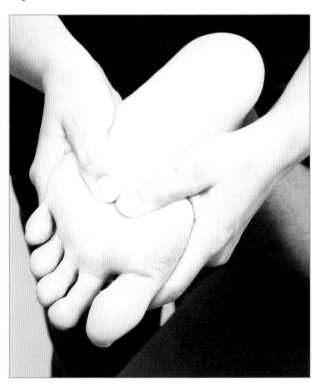

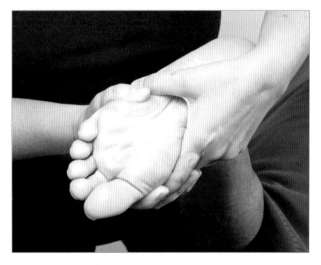

Finally, don't neglect the side of the palm and foot—the edge closest to the little finger/little toe. You can use your thumb, fingers, or the flat of your palm to do this; start at the finger/toe end and work down to the wrist/heel end and knead

All of this massage can also be self-applied using the opposite hand and, if your Raynaud's is bad and massaging is painful, keep alternating your hands so that each side gives and receives massage in equal measure. If your hands are particularly dry because of your Raynaud's, use a rich hand cream to massage rather than a massage oil.

Repetitive Strain Injuries

Background to the Condition

Upper-limb pain and dysfunction caused by work of a repetitive nature is not a new phenomenon and has been well documented for over 300 years. Discussion of this gathered pace from the late 1970s, with countries from Australia to Russia, Japan, Finland, the US, and the UK reporting dramatic increases in musculoskeletal conditions. This was the time of widespread replacement of typewriters with computers and a consequent increase in the automation of work.[137]

Repetitive strain injury (RSI) is a general term used to describe the pain felt in muscles, nerves, and tendons following repetitive movement and overuse. There are some specific conditions that are referred to under this heading, including tennis elbow, carpal tunnel syndrome, and vibration white finger. RSI is also referred to as work-related upper-limb disorder, nonspecific upper-limb pain, and occupational overuse syndrome. Where appropriate these have been discussed in chapters on the individual conditions. RSI is also used to describe general pain not attributed to a specific condition, and that is the area addressed in this section.

The terms "occupational overuse syndrome" and "work-related upper-limb disorder" are a good indication of the nature of the condition. Hours spent at the computer, doing a repetitive manual job, carrying out high-intensity repetitive activity over a long period of time, poor posture or having to work in an unnatural position, stress, and working in cold temperatures all add to the risk of RSI. The term can be deceptive too—hours spent texting, gaming, or recreationally on the computer or tablet can take their toll on our bodies. Studies in Australia have looked at the impact of extensive computer use by children in school, and the effects on musculoskeletal health.[138]

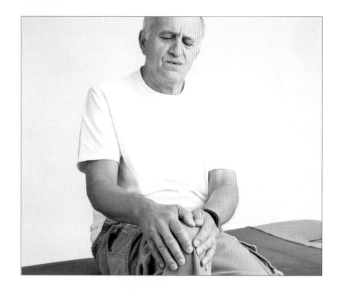

---

[137] http://www.rsi.org.uk/whatis/prevalence.html

[138] http://www.ncbi.nlm.nih.gov/pmc/articles/ PMC1936962/

The main cause of RSI is frequent and repetitive movements of a specific part or parts of the body, but there may be more than one contributory factor. Using a mouse on a computer may be a problem, but bad posture sitting at the computer on a work station that is too low for the individual, a cold office, stress, and not taking enough breaks can all become contributing factors. Some of these factors are within the employer's control, others are within the employee's control, but within any workplace there can be some people who will develop problems and others who do the same task every day who will not develop problems. In many countries there is now a requirement for employers to address issues that cause harm in the workplace but, despite a growth in workplace ergonomics and an awareness of RSI problems, these injuries are still remarkably common. Within the UK, RSI-related injuries cost industry up to £20 billion annually through lost production.[139]

RSI subdivides into two groups. Type 1 RSI is where the disorder is a recognized medical condition, such as tendonitis, carpal tunnel syndrome, tennis elbow, rotator cuff syndrome, Dupuytren's contracture, and writer's cramp (this is not an exhaustive list). With type 2 RSI, either symptoms do not fit with those of a recognized medical condition and there is no visible inflammation or swelling, or the pain doesn't stay in one area. This chapter will look at ways to treat type 2 RSI.[140]

The earlier an RSI is addressed and treated, the greater the chance of the client making a full recovery. Left untreated the problem will often develop and become a chronic condition. The first part of addressing the problem is to stop doing the activity that is causing the problem. This may mean assessing a job to see how it could be done differently; altering work stations or work practices; resting from certain activities, including leisure activities, that could be responsible; and allowing the body chance to recover.

The condition mostly affects parts of the upper body, such as the forearm, elbow, wrist, hands, neck, and shoulders. The symptoms can vary but often include pain or tenderness—this can be either a sharp pain or a dull ache. There may be stiffness, tingling or numbness, weakness, and cramp.[141] Left unaddressed and untreated the pain may worsen until it is constant, even when not doing the activity that first caused it. Some people will find that they are unable to do routine or household tasks, and for many the constant pain may disrupt sleep adding exhaustion into the problems of pain.

Along with the work and lifestyle changes to prevent further injury, massage can be very helpful. BUPA, a large private health care provider, recommends gently massage and moving the affected limb to stimulate circulation to help prevent muscles from weakening.[142] As stress can be a contributing factor to RSI, massage to help someone to relax can also be helpful.

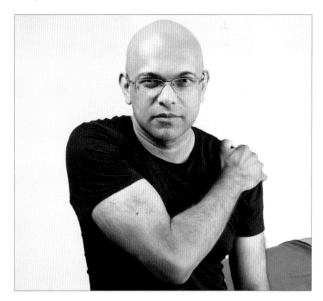

[139] http://www.repetitivestraininjury.org.uk/types-of-rsi.html

[140] http://www.bupa.co.uk/individuals/health-information/directory/r/repetitive-strain-syndrome-rsi

[141] http://www.nhs.uk/conditions/Repetitive-strain-injury/Pages/Introduction.aspx

[142] http://www.bupa.co.uk/individuals/health-information/directory/r/repetitive-strain-syndrome-rsi

Specific Contraindications

- If the pain is after an injury or trauma to an area, do not massage until the injury has been checked by a medical practitioner—you do not want to be massaging what turns out to be a broken limb.

- Do not massage over an open wound.

- Do not massage over an area that is swollen, red, or inflamed. This may indicate an underlying condition that may need medical treatment. If you massage on tissue that is already inflamed you are very likely to make the problem worse rather than better.

- If the client has another underlying medical condition, you should heed the contraindications for that condition.

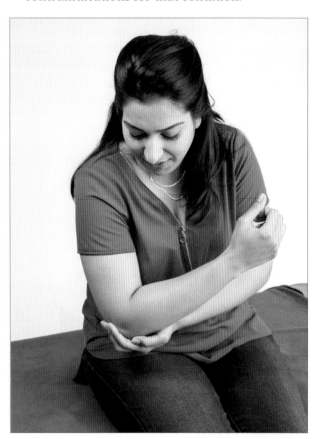

Massage Treatments

Massage can be very effective in treating RSI because with use, and, importantly, with overuse, muscles tighten and a tight muscle is more prone to injury. If a muscle is too tight its movement will be restricted and that will have an impact on the other muscles, and the skeletal structure, around it. Massage helps the muscle to "re-lax," literally to "return to looseness," allowing the body to return to its optimum state of fluidity and movement.

Massage can be given just to treat that specific area, so if a client has pain in the right hand, massage just to the right hand can be effective. However, the body is very interconnected so a problem in the right hand will cause problems in the right arm—the tight muscles in the hand pull and cause stress to the muscles of the arm, which has an impact on the muscles of the shoulder and on into the neck and back. So while as a first-aid measure you can treat just the right hand, follow it up with work to the whole of the upper body so that the problem is addressed in a complete way.

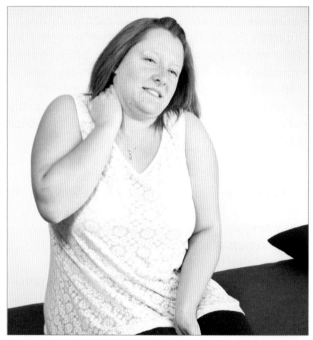

Even if the client is experiencing problems just in the shoulder, do remember that this will have started further out in the limb—a shoulder RSI will be from overusing the whole arm, so treat the whole hand and arm, not just the shoulder. When one side of the body becomes painful, we tend to overcompensate by making the other side work harder. We may start to open doors with the left hand and arm where we might usually use the right (or vice versa), so this unusual activity then starts to affect the left side too. If the pain is experienced in the neck it is important to work inward from both hands but also to work the head, face, and jaw before moving down to treat the neck. The head and scalp work will also be very useful in assisting the client to relax and to de-stress.

You can follow the treatment protocols in Chapter 2 for hand massage, Chapter 3 for foot massage, Chapter 4 for head massage, and Chapter 5 for back massage, and always try to track the source of the problem.

- For arm pain, start by massaging the hands.

- For shoulder, neck, or back pain, start by massaging the hands and the head and neck.

- For pain in the hips, start by massaging the feet.

- For pain in the upper back, start by massaging the hands and head.

- For pain in the lower back, start by massaging the back.

- If workplace stress is a significant issue, start by massaging the head.

By doing this you not only treat the area that hurts but you also treat the source of that muscular tension within the body.

This massage is safe to be carried out at home by friends or family, or you may prefer to seek professional massage help. Either way the focus of the treatment is to release any tension in the muscle to allow it to return to its natural flexibility and to encourage blood flow. Gentle exercise can also help, but be careful not to choose an exercise that will put any pressure on an already tender or injured part of the body.

Do remember that massage treatment is just one aspect of recovery; rest and identifying the root cause of the injury are critical in the long-term prevention of damage. Prevention, rest, and treatment need to go hand in hand in treating RSI.

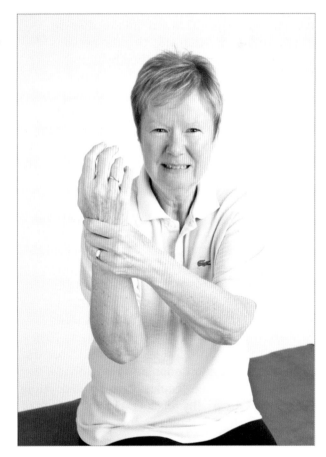

Restless Legs Syndrome

Background to the Condition

Restless legs syndrome (RLS), known by the medical profession as Willis–Ekbom disease, is a common condition affecting the nervous system. RLS is usually described by those living with the condition as an irresistible and involuntary need to move the legs, although other body parts may also affected, for example the arms.[143] According to the European Alliance for Restless Legs Syndrome (EARLS), RLS frequently remains unrecognized, misdiagnosed, and poorly treated.[144]

For people with RLS, the need to move the legs is overwhelming. Symptoms are usually worse late in the evening when they start to relax at the end of the day, and usually become even more severe at night so sleep is almost always affected by RLS. According to the National Institutes of Health National Center for Sleep Disorder Research in the US, RLS affects as many as 10% of Americans.[145] EARLS suggests that RLS occurs in 7–10% of the adult population worldwide.[146] RLS can lead to long sleepless nights and daytime fatigue, and invariably affects the quality of life of sufferers, including their employment, and those close to them,[147] such as partners who may be trying to sleep beside them.

RLS causes a creeping, crawling, burning, tingling, or aching in the legs, such that the individual feels a need to move the legs to relieve these unpleasant sensations. This movement helps to relieve the symptoms but they will often return as soon as the person stops moving; hence this leads to a nighttime of interrupted sleep and daytime exhaustion.

There are two recognized forms of RLS; primary or idiopathic, which accounts for 30% of the RLS population, and secondary or symptomatic RLS. For those with primary RLS, there is a strong genetic element but the root cause is still being explored; one major theory is that a deficiency in brain iron, particularly within dopamine-containing neurons, may predispose someone to develop RLS. A link between genetics and how the body stores iron suggests that iron metabolism may be a factor; this can then lead to a dysfunction of the dopamine pathways whose abnormal function causes the symptoms of RLS. Dopamine is necessary to produce smooth, purposeful muscle activity and movement and disrupting its function can cause RLS. As far as current medical research knows, RLS is neither a structural nor a neurodegenerative disorder, and most patients with RLS are neurologically normal except for their RLS.[148]

---

[143] http://www.rls-uk.org/

[144] http://www.earls.eu/about-rls/4575340792

[145] http://www.integrativehealthcare.org/mt/archives/2007/12/5_bodywork_tips.html

[146] http://www.earls.eu/about-rls/4575340792

[147] http://www.rls-uk.org/

[148] http://www.rls.org/document.doc?&id=1296

For a minority of the remaining 70% of RLS cases there may to be a link to other conditions, and these include chronic diseases such as kidney failure, diabetes, and peripheral neuropathy. Certain medications may aggravate symptoms; these include some antinausea drugs, some antipsychotic drugs, antidepressants that increase serotonin, and some cold and allergy medications that contain sedating antihistamines.[149] Treating the underlying cause will often alleviate the RLS symptoms. Pregnancy can cause temporary RLS and alcohol and tobacco can trigger symptoms for some people; however, for the vast majority of people there doesn't appear to be an underlying cause.

RLS is usually treated medically with drugs that increase dopamine—these do not suit everyone and in some cases have led to the development of obsessive–compulsive behavior, including gambling. Treatment is not usually continuous as more medication is needed with time as the body adapts to it, so a break is often needed in this treatment. Other medications include benzodiazepines such as clonazepam or diazepam. While these are generally prescribed to treat anxiety, muscle spasms, and insomnia they can give short-term relief from RLS, but they do have side effects that need balancing with the RLS symptoms.

Some doctors will prescribe opioids and anticonvulsants, but again these are not without side effects. Research is ongoing and more is being learnt about both the condition and how to treat it.

Massage has proved useful in managing symptoms for some people and will not cause any side effects; as such it is worth trying as part of the quest for finding an effective and individual treatment for RLS. A leading sleep expert in the US recommends massage as the front-line treatment for RLS,[150] while a paper looking at non-drug-related aspects of treating RLS[151] points to emergent evidence to suggest that massage helps in this treatment, although it was unknown whether this was because the treatment increased blood flow and muscle relaxation leading to an improvement in symptoms, or if the massage caused release of natural dopamine that led to the decrease. Either way, massage helped and has far fewer side effects than medication, so if nothing else, it's worth a try!

Specific Contraindications

There are no specific contraindications for treating someone with RLS but if symptoms are new or unexplained clients should first see their medical practitioner to find and address any underlying conditions.

If there is a known underlying condition then any contraindications for that condition would apply.

Massage Treatments

Massage treatments are best given in the evening when the symptoms are more problematic. Treatment can be given professionally or by friends or family members, and some treatments can be self-administered.

Begin any massage treatment for RLS by massaging the feet. If you are treating someone else then follow the protocol in Chapter 3 on foot massage for this part of the treatment. If you are self-massaging then you can do the foot work of this massage using a foot roller—just ensure that you don't miss out the toes as you work.

---

[149] http://www.ninds.nih.gov/disorders/restless_legs/detail_restless_legs.htm

[150] http://www.healthline.com/health/restless-leg-syndrome/expert-qa

[151] http://www.ncbi.nlm.nih.gov/pmc/articles/PMC3101885/?tool=pmcentrez

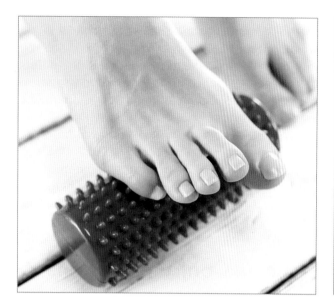
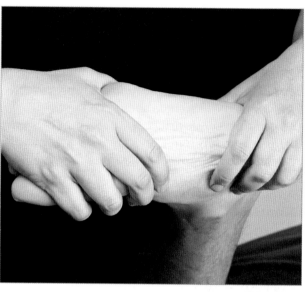

Foot rollers can be bought inexpensively online or a solid laundry ball will often suffice; just be careful not to stand on the roller or ball as you can damage the intricate bones of the foot, so use these tools while seated.

If you are working on someone else, your hands will be the best tools to use. The foot massage can be carried out with the client lying down and you seated, or the client can be seated and you can sit on the floor—the most important factor is that you are both comfortable and no strain is being put on anyone's back from the position in which you are working. Make sure you work the whole of both feet even if the RLS is mainly experienced on one side more than the other.

With the client either seated or lying facedown on a massage table with a face hole or face cradle, you need to work around the ankle and up into the calf.

To work the ankle, start by gently rotating the ankle; try to feel where there is any restriction of movement—this can be exhibited as a "clunkiness" in the movement—make sure you support the foot while you do this rotation by holding both the heel and the base of the toes, rotating in both directions. Now as you gently move the ankle use your thumb to press into the areas both behind and in front of the ankle, pressing and holding as you rotate; omit this part of the treatment if your client is pregnant.

Where an area is tight this may be tender but you should never be pressing hard enough to cause significant pain. Having worked both feet and ankles, you need to draw your attention to the calf.

The calf can be very tender to work so do so slowly, only building any depth once you have warmed up the muscle.

Begin by checking for any surface tension in the skin, fascia, and muscle by placing both thumbs together on the client's leg so that the tip of one thumb nail touches the tip of the other and, without letting go of your contact with the skin, slide your thumbs so that the thumb tips now lie next to the first knuckle, and then repeat in the opposite direction. This loosens up the surface layers. You need to work systematically up the back of the leg from ankle to just below the knee—work right around and across the whole back of the lower leg this way and repeat on the other leg.

Using a little massage oil to lubricate the skin, you should now aim to stroke upward from just above the ankle to just below the knee, being careful not to put any pressure on the back of the knee.

Begin with lighter strokes but deepen these as you repeat the move; you should be able to press quite deeply into the calf muscle so long as you

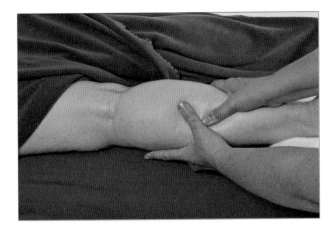

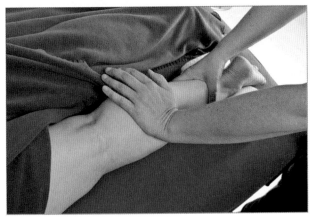

Working across the muscle fibers, so left to right and right to left across the leg, can help break up deep tension, but be sure to follow this up with long strokes back up the muscle afterward.

If we look at the anatomy of the upper leg, the hamstrings are the tendons that attach the large muscles at the back of the thigh to the bone.

The hamstring muscles—also referred to as the posterior thigh muscles, the semimembranosus, the semitendinosus, and the biceps femoris muscles—are the large muscles that pull on and work these tendons. Massaging this whole area can have a positive effect on RLS symptoms.

work slowly, and if you can synchronize your deep moves with the client's out breath that will allow you to work more deeply.

This is an area that is susceptible to cramp, so if the client gets cramp or feels it may be coming on, stretch the foot out so that it is flexed upward with the toes pointing toward the face and, once the cramp has passed fully, resume work but slow down and do not go as deeply. In the main belly of the calf you may find that the muscle is quite hard and resistant to touch—holding the muscle securely and shaking it can help to release this— if you can't get hold of the muscle then press with medium pressure with three fingers and then shake the muscle with your fingers.

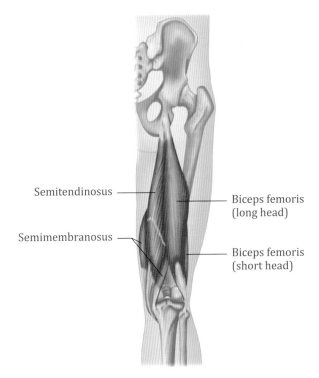

Semitendinosus

Semimembranosus

Biceps femoris (long head)

Biceps femoris (short head)

Posterior view

With your client still facedown, support the ankle with a rolled-up towel or cushion, as this helps to take pressure off the knee as you work on the back of the thigh.

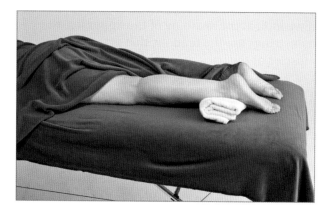

Ideally you would be working this area with your client on a professional massage couch with either a face hole or face cradle, but it is possible to use any other firm surface and allow your client to lie with the head resting sideways on a cushion. However, if you do this, make sure that they frequently change the direction the head is facing to avoid any pressure on the neck.

Begin with the same cross-frictional surface work that you carried out on the calves, either using your thumbs or, if the person you are working on has large legs and you have small hands, then you can use your whole hands for this by placing your hands palm down with your fingers pointing together and moving your whole hands from side to side. You will not be able to move a full hand's width without leaving the skin, but you will be able to move one or two fingers' width with each movement—be sure to work in both directions to fully release the skin and superficial fascia and muscles.

After the initial work you can, again, use oil to work more deeply into the whole of the back of the leg using the upward strokes and shaking movements that you have carried out on the calf.

Having worked the whole of this area, it is helpful to do some assisted stretches before moving onto the front of the legs and the hips. Ask your client to bend the leg back as far as possible; some people will naturally be able to touch heel to

buttock in this stretch, other people will be a long way out. The starting position isn't so important but it is good to note it to see if you can increase the stretch with the client. You can assist the stretch by supporting the foot at the ankle so that no pressure is being placed on the foot, and as the client tries to touch heel to buttock support the stretch by applying gentle pressure.

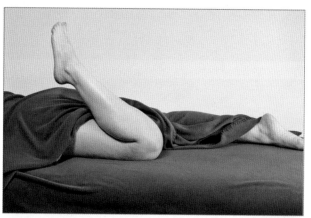

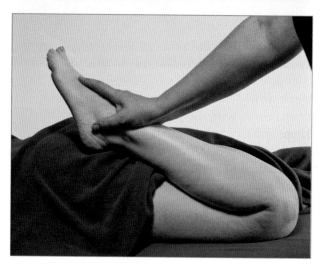

There should be no pain felt in the knee at this stage—if there is or if the client has a history of knee problems or has MS, avoid this stretch.

Next ask the client to push up with the foot as though trying to straighten the leg and push you away—you should apply counter-pressure to try to stop them, hold for five to ten seconds and release, and gently repeat this up to five times—remember, do not put too much pressure on, as this is a gentle assisted stretch.

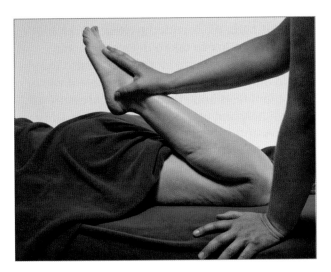

and draping for this, and there is no reason why the treatment cannot be completely successful through clothing and draping. Start by warming up the whole of the area by making circular motions with the flat of your fist—do this on both sides of the buttocks.

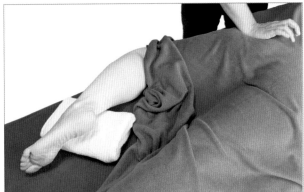

Next ask your client to turn to lie faceup and work gently with the same thumb-to-thumb surface release techniques up the whole of the front of both legs. Working either through clothing or using a little oil skin to skin, work up from the outer edge of the ankle to just underneath the knee on the muscles that come up the outside of the shin. You can work upward toward the heart and you can also work across the muscle using cross-friction; again, always finishing with working back up the muscle following its length.

Skipping over the knee and then supporting the knee with a rolled-up towel or small cushion, you can then work the top of the thigh. If you are working on a friend or family member, stick to the outside of the thigh, if you are professionally trained then gentle inner-thigh work can also be helpful here, but the front of the body work does not need to be as deep as the back of the body work—the calves, hamstring, and piriformis areas appear to have a much greater impact on RLS than work to the front of the body.[152]

The final area to work is the hips; you can warm up the whole of this area by working on the gluteal muscles—these are a collection of three muscles in the buttocks. The client may feel more comfortable with you working through clothing

You should also work the sacrum, the area at the base of the spine. The sacrum is a flattened bony area at the base of the spine, and if you feel across this area with your fingers you should be able to find the edges of the sacrum. It is safe to massage with gentle to medium pressure over this area; if you are new to massage only use gentle pressure. Using thumb pressure, work your way along and across the sacrum so that you cover the whole area with a press-and-release action, holding each press for five to ten seconds.

You should also be able to feel the bottom edges of the sacrum—these will be angular coming from the base of the sacrum (the top of the intergluteal cleft), moving upward and outward in the direction of each hip. With the flat of your thumb gently roll off the edge of the sacrum.

Having carried out the initial work you can ask your the client to lie on his or her side, use a pillow to support the head, and have the leg closest to the table out straight and the upper leg bent upward and forward in front of the body—this is the similar to recovery position in first aid.

Place the flat of your hand on the top of the client's leg so that your middle finger follows on the line of the femur (leg bone) and so that the base of your finger is on the head of the femur. Curl and spread out your fingers and press into the fleshy part of the leg; you will be working the area between the sacrum and the leg—note where your middle three fingers rest.

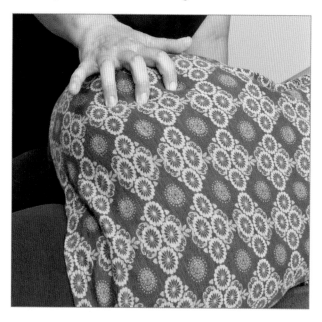

The points where these fingers rest are the three points that you are going to press into. If you are professionally trained in massage or other bodywork you can use your elbow to apply pressure here; if not, use your knuckles, placing two or three knuckles together to gain extra strength. Work with the client's breath, asking him or her to take a deep breath and then applying pressure on the out breath. You should only be working on soft tissue—if you or your client feels bone then take the pressure off immediately and feel for the softer areas. Once you have applied the pressure, hold it there. This will be uncomfortable for your client but it should feel like "good pain"; that is, it feels like it is doing something positive. Hold the pressure until the client feels as though you have released it—even though you haven't—this is the muscle releasing and is what you are aiming to achieve. Repeat for all three points on both sides.

The calf, hamstring, and hip work is more difficult for self-massage, although you can use a firm foam roller or tennis ball and experiment with the techniques. You can also use these self-massage techniques to help alleviate the symptoms during the night, which is when it is particularly useful to keep a foam roller by the bed.

Some people have also found that using a magnesium oil spray on the legs can be beneficial,[153] and this is readily available over the counter and is useful if your magnesium levels have been tested and are low. Despite its name, this isn't an oil, so would need to be used in addition to a massage oil if used during treatments.

---

[153] http://www.rls-uk.org/treatment/4567435170

Rotator Cuff Injury

Background to the Condition

While this chapter addresses rotor cuff injuries as a whole, there are three different conditions that can affect the rotator cuff: rotator cuff tendonitis, rotator cuff impingement syndrome, and a rotator cuff tear. These are common injuries and, if minor, are usually treated with a mixture of rest, medication, and rehabilitation exercises and massage. For rotator cuff tendonitis, use the advice given in the chapter on tendonitis where the condition is covered in more detail.

The rotator cuff is a group of four muscles around the shoulder joint with tendons that attach to the "ball" of the humerus, the upper-arm bone. These muscles and tendons control the movement of the shoulder and allow a person to lift and rotate the arms while holding the ball of the humerus firmly in the socket of the shoulder.

In the early stages of a rotator cuff tear, massage would be contraindicated, and depending on the severity of the injury surgical intervention may be necessary. A rotator cuff tear can be very minor or it can be a complete tear where tendon has been torn away from the bone. A rotator cuff tear will lead to limited movement; something as simple as brushing hair can be painful, difficult, or impossible. There will be pain, and while this can range from mild to moderate or severe, it is likely to increase at night if the person with the injury tries to lie on the affected shoulder.

There is likely to be swelling—this is the body's response to injury—and this swelling may be visible or not. Where the swelling is internal there may be a clicking, popping, or cracking sound when the shoulder is moved. If a client presents with these symptoms he or she should be referred to a medical practitioner for further

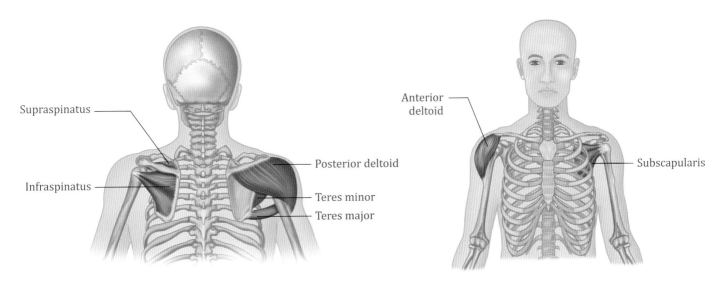

Supraspinatus

Infraspinatus

Posterior deltoid

Teres minor

Teres major

Anterior deltoid

Subscapularis

investigation to determine the extent of the injury, and there may be a referral to see a specialist surgeon. If the tear is minor, then as recovery progresses massage can be used to relieve the tension in the muscles both above and below the injury, but not on the rotator cuff itself until the tear is fully healed.

Rotator cuff (or shoulder) impingement syndrome is a very common cause of shoulder pain and can be a precursor to tendonitis or a more serious tear in the rotator cuff. People who undertake repetitive motions with their arms raised are most likely to suffer from this; sports such as swimming or tennis, or occupations such as painting and decorating, working in a warehouse, and nursing increase the likelihood of developing a this syndrome. Sleeping with an arm in an upright position and smoking[154] are also significant risk factors.

With impingement syndrome the pain is persistent throughout the day and will affect everyday activities. Simple things like reaching up behind the back or overhead are likely to cause pain. Left untreated, impingement syndrome may result in rotator cuff tendonitis and inflammation of the bursa. Left untreated for a long period of time, the rotator cuff tendons can be worn away by the constant rubbing so that they thin and may tear completely, leading to other complications.

Treating the condition in the early stages is a much simpler and quicker solution. It is important not to try to just "work through" this pain; other areas of the body will take the strain and muscles will be used outside of their normal capacity to compensate, and biceps ruptures are not unknown as a side effect of a shoulder impingement.

The rotator cuff comprises four muscles— the subscapularis, the supraspinatus, the infraspinatus, and the teres minor—and their respective tendons. A shoulder impingement occurs when the tendons of the rotator cuff become impinged as they pass through the narrow bony space called the subacromial space within the shoulder joint.

The impingement, or restriction, irritates the tendons causing inflammation and pain; as the inflammation causes swelling of the tendons the restriction increases and so too does the rubbing on and pain in the tendons. Without rest and treatment this cycle continues until the tendon begins to get rubbed and can eventually be torn apart.

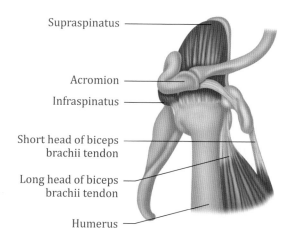

Supraspinatus

Acromion

Infraspinatus

Short head of biceps brachii tendon

Long head of biceps brachii tendon

Humerus

There are different stages in the progression of the injury and some of these are more likely to occur at different ages than others.

Stage 1 injuries are much more common in clients 25 years old or younger, symptoms are likely to be acute, and medical attention is advised to rule out complications. Stage 2 more often affects patients aged between 25 and 40 and this is linked to progressive degeneration in the rotator cuff. Stage 3 is more common for clients who are 40 and over, where tears in the tendon can occur along with bone spurs that may need surgical treatment. If the pain is accompanied by redness and swelling, a temperature, or severe pain the client should

---

[154] http://www.wjgnet.com/2218-5836/pdf/v3/i1/5.pdf

be referred for medical checking straight away. If this is not the case but the conservative treatments offered here do not help after six to eight weeks, then the client should, again, be referred to check that no complications exist.

A shoulder, or rotator cuff, impingement, is normally diagnosed by taking the medical history of the problem and X-ray or other imaging.

Specific Contraindications

• If the symptoms first arise after an injury, massage is contraindicated until the injury can be medically assessed.

• In the early stages of a rotator cuff tear, massage is contraindicated.

• Where there is swelling; heat; or a clicking, popping, or cracking sound when the shoulder is moved, massage is contraindicated.

• If the pain is accompanied by fever the client should be referred for immediate medical attention.

Massage Treatments

The first stage in treatment is to rest the shoulder: this means a complete break from the activities that are causing the problems. It may mean a change in work for six to eight weeks or not taking part in a certain sports for the same amount of time. Some medical practitioners will recommend nonsteroidal anti-inflammatory medication; while these can be bought over the counter, they may be best used under medical supervision since they can have significant side effects.

Both cold and heat can be useful; some people find that icing the area can help to relieve inflammation and pain, particularly in the early stages of treatment. It is also important to begin to gently stretch the area out by raising the hand up and behind the back, but this should be done carefully, gently, and when the muscles are warmed, and never straight after icing. A warm shower or stretching in a warm room will assist the healing process and this is the best environment to begin to stretch the muscles. It is important to remember that while you should avoid the repetitive motions that have caused the problems, completely immobilizing the shoulder will cause stiffness in the joint and surrounding muscles and fascia.

Massage can be an important part of this healing process but, as with any inflammatory condition, massage on the actual area itself should be avoided; massage work can be done below and above the area of inflammation, but not on it.

Begin your massage treatment at the hands and arms, paying specific attention to the little finger and the thumb but not ignoring the other fingers. Follow the instructions for detailed hand work given in Chapter 2. You can also use these instructions to work up from here to massage the muscles in the forearm and, in long strokes, up both the front and the back of the forearm moving from hand to elbow, avoiding working directly over the joints. Use a little massage oil to lubricate the skin for these longer strokes.

Moving up the arm there is a need for more caution, especially around the biceps area. If the biceps is very tender to the touch, avoid massaging this area and move on to massaging the shoulder and front of the chest (see overleaf). This area can be very tender, particularly for many women, specifically on the deltoids; if the biceps is not unduly tender then you can also massage the upper arm. Begin by warming up this area with long strokes from elbow to just below the shoulder—it is important not to work right up to the shoulder so that you do not irritate an already inflamed area. Instead, focus on the biceps and triceps, the brachioradialis muscle on the outer forearm, and the deltoids at the very top into the shoulder.

Posterior view

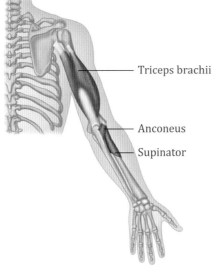

Triceps brachii

Anconeus

Supinator

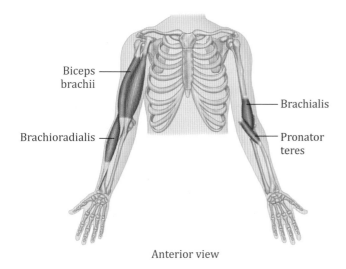

Biceps brachii

Brachioradialis

Brachialis

Pronator teres

Anterior view

The aim of this massage is to release the muscles in the arm to alleviate any residual tension that would pull on the tendons implicated in a shoulder impingement, even when those muscles are not specifically being used. Residual tension is tension that is there when the muscle is not being used and this is what, in your massage, you are seeking to clear.

Working these muscles below the shoulder can have a significant positive impact on the impinged shoulder, and it is also worth working on the muscles above the inflammation too. For the shoulder joint this means, initially, head and neck work: this massage is detailed in Chapter 4. Back massage can also be useful, but you must be careful that having your client facedown does not put undue pressure on the shoulder joint, so support this with a small cushion or loosely rolled-up towel if necessary. It is worth considering work to the front of the chest along the pectorals and the front of the deltoids with the client lying faceup. Be careful how you work this area. It should be slow and deliberate work; if you need clients to move their arm, ask them to move it so that it can be at their own pace and supported by their other hand as necessary—don't try to move it yourself or assist in stretches that could risk forcing the joint at all. Work across these muscles can be a simple press, hold, and release action, always within the client's tolerance and using slow movements so that the client feels in control of the treatment and so relaxes into it.

Be gentle with your warm-up, use oil and long, slow, flowing motions to encourage good blood flow throughout the muscles. If they are not too tender, work across the muscles of the upper arm as you did the forearm. You can use the palm of your hand for this work as your thumb may be too uncomfortable for your client.

Even though you will be working slowly and carefully with this treatment, the impact of it can be very positive for the client; as with any area that is causing a significant amount of pain, the client will guard the area to protect it, so be sure to work slowly and gently to work with, not on, your client.

Scar Tissue

Background to the Condition

Scar tissue forms when there has been some kind of trauma or injury to the body. This may be as a result of surgery; an accident; or when a muscle has been overstretched, torn, or sprained. While the surface of a scar may be visible to the eye, much more scarring takes place below the top layers of the skin.

Rather than replace damaged skin or muscle with new skin or muscle, the body is able to quickly repair itself, but with scar tissue. Scar tissue is collagen based, and these collagen fibers attach themselves to the edges of the damaged tissue and join it together, allowing the damaged tissue to heal. The new tissue is less flexible and more brittle than normal tissue so it is also more likely to be reinjured, and as the fibers are short they can restrict movement.

When scars form on the skin they can be felt as raised and hard lines. If they are in places that normally need to flex, for example on the hands or feet, then movement can be significantly restricted. Scars around larger joints can restrict the movement within those joints. Likewise, scars within the muscle can result in less movement and increased pain within that joint. Surgical scars or accidents resulting in open wounds will give both deep skin and muscle scarring, which can amplify the restriction. Added to this is the impact of scarring on the fascia that surrounds and interacts with muscle, connective tissue, organs, and skin. A complex picture can soon build.

There are two stages to scarring, and massage treatment in the two phases will differ; it is therefore important to know the age of the scar as well as the original cause of the injury. Surgical scarring is likely to be "neater" than scarring caused, for example, by being involved in a car accident, so the scarring felt in the latter example may go far beyond the boundaries of the scar visible on the skin.

The age of the scar is also relevant to how the treatment will proceed. A new scar is in its immature phase and initial healing is still taking place. An immature scar will be red and raised. It is likely to be very painful—even without being touched—and it can be itchy or oversensitive as the nerve endings start their healing process. In this phase the scar is being made through collagen production as the body tries to pull the damaged surfaces back together. This happens fairly quickly, and with surgery the external stitches will usually be removed within 14 days to prevent the body reacting against the stitches and causing an inflammatory response that could make the scarring worse. However, at this stage, the scar less than 15% of its final strength,[155] and for this reason dissolvable stitches are likely to be in place far below the surface to hold the wound together at a deeper level for the first three to four months.

---

[155] http://practicalplasticsurgery.org/docs/Practical_15.pdf
http://www.integrativehealthcare.org/mt/archives/2007/07/six_massage_tec.html
http://www.massagetoday.com/mpacms/mt/article.php?id=14020

Scar tissue will never be as strong as the original tissue so reinjury will always be a risk. Scar tissue will also be less flexible and more pain sensitive than normal tissue.

By 6 months the scar will have gained 50% of its ultimate strength, but it will take 12 months to reach its full strength. At 3 to 18 months the scar will stop producing collagen (depending on the size of the scar) and it is then considered mature. At 12 months the scar will normally have developed its final appearance, though improvements may still continue and in children the improvement can continue for several years. The scar should by now be finer and more akin to the natural skin tone. Deeper scarring that does not have a surface scar to judge by still takes the same long healing time, and care needs to be taken with work in the initial stages even though there is no visible scar.

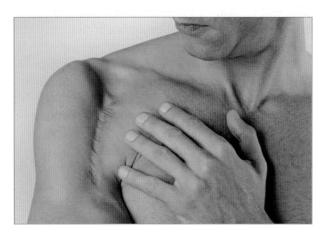

Scar tissue can restrict movement by tightening the skin, binding together the sliding surfaces of the muscles, and knitting together joints, fascia, and connective tissues in ways that they are not designed to be bound.

Treating a scar and scar tissue with massage can be very beneficial: it helps to elongate the collagen fibers to allow greater movement, it helps the fibers to align with the direction of the muscles, and it helps to soften the scar. The body's response to protecting an injured area is to shorten the muscles in that area, so the massage also begins to assist by stretching the muscles to regain their usual mobility.

Specific Contraindications

There are a number of contraindications that should be taken into account.

- Never massage a scar where there is an open or weeping wound. Doing so can easily introduce infection into the wound and can reopen it, slowing down healing and leading to thickening of the scar.

- Wait until any external sutures have been removed—again, these are a point where infection might be introduced; while they are in place the scar is new and vulnerable and could be damaged through massage.

- If the skin around the scar is red and hot then it suggests that an infection is present in the wound and the client should be referred to a medical practitioner to see if antibiotics are required and for the wound to be examined. The same applies if the client has a temperature or is feeling unwell.

Massage Treatments

Assuming all is well then very gentle massage can begin two weeks after the initial injury, provided that there are no open or weeping wounds. However, massage at this time needs to be very gentle. The hygiene of the person giving the massage is very important, with thorough hand washing and the use of antibacterial hand wash. The reason for massage being very gentle at this stage is that the wound only has 15% of its final strength and that strength will be less than an uninjured part of the same person's body. This is a finger-light movement—at this stage you are *not applying any pressure* to the scar—and it is a stroking rather than a deep movement. Applying pressure at this stage could delay the healing process and cause additional scar tissue to form, which would, longer term, leave a bigger scar.

The area around the scar may be slightly (or very) puffy as lymphatic drainage and circulation in the area may have been restricted following the injury. Gentle lymphatic drainage can assist and is a good first step. Working upward toward the heart, very gentle circular movements over and around the scar will help this drainage to take place. Then place two fingers together at a point approximately one inch below the scar, hold the finger furthest away from the scar still, and stroke upward with the other finger, stopping approximately half an inch before the scar. Then repeat the gentle circular movements across the scar up to the top of the scar. Place the two fingers half an inch above the scar and, using the finger furthest from the scar, stroke upward away from the scar. The pressure above and below the scar can be a little firmer than over the scar but still work very gently as the whole area will be traumatized. Repeat this whole sequence three times twice a day. None of these moves should hurt or make the scar any redder than when you started.

These initial massage treatments should be continued daily for at least six to eight weeks to have maximum effect.

Once the scar has reached a mature stage (after 12 months) or, indeed, if you are working on an old scar or an old injury you can be much more vigorous in your moves and add the following two treatments. In deeper scarring, adhesions can occur. Adhesions are bands of scar tissue that form to keep a wound stable, and they will attach to any tissue that they come into contact with. Pelvic adhesions are quite common after gynecological surgery or trauma, or after stomach and related surgeries. Abdominal massage is addressed elsewhere in this book, and abdominal massage should only be carried out by a trained and qualified practitioner. Adhesions can develop in most parts of the body when there has been a trauma or injury, and joints can become obstructed in their movement because of these adhesions. Massage can help to release adhesions and allow the free flow of movement to take place again.

Deep transverse friction massage across the scar and its surrounding areas can help to break up "stuck" tissue and old scar tissue. This may be uncomfortable for the client and you should never move beyond the person's tolerance levels. Work vigorously in the opposite way to how the muscle fibers lie (warm up the muscle first), working across the muscle rather than up and down it. This will increase blood flow to the area and will help the fibers to align. Finish with deep strokes in the direction of the muscle or scar.

Stretching is the final treatment and something that you can encourage your client to continue with at home. Stretching out the area will help lengthen the scar tissue, which in itself will increase mobility. Keep the stretch for 15–20 seconds and gently massage following the direction of the muscle after each stretch. Only stretch within the natural range of movement of any joint or limb and never put pressure behind any joint.

Using a massage oil to help lubricate the skin while you massage can be useful for both the lymphatic drainage massage and the deep transverse massage. Aloe vera has been used by some traditional cultures to help scars to heal and can have a positive impact on the appearance of the scar, helping it to soften and become less red. When using any product on an immature scar, be very careful as regards hygiene. Aloe vera can be harvested straight from the leaf of the plant but you can also buy it commercially if you don't live in a climate that suits the plant. It is produced in capsules at 99.9% purity (pure aloe vera) and the top of the capsule can be snipped off to release the gel, but dispose of the capsule after one use to avoid any risk of infection. If you are using oil, use a very neutral oil such as grape-seed and always from a sealed bottle where hands do not come into contact with the product. Avoid using cream from a jar where bacteria can be introduced from the hands and then multiply within the product. Hygiene always has to be the top priority when working with immature scars.

These treatments can either be carried out by a professional or at home by a relative, friend, or carer, and, depending where the scar is, by the "patient" themselves. They are best repeated often for maximum effect and over a prolonged period of time.

Sciatica

Background to the Condition

Sciatica is an umbrella term given to any sort of pain that is caused by irritation or compression of the sciatic nerve; this can include leg pain, sometimes accompanied by tingling, numbness, or weakness. It originates in the lower back and travels through the buttock and down the large sciatic nerve behind the thigh and radiates down below the knee. Sciatica is not a diagnosis in itself, it is rather a symptom of an underlying problem.

The sciatic nerve is the largest single nerve in the body and is made up of individual nerve roots that branch out from the spine starting at L3—these combine to form the sciatic nerve. The nerve then branches out in each leg to supply the various parts of the leg (thigh, calf, foot, toes, etc.).

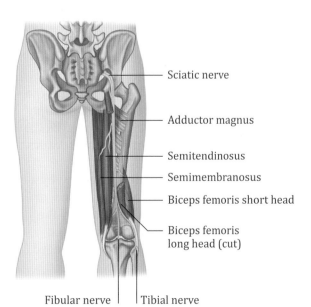

Sciatic nerve

Adductor magnus

Semitendinosus

Semimembranosus

Biceps femoris short head

Biceps femoris long head (cut)

Fibular nerve   Tibial nerve

It is important to differentiate what "type" of sciatica the client is suffering from. *Axial* sciatica (where the nerve root is impinged at the lumbar spine) and *appendicular* sciatica (where the nerve entrapment is elsewhere in the nerve, not in the nerve roots) need slightly different massage treatments.

One of the common causes of sciatica is a herniated disc (also known as a slipped or prolapsed disc); this puts pressure on the nerve causing the sciatica symptoms (an axial sciatica). This is not, however, the only cause; the incidence of sciatica increases with age owing to two age-related conditions: degenerative disc disease, which irritates a nerve root and causes sciatica, and lumbar spinal stenosis, which causes sciatica due to a narrowing of the spinal canal.

Piriformis syndrome is also a common cause of sciatic pain, where the sciatic nerve is compressed by the piriformis muscle.

There are a number of reasons why this can happen. If it is as a result of a new trauma or injury, then the client should see their medical practitioner to check this is not something that needs immediate attention; in the majority of cases it is likely that the piriformis muscle has simply become too tight and this puts pressure on the sciatic nerve giving the symptoms of sciatica. If the sciatica arises from piriformis syndrome, the symptoms will usually become worse after prolonged sitting, walking, or running but may feel better after lying down on the back.

Other, more rare, causes can include irritation of the nerve from adjacent bone, tumors, muscle tightness, internal bleeding, infections, injury, and, for some women, pregnancy.

Nerve entrapment by the piriformis muscle is probably the most common cause of appendicular sciatica, accounting for up to 70% of these cases,[156] and there are simple tests that can be done to establish if this is the case. As ever, if your client is in any doubt a medical opinion should be sought, this test is only one of many that can be carried out for sciatica. Appendicular sciatica is characterized by increased pain from sitting, walking up stairs or inclines, the direct pressure of sexual intercourse in women, or with resisted active external rotation of the femur.[157] This can be tested by asking your client to sit toward the edge of a chair and lift the leg of the affected side with the knee bent, as far toward the chest as is comfortable. If this increases the pain it indicates that the problem is more likely to be in the piriformis, or possibly the hamstrings.

When this is the case then deeper work is indicated in order to release the muscle tension that is putting pressure on the nerve.

Specific Contraindications

Massage is contraindicated if any of the following symptoms accompany the sciatica: weight loss, any loss of control of the bladder or bowel, if the pain or symptoms increase rather than decrease, or if the pain is too severe for self-management. If any of these symptoms occur, the client should see a medical practitioner.

Massage Treatments

There are a number of massage treatments that can help alleviate the symptoms. It is important to differentiate what type of sciatica you are dealing with in order to treat correctly. If you are in any doubt, err on the side of caution and work with the simpler and gentler treatment given for axial sciatica.

As lower-body tension can be rooted in tension in the feet, it is important to work the feet prior to working deeply into the legs. You can follow the directions for this as detailed in Chapter 3.

Having completed the foot work, start by warming up the back of the leg muscles with long strokes that gradually deepen. Use massage oil to lubricate the skin; if your client is very hairy you will need more oil as the hair will absorb the oil. Having warmed up the muscles, use your thumbs to crisscross the muscles to help release fascia and surface tension, always working upward toward the heart. Once you have worked on the calves, move to the thighs, avoiding contact with the area behind the knee. Warm up the outer thigh muscles and complete the crisscross work up the outside of the upper leg. Once you have warmed up one leg, repeat this work on the other.

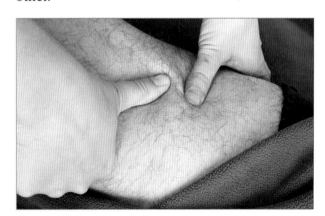

---

[156] http://www.massagetherapy.com/articles/index.php/article_id/2064/Assessing-Sciatic-Pain.

[157] http://www.abmp.com/textonlymags/article.php?article=668

You are now ready to do some deeper work, specifically to the outer leg starting above the ankle. Standing to the side of your client, level with his or her ankles, you can either use the flat of your thumb, the flat of three or four fingers together, or the flat of your palm for this work, but always support the hand you are using with your other hand as shown in the photographs.

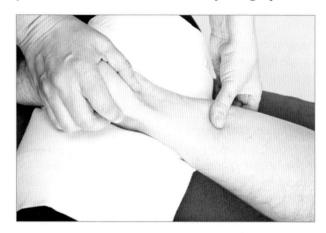

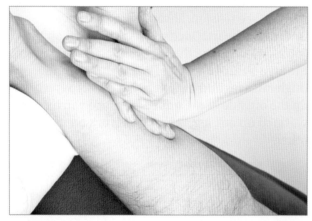

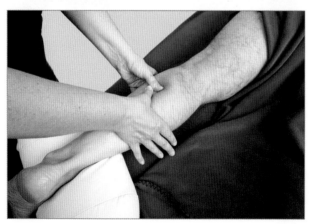

Gradually work up the leg, pressing into the muscle as you slide slowly up it, always within your client's tolerance and stopping before you get to the area behind the knee.

Repeat this four or five times, each time working more deeply. If you find one area of the muscle that feels tighter (more resistant) or more tender than other areas, hold static pressure on this spot and you will begin to feel the tension releasing and the muscle relaxing. Your client should also report a decrease in the tenderness experienced. Without working on the area to the back of the knee, repeat this process on the upper leg, working only on the center and outer leg and avoiding the inner thigh.

If you are working with a client with appendicular sciatica, you can carry on to work the sacrum and gluteal muscles (glutes) as detailed below. If your client has axial sciatica then you should not do this deeper work; an adaptation of this treatment is detailed after these directions.

You now come to work on the sacrum. Start with your client facing downward, and feel for the sacrum. It is located in the lower back and you should be able to feel both the flat of the bone and the edge of the bone.

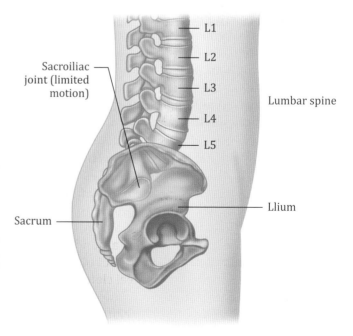

Use your fingers to feel around the sacrum and test to see if the skin moves freely across this area. If it does not, start by making small circles across the sacrum by placing three fingers together and pressing onto the sacrum so that you are securing the skin against your fingers.

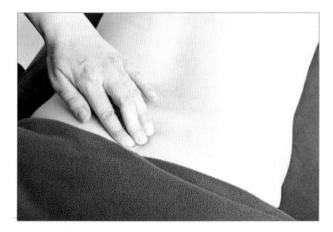

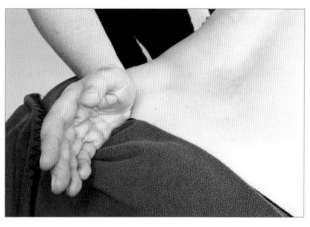

For Appendicular Sciatica Only

Having carried out the sacral massage, ask your client to lie on his or her side, providing a pillow to support the head. Ask your client to keep the leg closest to the table straight and bend the other one upward toward the chest, using a pillow to support the knee to prevent it rolling forward and putting any pressure on the spine by twisting.

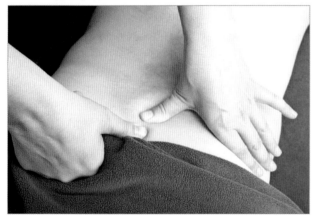

Without lifting your fingers or changing the spot on the skin where you are pressing, move your fingers around to make small circles, working three or four times in each direction. Move across the whole sacrum with this motion, making sure you work right to the edge; you should be able to feel the edges under your fingers as the solidity of the bone gives way to the softer flesh of the glutes and buttocks. Once you have worked your way around the whole sacrum, move to its edges and, with the heel of your hand, slowly roll off the sacrum, working all the way around it (with the exception of the bottom point of the sacrum, which finishes in the intergluteal cleft, as this intrudes too much on privacy). You can carry out all of this sacral work through clothes or a towel.

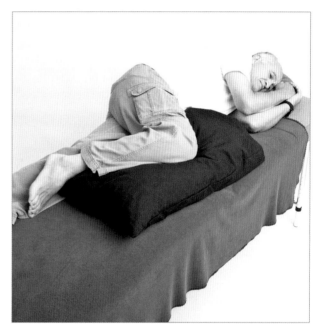

Place your open hand at the head of the femur—you will feel this at the very top of the leg—place your palm on the top of the head of the femur, and spread your fingers outward. The area under your fingers is the area you are going to work.

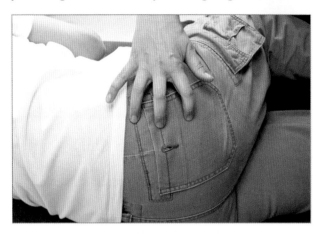

This should feel soft to the touch but there may be tender and tight areas within it. If you are a friend or family member giving a treatment, use the flat of your knuckles for the next move; if you are a trained professional you can use your elbow. Try to feel the more resistant areas by applying gentle pressure, these will also be the more tender spots. such Ask your client to take a slow, deep abdominal breath and on the out breath press slowly and deeply into the muscle.

Ask your client to let you know when this starts to become painful and stop at that point (or professionally working to the maximum depth your client is happy to work to), hold the pressure without moving or otherwise changing depth or position. There should not be any pain in the back so if this is reported, stop immediately. After 30–60 seconds you will feel the muscle under your hand or elbow relax and your client will report that it no longer hurts. Slowly release the pressure and feel further down and repeat, so that you have treated all three points. Carefully assist your client to turn over and repeat on the other side.

For Axial Sciatica

Begin with the same foot and leg treatment as detailed above, but the sacral work should be gentler. Your client can still be lying facedown if you have a table with a face hole, but support the legs with a pillow or cushions placed underneath the lower legs—this helps to take any pressure off the spine.

Depending on how mobile your client is you may be able to complete the work into the hips as detailed above, but for axial sciatica you need to work more lightly, using gentler pressure with your thumb or knuckles rather than using your elbow. For axial sciatica try to limit your treatment to around 30 minutes so that the client is not lying facedown for too long.

Massage for axial sciatica can give some relief but this may be very temporary as it is not addressing the root cause of the problem; however, even this temporary relief is usually very welcome.

Scoliosis

Background to the Condition

Scoliosis is a back condition where the spine is curved either to the left or to the right side. A curve of up to 10 degrees is considered within the normal spinal range, so scoliosis is only diagnosed when a curve reaches 11 degrees.

Although the catch-all term "scoliosis" is used, it reflects at least six different conditions. *Idiopathic scoliosis*, where the cause of the curvature is unknown, accounts for around 80% of all cases (idiopathic comes from the Greek and means "of unknown cause").

Congenital scoliosis develops before birth and is caused by a defect in the formation of the spine. The vertebrae may fail to separate or parts of the vertebrae can be missing, leading to one side of the spine growing more than the other, causing the spine to curve.[158]

The term *neuromuscular scoliosis* is used to describe curvature of the spine in patients with any disorder of the neurological system. Common categories include cerebral palsy, spina bifida, muscular dystrophies, and spinal cord injuries.[159] People with this form of scoliosis may also develop kyphosis, where the upper back

also becomes rounded. This form of scoliosis is usually degenerative and gets worse with time. As muscles weaken, the spine is under more pressure and collapses. For wheelchair users this can lead to difficulty in getting comfortable and can cause recurrent chest problems as the lungs are compressed.

Scheuermann's kyphosis is a structural curvature of the thoracic or thoracolumbar spine that normally develops before puberty and deteriorates during adolescence.[160] This condition affects men and women equally. There is often a delay in diagnosing Scheuermann's kyphosis as when it first comes to light during adolescence it is frequently mistaken for postural kyphosis, linked to bad posture. Scheuermann's kyphosis is not posture related.

Syndromic scoliosis is scoliosis that occurs as part of another recognized syndrome. For example, people diagnosed with Marfan syndrome, Rett syndrome, or Beales syndrome are likely to develop scoliosis.[161]

Finally, *degenerative scoliosis* occurs in adults, either as a development of a previous mild scoliosis or as the result of arthritis or degeneration of the spine. Degeneration can be

---

[158] http://www.sauk.org.uk/about-scoliosis/types-of-scoliosis/congenital-scoliosis.html

[159] http://www.sauk.org.uk/about-scoliosis/types-of-scoliosis/neuromuscular-scoliosis.html

[160] http://www.sauk.org.uk/about-scoliosis/types-of-scoliosis/scheuermanns-kyphosis.html

[161] http://www.sauk.org.uk/about-scoliosis/types-of-scoliosis/syndromic-scoliosis.html

mild or more severe; surgery is an option for pain relief but decisions have to be made on a case-by-case basis, balancing the benefits against the risks of spinal surgery, particularly in patients over 40.

Medical treatment of scoliosis has traditionally been surgery or bracing. There is emergent evidence from trials that some patients have seen an improvement in symptoms (a decrease in both pain and the angle of curvature) from chiropractic treatment,[162] and there is a growing body of patient-led evidence to say that symptoms have been improved by other complementary treatments. Some find yoga very helpful in keeping the surrounding areas moving and flexible, while for others acupuncture and massage can be effective in treating the surrounding soft tissue, which is under strain owing to the scoliosis.

Other integrated physical therapies, including the Schroth Method, that combine treatments and exercise are also showing promising results in improving not just the pain but also the scoliosis itself.[163]

Massage has long being recognized as helpful in treating the muscular pain that accompanies scoliosis and this is the area that will be concentrated on in this chapter. The Scoliosis Association UK say of massage: "Curvature of the spine causes the muscles in the shoulders and around the spine to misalign or become stretched or compressed. In turn this malalignment causes tension or muscle spasms. Massage therapy can help unlock some of this tension."[164]

Specific Contraindications

There are no specific contraindications for scoliosis as each person will be different in the severity of the condition and how it is managed both personally and medically. It is important to take into account any other medical conditions and the contraindications for those conditions. However, if a client has had spinal surgery in the last 12 months or has been undergoing treatment with a brace then massage on the back, side, or front of the body should only be carried out in discussion with the supervising medical practitioner. Massage to hands and arms/feet and legs should not present any challenge to the other treatments. If the client has osteoporosis, omit the part of the treatment that works on the intercostal muscles between the ribs.

Massage Treatments

How massage is approached will depend very much on the severity of the scoliosis. Some scoliosis will cause the pelvis to be tilted and for this it is important to start by massaging the feet and up the legs and then to move to the hands, arms, head, shoulders, neck, back, sacrum, and hips. The work is carried out in this sequence so that all areas that may induce tightness of the muscles around the spine are loosened first, ensuring nothing else is pulling on those muscles and causing added strain and tension. It might be tempting to go straight for the back muscles as this is where the problem presents itself, but if, for example, the client spends a lot of time sitting using a computer in their job or home life then the hands, arms, and shoulders will likely be tight from that work, and the tension in these muscles affects the muscles in the back. You will therefore get much better results by first freeing these muscles.

[162] http://www.ncbi.nlm.nih.gov/pmc/articles/PMC3259989/

[163] http://www.scoliosissos.com/clinic/overview.shtml

[164] http://www.sauk.org.uk/about-scoliosis/complementary-therapies/massage.html

Likewise, if the pelvis is tilted then that will cause asymmetry in the legs, which will affect all the leg muscles and upward into the glutes, pelvis, and lower back. Treating the client holistically will yield much better results.

There are two key aims of massage for scoliosis: the first is to ease continually overstretched muscles to allow them to relax and reduce the muscular strain on the spine, and the second is to increase flexibility and reduce pain in the whole body.

The scoliosis may be a single C-shaped curve or a double S-shaped curve. A curve that goes to the right is described as *dextroscoliosis* (dextro = right) and a curve to the left is described as a *levoscoliosis* (levo = left). A left curve almost always occurs in the lumbar spine; if this occurs in the thoracic spine it warrants further investigation, and massage should not be carried out until after these investigations are complete.

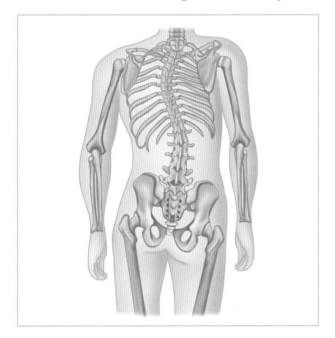

There are specific terms used to describe the location of the curves: a thoracic scoliosis is curvature in the middle (thoracic) part of the spine, and this is the most common location for spinal curvature. A lumbar scoliosis is curvature in the lower (lumbar) portion of the spine, and a thoracolumbar scoliosis is curvature that includes vertebrae in both the lower thoracic portion and the upper lumbar portion of the spine.[165]

While all of this is important, it is also critical simply to look at your client's back and to see where the curves are and how they are pulling on other structures, including the shoulders, arms, ribs, and hips. Understanding how the scoliosis affects the rest of the body will help you focus your treatment and make it more effective.

It is worth investing time in treatment with an overall fascial release. To encourage the fascia to release there are two useful techniques that can be used simply and effectively. The first is to roll the skin; practice this move on yourself first so that you are confident using it on your client. Pick up the skin between your fingers and simply roll it so that you are moving across the area you are working on. You don't need to work in any particular direction and it's better if you change direction frequently; unless the client has very dry skin, avoid using oil as it will be difficult to grasp the skin once oiled.

Next, using your thumbs, place your thumb tips together on the client's skin and, without releasing your grip, slide your thumbs so that the tip of the nail and the first knuckle are parallel. You are eventually aiming to work across the whole of the body in this way but you may need to break this down into shorter treatments working on different areas at different times so that you do not overwhelm your client. Further details are given about these techniques in the chapter looking at fibromyalgia.

[165] http://www.spine-health.com/conditions/scoliosis/scoliosis-types

You can choose where you start your treatment, either following the instructions in Chapter 2 for the hand and arm work, Chapter 3 for the feet, or Chapter 4 for the head massage work. You need to work all of these areas in detail so it is simply a matter of personal choice for you and your client which of these you start with.

Hip work should be carried out only after the legs have been treated, and you can use the directions for the sacrum and hips found in the section on pregnancy; this more conservative and supported hip work is suitable for treating clients with scoliosis. Having worked the hands, arms, feet, legs, and hips, along with the head and neck, you are now ready to massage the main torso.

The intercostal muscles below attached to the ribs are involved in moving and stabilizing the chest wall during respiration. Specifically, they are responsible for the expansion and contraction of the rib cage during breathing; the internal intercostals contract and pull the ribs inward during exhalation, and the external intercostals lift the ribs away from the torso during inhalation. These muscles form a muscular web between the ribs,[166] and they become the posterior intercostal membranes that are attached to the spinal column; treating these muscles can have a direct and positive impact on the spine.

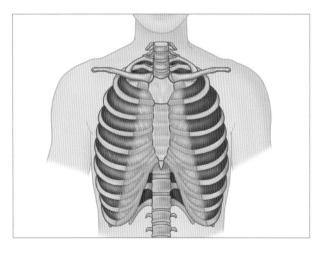

With your client lying faceup (supported by pillows where necessary) ask him or her to raise the arm on the side you are going to be working on first so that it rests above the head. You can give this treatment with the client clothed or through a thin blanket or sheet. Gently feel for the ribs, miss the gap between the bottom rib and the rib above it and start your treatment on the next rib up.

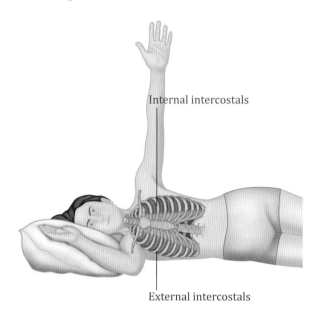

Internal intercostals

External intercostals

Feel for the gap between the ribs and place the flat of your little finger, curved to follow the ribs, into this gap. Ask your client to take a deep breath, apply very gentle pressure with the inhalation, and hold it for the exhalation, releasing it when the exhalation is complete. Move up a rib, and continue this treatment up the whole of the front of the body.

---

166 http://www.handsonhealthnc.com/why-your-side-may-hurt-2

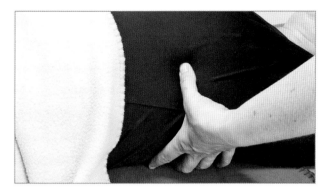

Ask your client to roll onto his or her side so that you are working on the same side of the body, and then repeat this treatment moving up the side of the ribs, again missing the bottom rib and always working slowly, with the client's breath, and gently. It is easy to cause pain and bruising in this area so gentleness is called for. Once you have completed one side of the body, start again on the other side with your client first faceup and then on his or her side.

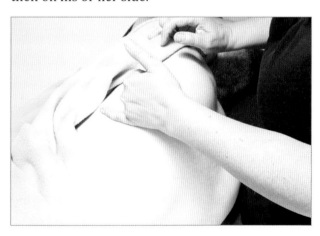

Ask your client to lie facedown. This treatment is best carried out using a massage table with a face hole or face cradle so that you do not put any pressure on the neck, but if you don't have this and are working on a family member or friend, adapt the massage so that the client is lying in the side position with the head supported, and swap sides as you work on the different sides of the spine, always working on the side of the spine that is upward.

It is important when you come to massage the back that you work the muscles down each side of the spine—both are implicated but for different reasons. Muscles on the outside of the curve will be stretched and under pressure from always being taut; muscles on the inside of the curve are never stretched so become tight and tender.

When massaging the back always work away from the spine so that you are never pressing inward onto the spine. Massage around the spine should never touch the spine itself and no direct pressure should ever be placed on the vertebrae or the spinous processes (this is the bone that can be felt when running the fingers down someone's back). It can be good for the client if you combine the light and deep moves, starting with the lighter ones.

Standing at your client's head and using massage oil to lubricate your hands, place a thumb either side of the spine and follow down the curve of the spine using light pressure; remember you are working on the muscles, not the spine itself.

You will feel the strong trapezius and erector spinae muscles, but do not be overly concerned with finding specific muscles at this stage—your aim is to warm up the whole of the back muscles. Be careful not to press onto the ribs so stay close to the spine; after three or four warm-up strokes you can begin to deepen your pressure a little, and continue with this work for another seven or eight strokes.

This should feel good to your client; if it is at all painful you are working too deeply so pull back a little. When you reach the curve(s) in the spine, just follow the curve and you will follow the flow of the muscles for that individual.

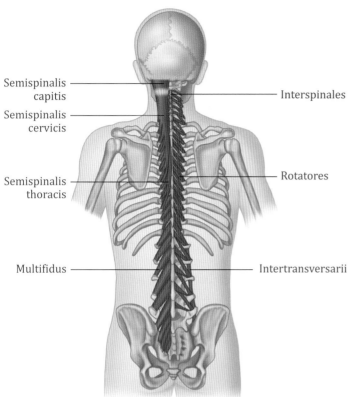

Semispinalis capitis
Semispinalis cervicis
Semispinalis thoracis
Multifidus
Interspinales
Rotatores
Intertransversarii

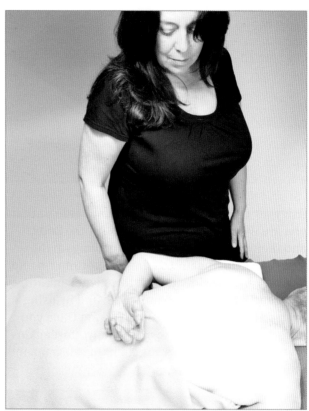

Ask your client to raise the arm behind his or her back, supported with a folded-up towel or small pillow under the front of the shoulder so that this does not become strained. The shoulder should rest in this position; if necessary support the arm with your hip so that the client can relax.

Starting at the edge of the spine, use your thumbs to sweep outward and underneath the raised shoulder blade, then work your way around and underneath the shoulder blade.

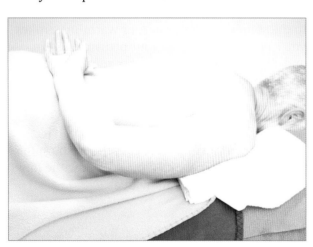

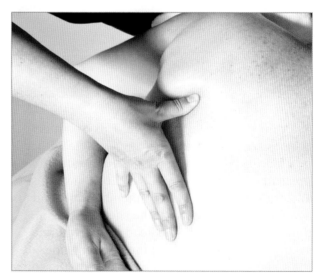

You may find that some areas are more resistant than others—hold your thumb pressure on these areas for 20–30 seconds and you should feel them start to relax. Repeat on both shoulders.

Having observed where the scoliosis curve is you can now work the muscles either side of these. You will see from the diagram that the muscles of the back are complex; do not be too overconcerned about which muscle you are working on, simply follow the curve of the spine wherever that is for the individual client. Start with the inner curve and, using a little massage oil, make small, light circular movements out from the spine toward the ribs. Work the whole area slowly and meticulously from where the curve begins to where it ends—this way you work the whole area. After you have completed the light work you can repeat these same circular motions but a little more deeply. Then repeat the same two moves on the outer edge of the curve.

Once you have completed the lighter and medium-depth work you can then start to work a little more deeply. Return to the inner curve and use your thumb to knead more deeply into the muscle on this inner curve; as you knead inward, hold your pressure for 20–30 seconds.

Your client should be aware of the pressure but you should not be causing any significant pain—if you do, release the pressure immediately and repeat the light pressure only (on both sides) to resettle the muscle. If the deeper work is tolerated, work each side of the curve in turn; you will naturally cover a bigger area with the outer curve. Having completed this, repeat the light circular movements on each side. If there is an S-shaped curve work both curves in turn. Finish this part of the treatment by using long strokes down the back with your thumbs either side of the spine; this should feel more relaxed and should feel amazing for the client.

You can finish the treatment with gentle head work but do not spend too long on this. The client needs to take time to get up and to get up slowly—to be up and moving as best they can within 15–20 minutes of the treatment—allowing the body to readjust to its new-found flexibility, and gentle movement exercises (the doctor or physical therapist is likely to have already given these) will help prolong the effects of the treatment. The results of a good massage treatment should include increased flexibility, decreased pain, and better sleep.

Shin Splint Syndrome

Background to the Condition

Shin splints is a term often used by runners, dancers, or those involved in impact sports to describe pain in the lower legs, but it is a term that can cover a number of different conditions. Some of these conditions respond well to massage therapy and for others massage is contraindicated. Most commonly (but not exclusively) it refers to one of the following conditions:

- Compartment syndrome

- Stress fractures of the tibia and/or fibula

- Anterior tibial tenosynovitis

- Posterior tibial tendonitis.

The first two conditions are contraindicated for massage; it is therefore important for the practitioner to recognize when someone presents with the possibility of these conditions.

Compartment Syndrome

This is a medical emergency and massage is obviously contraindicated. There are two types of compartment syndrome: chronic and acute. In the arms and legs, each muscle group, along with its respective blood vessels and nerves, is contained within layers of fascia. These contained sections of muscles, vessels, and nerves are known as compartments. The fascia surrounding compartments is incredibly strong and has limited flexibility (particularly if the fascia has become "stuck") so if an injury takes place within the compartment that causes bleeding or swelling then the pressure within that compartment can build up.

An acute case of compartment syndrome usually takes place after a trauma to that area, typically an accident of some sort. Left untreated this can lead to permanent damage to the muscles and nerves of the affected limb and medical/surgical intervention is necessary.

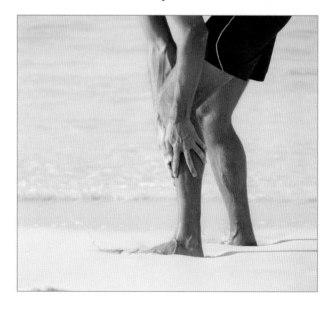

Chronic compartment syndrome comes on much more slowly and is less of a medical emergency, but still needs treatment, and massage would be contraindicated. A person with chronic compartment syndrome will often get cramp in the affected area during exercise, the muscle might visibly bulge, and, when it is the leg that is affected, there may be problems in moving the foot freely. If a client or friend refers to you for massage with these symptoms, he or she should be referred to a medical practitioner and you should not massage. If the symptoms present following a trauma then you should refer the client to the nearest emergency room.

Stress Fractures of the Tibia and/or Fibula

Stress fractures of the tibia and fibula are suffered not only by athletes who train to an extreme, but also those who have poor running footwear, those who have rapidly increased their training regime or who have changed to a harder surface to train, those who have an underlying disease that compromises bone density, and those who have flat or very inflexible feet. While massage can help prevent stress fractures by keeping the feet supple and the muscles of the leg loose, it is contraindicated when a fracture has occurred.

Stress fractures are breaks in the bone and typically will give pain in the lower third of the leg, and there may be tenderness and swelling locally in this area. The pain is present not just when running or training but in everyday activities and it will usually only be in one leg; however, all of these are "mays" and it is possible to have stress fractures in both legs and have no swelling or tenderness and the only absolute way to know is for the sufferer to be checked out medically. If in doubt refer the individual to a doctor.

Anterior Tibial Tenosynovitis

Anterior tibial tenosynovitis is a shin splint injury usually associated with sports where the foot is repetitively or forcefully pushed upward; affected sports people include sprinters, hill runners, snowboarders and skiers, and those exercising on uneven surfaces. For some people the pain will only be experienced when the ankle is flexed upward toward the body, while others will feel it after exercise when the leg is resting. Pain can be more intense after a long rest period (overnight or after sitting for a long time) and the sufferer will often talk about there being a dull ache. Pain usually starts at the front of the ankle and worsens over a couple of weeks, with the pain radiating upward from the front of the ankle to the lower leg.

The tibialis anterior muscle (below) is a large muscle running down the outside of the shin and its tendon inserts at the base of the metatarsal of the first toe; it is responsible for much of the movement of the lower leg at the inner ankle. Anterior tibial tenosynovitis occurs when this tendon sheath becomes inflamed or damaged.

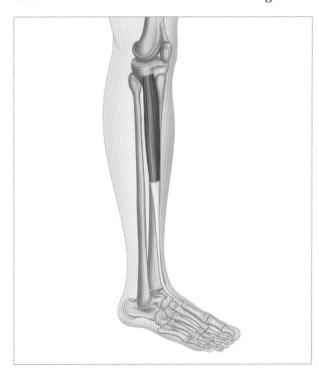

Rest is one of the key success strategies in recovering from anterior tibial tenosynovitis—the inflammation needs to settle for natural healing to take place. Icing the area regularly will also help to reduce the inflammation in the initial stages. While the tendon is inflamed this is the only recommended treatment; massage will help, but wait until the initial inflammation has resolved. For someone who is just about to start or increase a training program, then massage is a great preventative treatment.

Posterior Tibial Tendonitis of the Ankle

The posterior tibial muscle (below) attaches to the back of the shin bone and the posterior tibial tendon connects this muscle to the bones of the foot.

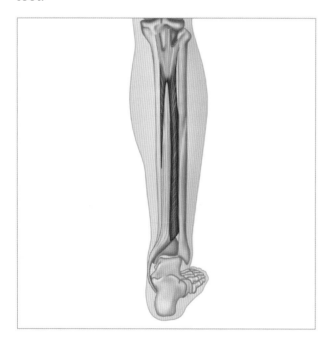

This tendon passes down the back of the leg, close to the Achilles tendon, and then turns under the inner side of the ankle and attaches to the bone of the inner side of the foot. When this area becomes damaged it can take a long time to heal as it is in an area of the foot that does not have a large blood supply. One of the key symptoms is that the arch of the foot flattens and the toes point outward; there will also often be tenderness and an inability to stand on tiptoes in the affected foot. One of the key tests is to ask the person to go up on the toes of each foot in turn; when he or she cannot stand on one leg and raise the heel, the problem is usually with the posterior tibial tendon.

It is more common in women and in those over 40 years of age. Some underlying health conditions, such as diabetes, arthritis, and hypertension, also increase the likelihood of posterior tibial tendonitis occurring. Treatment is usually focused on orthotics, inserts into the shoe, or arch supports, and sometimes orthotic boots or a cast will be worn; surgery may be a consideration for some people.

Specific Contraindications

Compartment syndrome—problems following a trauma should be referred for urgent medical assessment and massage is contraindicated. Stress fractures of the tibia and/or fibula—if pain is present not just on exercising, this should be referred for medical checks and massage is contraindicated until it has been confirmed that no stress fractures are present.

Omit working either side of the Achilles tendon at the heel if your client is pregnant.

Massage Treatments

Anterior Tibial Tenosynovitis

Treatments for this condition can sound very complex but you basically need to loosen up the foot and then work into the lower leg. This treatment is best carried out in conjunction with stretches and strengthening exercises, which the client's physiotherapist or doctor can prescribe. The best starting point is to work the foot and you can follow the instructions for foot massage in Chapter 3; this ensures that any tension in the foot is not contributing to the problems further up the leg. It will easier to carry out this treatment if your client is lying facedown. If you do not have a massage table with a face hole, you can do the foot work seated first, to avoid too much time spent facedown with the head turned to one side.

After you have worked the foot, it is beneficial to work up the back of the leg; although the problem lies in the front of the leg, clearing any tension in the back will help to release the front and this time will not be wasted. These instructions are similar to the calf work for treating plantar fasciitis. Start by warming up the calf muscles by using a little massage oil and starting at the area at the back of the heel—not the heel pad but the area below the ankle on the very bottom of the back of the foot. Starting here, squeeze the back of the heel with short movements, holding for just two to three seconds at a time, being careful not to pinch the actual Achilles tendon—you are working further out from that into the connective tissue that surrounds it, so squeeze rather than pinch. You should omit this part of the treatment if your client is pregnant.

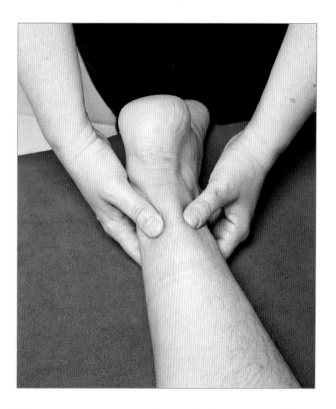

The next two paragraphs apply also to posterior tibial tendonitis; in that section where you are referred to the anterior tibial tenosynovitis section for massaging the rest of the lower leg, this is the part to follow.

As the Achilles tendon is integral to the calf, you now need to focus on releasing the back of the leg. Be careful to warm up the calf muscles first, using both hands and starting with gentle movements, only moving deeper into the calf as the muscles warm and begin to release; otherwise it will be painful and may start to cramp. You can do this by kneading the muscles and using long strokes up the leg, focusing particularly on the outside of the leg. The inner calf can bruise very easily so be more careful and gentle when massaging this area. Stretching the foot as part of the treatment will also help, gently bringing the foot upward as if pushing the toes toward the face, while keeping the foot flat and supported with your hand. Hold for five to ten seconds and slowly release, repeating this stretch three or four times.

Once you have warmed up the area you can begin to work more deeply, holding the leg with your thumbs at the center just above the heel and stroking upward and outward, using your thumbs to work more deeply into the Achilles tendon as you go. You will need to repeat this move three or four times as you work up the calf to ensure you cover the whole area. Work slowly as this area is inclined to cramp if you work too deeply or too quickly. Finally, shake the calf muscle using your fingers—this will help to resettle the muscle after the deeper massage.

You are now ready to ask your client to turn to be faceup so that you can work the front of the lower legs. You will see on the diagram below that the tibialis anterior tendon attaches to the foot close to the inner ankle and that the muscle goes toward the outer knee.

You need to massage that whole area. Begin just forward of the inner ankle and press and hold the point just in front of the ankle.

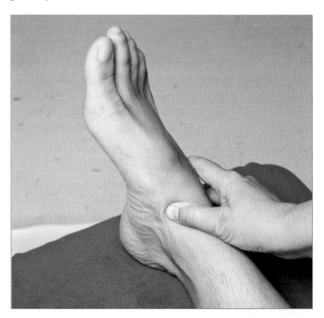

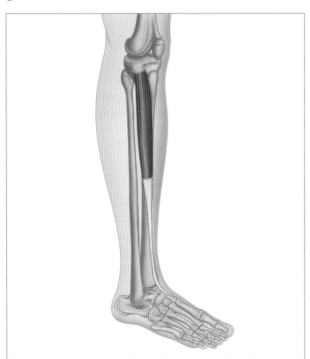

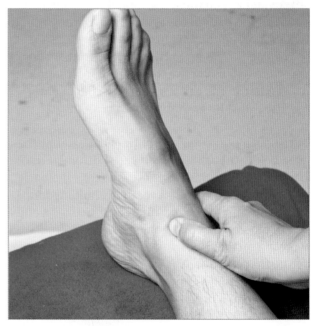

This area is likely to be very tender so work slowly and carefully. As you press, slowly move your thumb just half an inch to an inch upward and toward the center so that you are following the tendon. Continue with this movement, releasing after you have moved the half an inch to an inch, and then replacing your thumb at the point where you left contact with the leg, before reapplying the pressure and moving another half an inch to an inch. Depending on the size of the client's leg you may need to repeat this move three or four times until you find that your thumb is resting at the midpoint of the front of the leg. Repeat these moves three times, moving from ankle to midshin in your staged moves each time.

You are now ready to work the outer part of the front of the leg. Start at the ankle and, using massage oil (you will need more oil if the client has hairy legs), place your hand so that your thumb is pointing upward and, with your thumb, stroke and knead the muscles at the outside of the leg—as you move up the leg you will be working on the tibialis anterior.

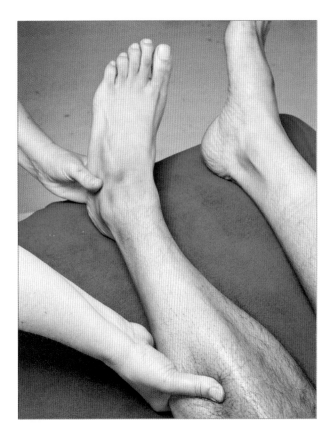

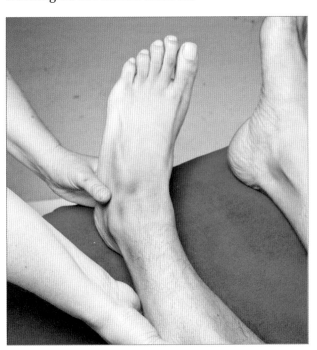

To balance the treatment you should work both legs, although you may want to spend more time on the one that is problematic.

Posterior Tibial Tendonitis

As this condition develops it can progress from being posterior tibial tendonitis to posterior tibial tendon dysfunction. When this happens surgery may be required to restructure the foot. Massage treatment, along with strengthening exercises and the use of podiatry inserts, can help arrest this development so it is important to work in conjunction with a physiotherapist, podiatrist, or gait specialist. Left untreated, some cases will require surgery as the actual structure of the foot will change, bones will misalign, and the foot will flatten, but rest and treatment at an early stage can help to avoid this.

Rest and ice are the first key treatments—it is vital to discourage the client from trying to "work through" the pain barrier or further injury can take place. It is important to start the treatment by working the bottom of the foot where the tendons insert (below). As with all inflammation, do not work an area when it is in an acute stage, if there is any inflammation or additional heat in the area.

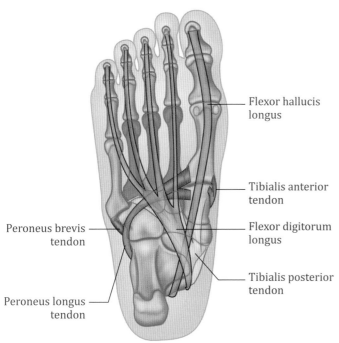

Flexor hallucis longus

Tibialis anterior tendon

Peroneus brevis tendon

Flexor digitorum longus

Tibialis posterior tendon

Peroneus longus tendon

One of the key aims of massage for this condition is to lengthen the muscles that are beginning to shorten; the area is likely to be tender but to be effective you need to work deeply; although, as ever, only within the client's tolerance.

Start by working the whole of the foot as described in Chapter 3, paying special attention to the big and second toes so that the foot starts to feel floppy and warm. The toes should be soft and pliable. It may take several sessions to do this; don't be tempted to work deeply into the calf until you have really released the foot—you can do warm-up to mid-depth work but wait until you have the foot flexible to go more deeply, even if this takes several sessions.

If you can, work every two to three days to begin with to build on the progress you make at each session. Don't ignore the side of the foot as the tendon that attaches the muscle you need to free runs up the inside edge of the foot, starting approximately halfway between the big toe and the ankle.

The area around the ankle will be tender; remember to work both sides of the ankle as tension on the outside of the ankle may also hold the inside ankle tight, and your aim is to free all areas to allow the muscle and tendon to move more freely. Start this work by gently rotating the ankle with your client facedown, rotating it three or four times in each direction. Support the foot with your hands as you do this, and do not force the ankle to move more than it naturally and easily does.

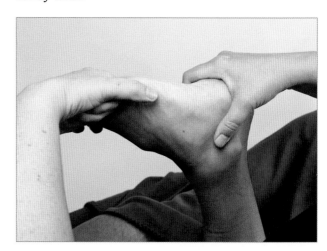

Next, supporting the foot and resting the leg on a pillow or your own leg and holding the foot securely as shown in the photograph, you need to trace up from the outer top knuckle of the big toe to about two inches above the ankle bone, following the line of the tendon as shown in the illustration.

This area will be very tender so work gently and slowly—if you work too deeply your client will pull away from you and may bruise. As you repeat the treatment you will be able to very gradually go deeper, but this will be a very gradual process.

Finally, massage the rest of the lower leg following the instructions above for the anterior treatment, but you can omit the work on the inner calf as you have already addressed this in a more specific way. This will not be a quick fix treatment but it can be an important part in the repair and rehabilitation of this injury.

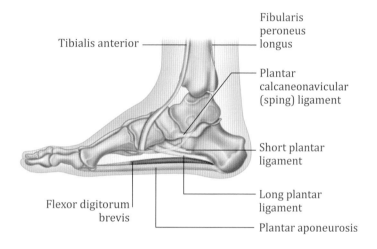

Tibialis anterior

Fibularis peroneus longus

Plantar calcaneonavicular (spring) ligament

Short plantar ligament

Long plantar ligament

Flexor digitorum brevis

Plantar aponeurosis

Sinusitis

Background to the Condition

Sinusitis can be either a bacterial or a viral infection[167] that results in inflammation of the lining of the sinuses. The sinuses are found within the facial bones, and are small air-filled cavities behind the cheekbones and forehead.

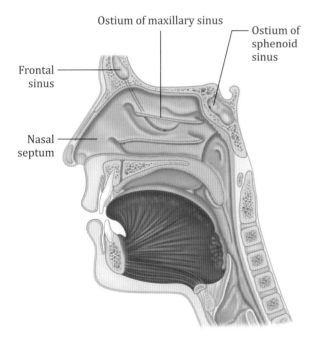

Ostium of maxillary sinus
Ostium of sphenoid sinus
Frontal sinus
Nasal septum

Sinusitis can be either acute or chronic. Acute sinusitis will usually be experienced as a high temperature, pain and tenderness in the face, and a blocked nose or nasal discharge. It will usually start very quickly and lasts between one and four weeks. It can often self-resolve but some cases may need intervention with antibiotics.

Subacute sinusitis lasts between four and twelve weeks, whereas chronic sinusitis is defined as where the problem has gone on for longer than twelve weeks. Sinus infections often develop after a person has had a cold or flu, but can also be caused by (often undiagnosed) problems with the teeth. People with hay fever and other allergic conditions are more susceptible, as are smokers, those with a compromised immune system, people with blockages in the nose, and those with cystic fibrosis, and it has a higher rate of occurrence during pregnancy. A visit to a medical practitioner will help to rule out any underlying conditions that may need separate treatment. In a very small number of cases there can be serious complications[168] that need urgent specialist medical attention (see Specific Contraindications, below). As with any condition, if the client is concerned about the symptoms, he or she should be encouraged to consult a doctor.

---

[167] FAACI position paper on rhinosinusitis and nasalpolyps executive summary. W Fokkens et al., *Allergy*, 2005, 60: 583–601.

[168] KW Ah-See, and AS Evans. Sinusitis and its management. *British Medical Journal*, 2007, 334: 358–361.

The pressure that builds up in the sinuses can create a great deal of pain and this can be a very debilitating condition. Anyone who has suffered with the problem for longer than a week or two is likely to be very keen on finding treatments that will help alleviate the suffering. Massage can be very effective in treating symptoms and helping with pain relief.

Specific Contraindications

If a client presents with swelling or drooping of the eyelid, loss of eye movement, sudden changes to vision, fixed or dilated pupils, severe headache, or altered vision, do not massage and refer the client to an emergency doctor.

As you are working on the face you need to ensure that your fingernails are cut very short to avoid any scratches.

Massage Treatments

Sinus massage always works outward from the center of the face. You can start either at the forehead or at the nose, but if your client is at all anxious starting with the head will have a natural calming effect. You need to use medium fingertip pressure and a small amount of oil—just enough that the fingers do not drag the delicate skin on the face but not so much that your client is left feeling or looking oily. Using a good quality base oil, such as grape-seed oil, will simply nourish the skin and not cause any problems with oily skin.

Find the midpoint between the eyebrows at the top of the nose and, using two fingers placed together, stroke outward following the line of the eyebrows.

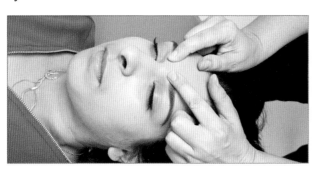

Each stroke needs to be around an inch long, returning back over the last half inch for the next stroke—these can be quick moves as the aim is to stimulate the whole area. You need to stroke outward so that you are encouraging the sinuses to drain. You are working on the frontal sinuses—doing this can help clear the "foggy head" and headache associated with sinus problems. Next, move up half an inch and repeat the outward strokes, moving up and out constantly so that you cover the whole of the forehead area. Following this you need to work the whole area again but using small circular movements, again starting at the midpoint between the eyebrows and making small outward circles across the forehead toward the ears, then moving up half an inch and repeating this until you have massaged the whole forehead with both strokes.

Next you can move to the sphenoid and ethmoid sinuses. These are the sinuses that are situated on the inside of the eye socket toward the nose. Placing one finger on the inner point of both eyebrows, press and hold that point for one to two seconds, release, and move one finger width down and press again for one to two seconds.

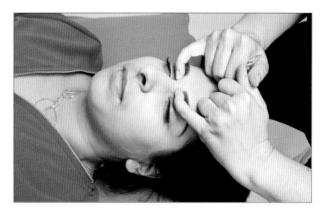

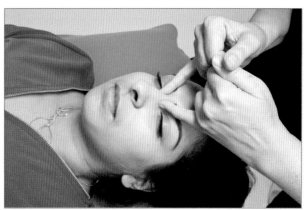

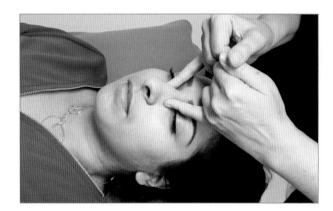
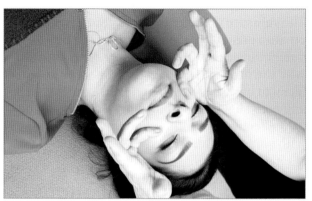

Move in this way down the whole of the inner side of the eye socket from where the eyebrow starts until you are parallel with the bottom of the eye. This is a small area and can be delicate, so work very precisely and carefully. Repeat this massage three or four times; your client should feel instant relief of the congestion in this area. It's worth having a glass of water to hand as the sinuses may drain into the throat as you work, and swallowing water may help with this process.

The maxillary sinuses are the largest of the sinuses and are in the maxillae, the bones of the front of the face that go from under the eyes either side of the nose down to and including the upper jaw. When inflammation is present, the upper part of this area is likely to be tender to the touch. With a drop of oil on your finger for lubrication, find the inner top part of the maxilla. You will be able to feel this approximately half an inch below the eye at the outer edge of the nose. Being careful not to put any pressure on the eye (you are working below that point but be careful not to slip), use finger pressure, one or two fingers only, apply light–medium pressure, holding for one to two seconds, releasing and moving further along that line toward the ear, following the cheekbones until you get to the ear.

Return to the midpoint and repeat the move slightly lower down, again moving outward across the face with your finger pressure. Repeat until you reach the area parallel to the bottom of the nose. Having worked this area with static finger pressure, now work with the small stroking movement that you used on the forehead, sweeping across the cheeks from the outer edge of the nose to the ear, working down across the whole area. Finally, using the same small circular movements that you also used on the forehead, treat the whole of the area again, working outward from the nose.

Once you have worked all of the sinuses, repeat the whole treatment starting at the frontal sinuses, down the sphenoid and ethmoid sinuses, and then again across the maxillary sinuses. A relaxing way to finish the treatment is to return to the frontal sinuses and finish the treatment by working this area again. In all of these treatments you should work both sides of the face at once, keeping equal pressure on both sides. In most cases these moves can be carried out by a qualified practitioner, by a friend/partner, or by the patients themselves—self-massaging the area two or three times throughout the day should help greatly.

One additional area that can help but cannot be self-administered is massage to the scalp and head. Specialist cranial sacral therapy can help but if you are not qualified in this modality you can still help, either as a massage practitioner or concerned friend or partner. This massage helps by increasing the circulation in the whole area. You can follow the instructions given in Chapter 4 for this treatment. Unless your client has dentures, don't ignore the jaw work that is part of this head massage: while tightness in the sternocleidomastoid (SCM) muscle will not give rise to a sinus infection, it can cause sinus symptoms[169] by restricting the movement of the muscles and fascia that interact with the maxillary sinuses, and releasing the SCM can help to relieve the symptoms experienced. The SCM is the large ropey muscle that runs from the mastoid process (felt as a rounded bump behind your ear) to the joint between the collarbones and the sternum. It can affect, and be impacted by, the jaw; teeth grinding, waking with gritted teeth, or gritting teeth when concentrating or stressed all lead to a tightening of the SCM.

---

[169] http://www.dynamicchiropractic.com/mpacms/dc/article.php?id=44247

Temporomandibular Joint Disorders

Background to the Condition

Temporomandibular joint disorders (TJDs) are problems with the joint between the lower jaw and base of the skull. There are two temporomandibular joints (TMJs), one each side of the jaw, that allow the mouth to open and close; these are gliding joints. TJDs are also known as TMJ disorders and TMJ disease.

There are two types of TJDs: muscle-related TJD, which is the more common form, and joint-related TJD, and these conditions can often coexist. Muscle-related TJD is also sometimes called TJD secondary to myofascial pain and dysfunction. While it is not a serious condition in terms of it being a threat to life, it can have a serious impact on health. It is estimated that 20–30% of the adult population will have TJD problems at some point in their life.[170]

Muscle-related TJDs are more commonly caused by clenching the jaw and nighttime teeth grinding, which overworks the jaw muscles and puts the joint under pressure, while joint-related TJDs are caused by degenerative joint disease, rheumatoid arthritis, ankylosis, dislocations, infections, or tumors.[171]

Joint TJDs lead to a popping or clicking of the jaw joint, the jaw locking, pain at the side of the jaw joint (usually one sided), and headaches. Muscle TJD will lead to pain on both sides of the jaw joint, headaches, and a difficulty opening and closing the mouth. In addition, any of the following symptoms may also be present: pain in the shoulders, back, or neck; tinnitus (ringing in the ears); dizziness; blurred or double vision; vertigo and nausea; hearing problems; and pain in front of the ears.[172]

Treatments for TJDs include medications, mouth guards, splints, surgery, and even joint replacement, but the role of massage should not be overlooked and is recognized by medical practitioners.[173]

There are a large number of muscles around the head, neck, and shoulders and to get relief from muscular TJDs it is best to treat all of these. As stress and tension can be contributory factors to TJDs, massage work to relax both mentally and physically will never be wasted. Cross-reference the names of muscles used with the diagram, if necessary, to ensure that you work all of the areas.

---

[170] http://www.nhs.uk/conditions/temporomandibular-joint-disorder/Pages/Introduction.aspx

[171] http://emedicine.medscape.com/article/1143410-overview#a0104

[172] http://www.fibromyalgia-symptoms.org/fibromyalgia_tempero.html

[173] http://www.fibromyalgia-symptoms.org/fibromyalgia_tempero.html

Specific Contraindications

- If your client has dentures, they should be removed before the treatment.

- If your client has had recent dental surgery, wait until everything has fully healed before treatment.

Massage Treatments

Begin your treatment by working on the head, following the protocol for head massage in Chapter 4.

Next you need to work on the orbicularis oculi muscles (below) around the eyebrows.

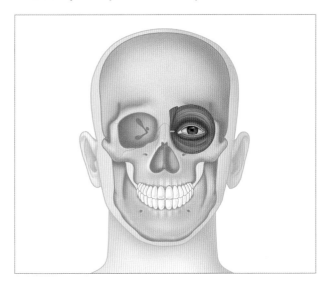

Use the eyebrows as your guide and work very carefully and precisely to avoid putting any pressure at all on the eyes themselves. You can use your index fingers for this but, if you can, use your little fingers as this will avoid working too deeply; it is important that you have short nails for this to avoid scratching your client. Start on the very inside of the eyebrows close to the nose. Press down with equal pressure on both sides and hold the pressure for four to five seconds, release and move a finger width out along the eyebrow, and reapply the pressure. Do this across the full length of the eyebrows and repeat the whole process three times. You may find that

your client reports that this is tender on the first set of moves but this should decrease as the muscles relax with the repeated moves.

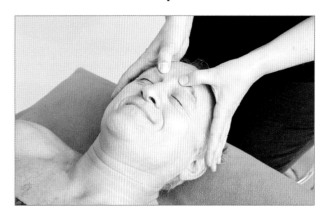

Next, use your three middle fingers placed together to work on the auricularis superior (below)—this is the thin fan-shaped muscle just to the front of the ear. Place your three middle fingers at the front of the client's ear so that they are in a line, press with light to moderate pressure, and, without moving your fingers off the skin, slowly circle your fingers three or four times and then repeat in the other direction.

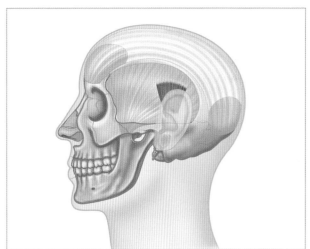

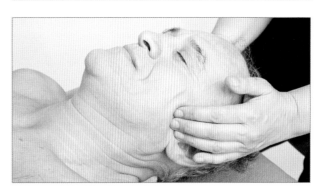

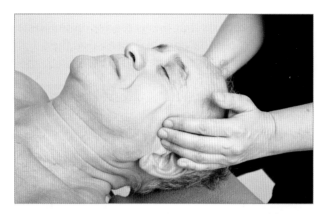

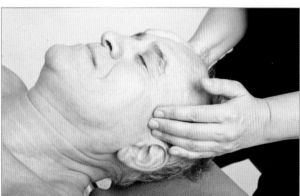

Begin by using your fingers to circle in both directions over this area to release any surface tension. Having warmed up the area, find the notch that will be around one inch in front of the ear on the underside of the cheekbone; if you have trouble locating this on your client first find it on your own face—once you know where it is it becomes relatively easy to locate.

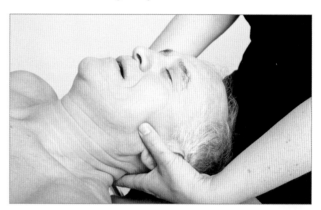

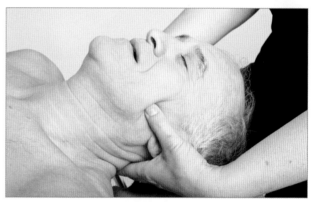

Next, move forward of the ear to work on the masseter muscle (below)—pound for pound this is the most powerful muscle in the body. This muscle can be found on the underside of the cheekbone and attaches to the side of the jawbone.

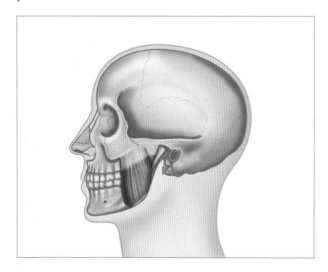

Ask the client to relax the jaw by letting the mouth open and teeth fall slightly apart. Encourage your client to take a deep breath and on the out breath press into this point on both sides with equal pressure. This muscle can take deep pressure, and although it can be tender it is a "nice" tenderness in that there is a sense that it's doing good. This is also a move that your clients can do at home between treatments, just encourage them also to do the gentler circling warm-up work first.

It is also important not to underestimate how tension in other muscles can cause a knock-on effect into the muscles of the face and head; a treatment for TJD is not complete without also working the neck. If you are working on a friend or family member rather than professionally, it can be daunting to work the neck and there is a fear of doing damage; you can, however, work this area very safely so long as you follow some simple guidelines. At the front of the neck is the very powerful sternocleidomastoid (SCM) muscle (below); this is a thick ropey muscle that is responsible for turning the head.

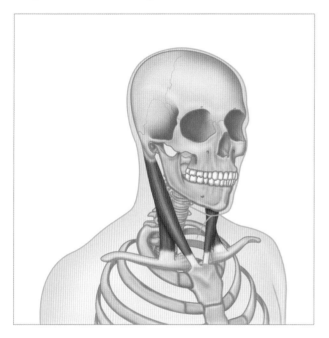

Its name comes from the bones it attaches to: sterno comes from sternum, or breast bone; cleido is the clavicle, or collar bone; and mastoid is the mastoid process, which is behind the ear. You can work this safely by asking the client, while he or she is still lying faceup, to turn the head to one side. The SCM will be raised on the side facing up. Use a little high-quality massage oil and, starting at the top behind the base of the ear, run your fingers down the length of the

muscle to where it disappears underneath the collar bone—that is the SCM. Make sure that you stay at the back of the muscle, closer to the back of the neck, as it is important that you do not slip forward of the muscle and put any pressure onto the front of the neck—visualize that you are going to massage the back of the muscle.

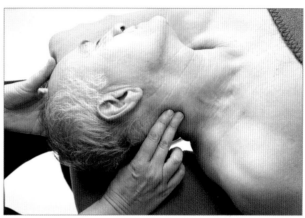

Massage down from ear to collarbone three or four times with gentle but increasing pressure, working very slowly; if you work too deeply or too fast you will feel the muscle tighten to your touch, and if this does happen you need to lighten your pressure and slow down. Always work downward from ear to collarbone.

Next, you are going to do the same movement but with the flat of one finger, usually the index finger. Stop every inch or so and apply a little more pressure (check with your client that this is not too much), and hold the pressure steady until the muscle begins to relax. This may take one or two minutes but just stay steady onto the muscle; this should never be so deep that it causes your client pain. Move an inch down and do this again, and repeat the same process all the way down the muscle—if the muscle relaxes quickly, move onto the next point. Ask your client to turn the head the other way and repeat the same treatment on that side.

Finally, if you have a massage table with a face hole, ask your client to lie facedown so you can work the muscles on the back of the shoulder and the neck. If you do not have a massage table, adapt this part of the massage to work with your client seated. Someone with a TJD is likely to have tight and rounded shoulders and these are muscles that need to be relaxed. You will get much better results if you also work the hands and arms as detailed in Chapter 2.

Working on the basis that prevention is always better than cure, there are also some self-help aspects to improving or curing TJDs and you can use these on yourself or advise your client to use them. The person with TJD problems should avoid chewing gum and toffees, trying to rest the jaw by eating only soft food when the problems flare up. Gently stretching the jaw while applying a warm or cold flannel to the jaw (use wet rather than dry heat) will help, but avoid opening the jaw too wide, including trying to get enough sleep so that yawning is kept to a minimum. If a client is having dental work, the dentist should be informed that the client will need to close the mouth at regular intervals. If a client is stressed, deliberately relaxing the jaw to avoid clenching it will help, and resting the chin on the hands should be avoided as this puts pressure on the TMJ. If the problem does flare up it is possible to help by self-massage of the whole jaw area; if you are self-treating don't worry too much about which muscles you are working on—when you hit the right spot it will be a good pain that will bring about relief as the jaw muscles learn to relax.

Tendonitis and Tenosynovitis

Background to the Condition

Tendons are tough bands of fibrous tissue that connect muscles to bones. We need them for movement—when a muscle connected to a bone contracts, it transmits this force through the tendons, causing the bone to move. Tendons are different from ligaments: tendons attach muscle to bone, and ligaments connect bone to bone. Tendons can succumb to a number of injuries, usually either from overuse or from a direct, often sports-related, injury. A complete tendon rupture or tear will generally present very suddenly and very painfully, and will result in a loss of movement that will need immediate medical attention—massage would be contraindicated in this case. Two other common conditions of tendons are tendonitis and tenosynovitis, and it is these that this chapter will focus on.

When a tendon becomes inflamed this is referred to as *tendonitis*. Some, but not all, tendons are in protective sheaths; this sheath is lined with a membrane containing synovial fluid, which helps the tendon to move easily and minimizes friction.[174] When these sheaths become inflamed it is known as *tenosynovitis*. You may also hear of *tendinosis,* which refers to a chronic degeneration of a tendon without inflammation, where the main problem is failed healing of repeated minor injuries rather than inflammation, and *tendinopathy*, which is a more general term for a tendon disease or injury, without specifying the type.[175]

We will focus here on tendonitis and tenosynovitis, the two inflammatory conditions. Both are commonly caused by the overuse of the affected tendon, are injuries that usually occur over time, and can either be sports related or a form of repetitive strain injury. Tendonitis and tenosynovitis commonly occur together and are more prevalent in middle-aged people. Tenosynovitis on its own can also be a symptom of arthritis, particularly rheumatoid arthritis, although when this is the case pain and swelling in the joints would usually be found.

Specific Contraindications

It is important to stress that since both conditions are caused by inflammation, massage directly over the area is contraindicated—but you can assist recovery by working above and below the area affected. If onset of pain is sudden, following an injury, wait 72 hours before starting any treatment to allow the initial healing to take place.

---

[174] http://www.nhs.uk/conditions/tendonitis/Pages/Introduction.aspx

[175] http://www.patient.co.uk/health/tendonitis-and-tenosynovitis

Massage Treatments

Rest is critically important in recovery: the tendon and its sheath need time to self-repair. Ice will help ease the inflammation and pain, and for those who want to use medications then nonsteroidal anti-inflammatory drugs can be effective.

Strengthening exercises for the surrounding muscles can be very helpful, as can releasing any tension held in the muscles, which can put a constant strain on the tendons and their sheaths. Remember you are working only above and below the affected area and never directly onto it.

Tendon problems can occur anywhere, but the most common areas for tendon problems are the shoulder, elbow (which is discussed in more detail in the chapter on tennis elbow), wrist, fingers, knee, and the back of the heel. Where you should and should not massage will vary depending where the tendon problems are, so we will briefly look at each of these individually.

Shoulder

Supraspinatus tendonitis (also known as "swimmer's shoulders") refers to inflammation of the tendon at the top of the shoulder joint. It causes pain when lifting the arm sideways or when lying on the shoulder to sleep. It is a particularly common injury in sports people and people whose jobs or leisure activities involve overhead work, and people who walk dogs who pull on their leads can also suffer from this injury.

In addition to the rest and ice generally prescribed for inflammation, you can also work to release any tension in the muscles in the hand and arm following the directions in Chapter 2. For optimum results work this area twice a week, applying ice to the affected shoulder afterward. Do not work directly into the shoulder.

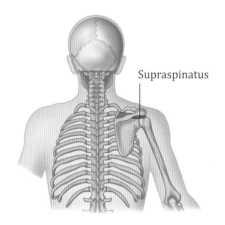

Supraspinatus

Wrist

Tendonitis of the wrist usually affects a single tendon, but it can involve two or more. It often occurs at points where the tendons cross each other or pass over a bony prominence,[176] and causes pain and swelling of the inflamed tendon. One particular form of wrist tendonitis is "de Quervain's tenosynovitis": most common in women aged 30–50, it is particularly prevalent in new mothers where the act of picking up the baby aggravates the tendon around the base of the thumb and wrist.

The standard treatments of rest and ice apply here, and massage can be applied to the fingers and thumb below the area inflamed and the arm and shoulder above it—again, following the instructions for hand massage as detailed in Chapter 2. Massaging the arm and shoulder will also help to relieve muscular tension that could put pressure on the tendons.

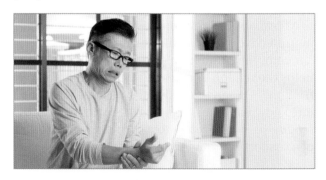

176 http://orthopedics.about.com/cs/handwristsurgery/a/wristtendonitis.html

Knee

Tendonitis in the knee is linked to the patellar tendon that connects the kneecap (the patella) to the shin bone. This problem mainly occurs in athletes whose sport involves repetitive jumping, giving it the nickname "jumper's knee." Along with pain the kneecap can look swollen, and moving the knee can result in a crunching noise. Rest and ice are indicated as the starting point for treatment.

Massage should avoid the knee but you can safely work the foot in detail following the directions in Chapter 3 on foot massage, and you can work on the upper leg in long and moderately deep stroking movements. If you are massaging with the client facedown, support the leg with a pillow under the ankle. If the client is faceup, support the leg with a pillow under the knee. Make sure you never put any pressure on the knee itself.

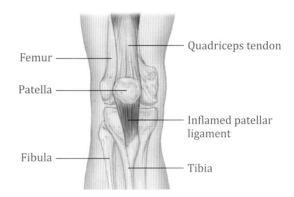

Femur
Quadriceps tendon
Patella
Inflamed patellar ligament
Fibula
Tibia

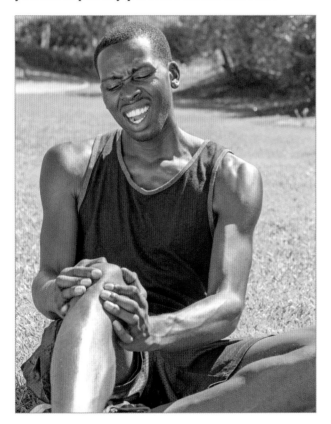

Heel

The other main area susceptible to tendonitis is the back of the heel—the Achilles tendon. There are two areas of the Achilles tendon prone to this problem: in the middle of the tendon (midsubstance Achilles tendonitis) and at its insertion into the heel bone (insertional Achilles tendonitis).[177] Insertional tendonitis is primarily a running injury and pain will be felt at the very back of the heel; symptoms will generally improve with use and are worse getting up in the morning or after periods of rest or sitting. Midsubstance Achilles tendonitis is by far the most common type, and is also prevalent in athletes, although obesity and lack of movement can also leave a person susceptible to injury from otherwise minor movement.

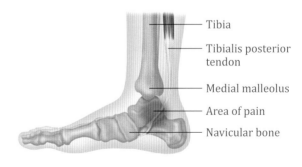

Tibia
Tibialis posterior tendon
Medial malleolus
Area of pain
Navicular bone

---

[177] http://www.londonfootandanklecentre.co.uk/conditions/achilles_tendonitis.php?gclid=CODHtfyj2LwCFUT3wgod8E4AYg

Treatment for this condition is very similar to that outlined the chapter on plantar fasciitis, and should focus on the toes and feet, paying particular attention to the sole of the foot but avoiding deep work across the center of the arch of the foot.

Tendon injuries will unfortunately take a number of weeks or even months to heal. If symptoms worsen, if movement or the strength of a joint is compromised, or if the inflammation is severe, visit a medical practitioner to rule out a rupture or other injury.

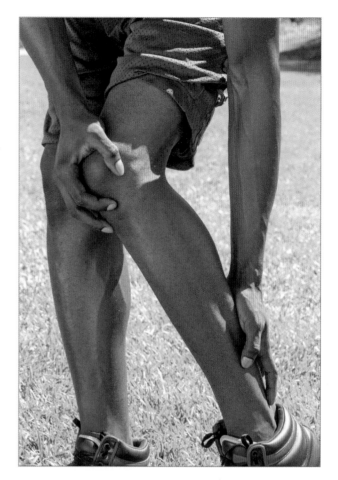

Tennis Elbow

Background to the Condition

Tennis elbow (top image, below), known medically as "lateral epicondylitis," is a problem with the tendons that attach the muscles of the wrist and fingers to the bone on the outer part of the elbow. Golfer's elbow (bottom image, below), or "medial epicondylitis," is very similar but affects the tendons on the inside part of the elbow. While it can be caused by inflammation of the tendons (tendonitis), it is not always so straightforward and the nerves, muscles, and joints around the tendons are often implicated.

Tennis elbow is a self-limiting condition in that it doesn't spread to anywhere else, no one dies from it, and, with rest and minor treatment, it will usually recover within around 12 months. This doesn't mean it's not real or painful. It is a very common complaint—the NHS in the UK estimates that as many as one in three people have tennis elbow at any given time.[178] It affects men and women equally, with the main age group suffering from this complaint being those in their forties to sixties, although there has been a rise in younger people suffering from this in more recent years from extensive texting or time spent playing on computer game consoles.

Although not always caused by playing tennis (nor golf for golfer's elbow), tennis elbow is a problem brought about by the overuse of the arm both in length of use and the strength of use—that is, how long and how hard the muscles have been used. While an ultrasound or MRI scan can be used to diagnose tennis or golfer's elbow, they are not usually needed as a diagnosis can be made simply from the description of the symptoms. If the pain is accompanied by tingling then further investigation is usually carried out to check for and rule out any potential damage to the nerve.

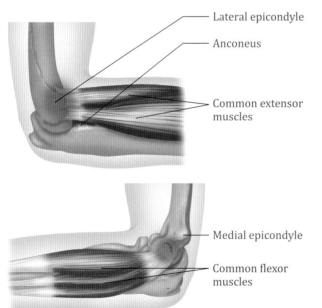

Lateral epicondyle

Anconeus

Common extensor muscles

Medial epicondyle

Common flexor muscles

178 http://www.nhs.uk/conditions/Tennis-elbow/Pages/Introduction.aspx

In tennis elbow pain is not always present all the time, but it will be more noticeable when lifting, twisting, or bending the arm or trying to hold small objects such as a pen or hair brush. The pain will be primarily felt on the outside of the top of the forearm, just below the bend of the elbow. Pain from golfer's elbow will be felt with the same activities but the pain is usually felt on the inner bottom part of the elbow. Pain for both conditions often starts with a sharp pain on impact or with strenuous use, which becomes more frequent with a dull ache felt much of the time.

Having a break from the activities that trigger the problem is the first line of recovery; this allows the area to recover and any inflammation to settle down. Some people will take nonsteroidal anti-inflammatory medications and the gel versions of these can be useful for this injury. Icing the area will help to reduce inflammation. While some people will find that an elbow support can be helpful, particularly if the pain is acute, it is important not to immobilize the elbow nor to stop using the arm completely. The area needs to be strengthened and the tendons stretched.

Gentle resistance stretches can be helpful in strengthening the tendon without putting any more pressure on what may be tight or tender muscles. Supporting the arm on your leg or a table top, simply raise the wrist toward the body and push against it with the other hand, trying to push the hands in opposite directions (one up and one down), so that the palms of the hands are pushed together. Hold for a few seconds and stretch in the opposite direction by folding the hand down and using the other hand to resist bringing the first hand back up. Repeat 10 times in both directions twice a day. The second stretch is even simpler: with your elbow on your knee or a table, flex your wrist backward until you can feel the stretch in your forearm, you can use the other hand to extend this stretch gently, and hold for 5–10 seconds. Repeat 10 times, twice a day. Be careful whilst performing these stretches not to put undue pressure on the wrist—you are aiming to stretch the tendons, not cause any

pain in the wrist. Other exercises to strengthen and stretch the area may be prescribed by a physiotherapist.

Specific Contraindications

The key contraindication is to not massage the area immediately around or inside the elbow as this may cause further irritation and inflammation.

If the pain is accompanied by tingling or loss of sensation the injury should be medically checked to rule out additional complications.

Massage Treatments

The good news is that there are some great massage treatments that can help to treat tennis elbow. First work the hands as detailed in Chapter 2, and you then need to bring your attention to two areas: the forearm and the neck, specifically the scalenus muscles.

If the arm is really too sore to be able to withstand much touch, begin with a regular ice-cube massage, once or twice a day for a week. This is not a deep nor technical massage and it can easily be self-administered by the client. First apply a little massage oil to protect the skin and then take an ice cube that has been out of the freezer for three to five minutes (this is important so that it is not too cold). The ice cube should be wet from the surface water melting; if it's not, wait a few more minutes. Never use an ice cube straight out of the freezer directly onto the skin. When the ice cube is wet, and having used some massage oil on the skin, use it to massage the area that is very tender. Work both up and down and across the muscle and be sure to work the whole forearm, both sides and from wrist to elbow. You will not be able to get much pressure with an ice cube but the important factor here is the application of ice to an inflamed area—but in a focused and controlled way. Massage until the ice cube has melted or until the area starts to be uncomfortable from the cold.

After this initial very tender phase has passed you can then work more deeply into the muscles. Work the under part of the forearm first as this will make the upper part of the forearm easier to release and it should be less tender for your client working this way. Once you have warmed up both sides with long strokes up the forearm, gradually develop your depth.

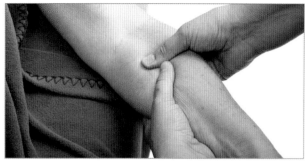

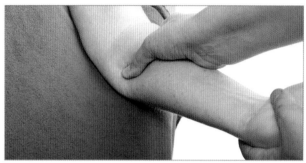

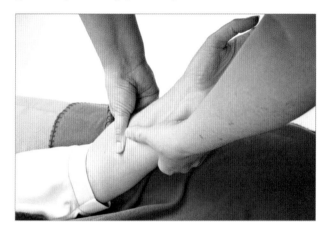

Hold the arm in both hands so that your thumbs meet in the center of the arm. Working on the under forearm, work upward from wrist to just below the elbow, moving your thumbs apart as you get toward the top of the forearm so that you move outward over the belly of the muscle as you work up the arm.

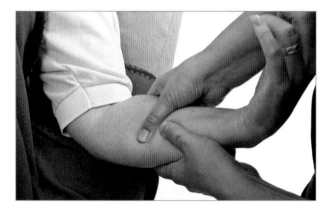

On the upper part of the forearm, keep your thumbs together as you come up the arm and stop about three finger widths (measure this by the width of your client's fingers, not your own) from the crease of the arm at the elbow. You will find that one spot here in particular is tender—this is the area that you now need to apply static pressure to. Press and hold with your thumbs.

Work only to your client's tolerance so that you do not overwork or damage the muscle. Ask your client to focus on breathing through this process, encouraging deep and slow breathing. Maintain a steady pressure on that one point, do not increase or decrease it, and ask your client to report when the tenderness of the point drops and only the feeling of pressure remains. This may take up to two minutes but the release that comes with it is worth the wait. This is something that the client can do at home or with a friend or family member. As long as you only work as deeply as the client can easily breathe through, then you will not do any harm and you should help to relieve the symptoms.

If you try this pressure on your own forearm you may become aware that the side of your neck (your scalenus muscles) suddenly feels more relaxed, particularly on the side on which you have been pressing. The two areas are interconnected by a complex series of muscles, tendons, ligaments, and fascia. You will therefore only benefit your client by also doing the head and neck work detailed in Chapter 4.

Most cases of tennis elbow will settle from an acute state in two to three weeks, with the full problem being resolved in a few months. It is rare for surgery or medical intervention to be required.

Tension Headaches

Background to the Condition

Tension headaches are the most common type of headache, they are experienced by most people during their lives, and they are the "everyday" headaches. The NHS in the UK estimates that about half of adults experience tension-type headaches once or twice a month, and about one in three get them up to 15 times a month.[179]

Tension headaches are known as primary headaches, meaning that there is no known underlying cause. A tension headache may feel like a tight band around the head or a weight on top of the head. The headache can be one sided but it is more usual for it to be on both sides of your head. The tension may spread down the neck and shoulders or feel like it's coming up from the neck and shoulders, and there is often pain or a sensation of pressure behind the eyes. A tension-type headache can last anything from 30 minutes to a week but most will last between one and a few hours.

While tension headaches do respond well to over-the-counter painkillers, taking these on a regular basis can lead to medication-overuse headaches. If painkillers are taken on a daily or almost daily basis to treat a run of tension headaches, stopping the painkillers will cause physical withdrawal symptoms, the primary symptom of which will be headaches. These withdrawal symptoms will last on average two weeks but the longer-term benefits of not using the painkillers are worth the relatively short-term withdrawal. If strong painkillers have been used for a long period of time, this withdrawal should be under medical supervision.

The exact cause of tension-type headaches is not clear but certain things have been known to trigger them, including stress and anxiety; squinting at papers or computer screens; poor posture; lack of sleep and tiredness; not drinking enough water or fluids, resulting in dehydration; low blood sugar from missing meals; bright sunlight; not moving around enough, allowing muscles to tighten; changes in the weather; having hair tied up too tightly; or being exposed to too much noise, or to noises at a certain frequency, or certain smells. Avoiding all of these triggers is very difficult for most people working and living in a public space, but knowing your own triggers can help you manage your headaches and deal with them more quickly when they do occur.

---

[179] http://www.nhs.uk/Conditions/headaches-tension-type/Pages/Introduction.aspx

Exercise, relaxation, and hydration are all helpful in treating tension headaches, along with taking a break from the computer, ensuring that blood sugar doesn't get too low, relaxing hair ties, and wearing correct glasses, but there are also some very useful massage techniques that will help to alleviate a tension headache once it starts.

Specific Contraindications

If someone is experiencing tension-type headaches more than 15 times a month for at least three months in a row, this is known as chronic tension headaches. While most people can manage the occasional headache, chronic tension headaches become more debilitating and can have a significant negative impact on life. If headaches are severe or if there is a significant increase in the number of headaches then it is worth considering a visit to a health care practitioner.

If headaches are accompanied by a very stiff neck, fever, nausea, vomiting, and confusion; or come on following an accident, especially involving a blow to the head; or if they are accompanied by weakness, numbness, slurred speech, or confusion, then emergency medical help should be sought as there could be an underlying condition that needs urgent medical attention.

Massage Treatments

Starting a treatment by relaxing the eyes can be very effective and is also something that can be self-administered. Cup your hands gently over the eyes (without pressing on the actual eyes) and hold for two minutes; you may find that vision is a little blurry immediately afterward—warn the client that this is normal as the eye muscles have relaxed, and it will quickly return to normal. If you are able to treat the headache in a warm room with dimmed lighting where the client can lie down, then encourage him or her to keep the eyes shut for the rest of the treatment. If you are self-administering the treatment in an office environment that would be more tricky!

Next, place one finger at the center of the eyebrows and without losing contact with the skin move your finger in small circles, repeat six or seven times, and then move along the eyebrow half a finger width so that each time you move you are covering half a new area, and half where your finger has just been.

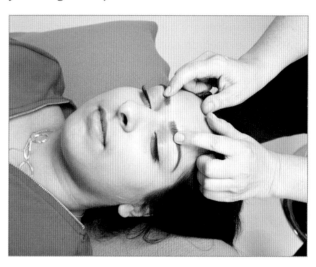

Work your way all along both eyebrows simultaneously. Again, this is a technique that can be self-administered, even in a work setting. Holding your fingers together so that they form a solid line, place them in the center of your forehead with your little finger close to the eyebrows and your index finger close to the hairline. Pressing down a little, pull your fingers outward, releasing the pressure as you get toward the temple. If you have dry skin or are working on a more elderly client, use a little massage oil or moisturizer so that you don't drag the skin. Repeat this move five or six times.

Placing your fingers about half an inch apart and just above the temples, press just enough to have a firm contact with the skin of the scalp and move your fingers in small circles without losing contact with the skin. Move in both directions so that you are freeing the tiny muscles around the head, and work backward from this position so that you cover the whole of the scalp. Next, place your thumbs along the midline of the head, starting at the hairline, and press for the count of three, release, and move your thumbs down to as far back on the head as you can comfortably reach.

You may find it beneficial to also follow the protocol for back massage detailed in Chapter 5 as there is a close relationship between tension headaches, neck tension and shoulder/back tension. At the very least you should include this very useful gentle stretch in your treatment.

Have your client lie face up on the massage table. The suboccipitals are a group of four muscles which are located on each side of the back of the neck, just below the base of the skull (see Chapter 5). These muscles connect the skull with the top two vertebrae of the neck and are responsible for both turning and tipping the head.

If you are not working professionally in massage and do not know how to locate these muscles, place your own fingers underneath your skull towards the top of your neck and you will feel two ropey areas either side of the spine; you are looking to place your fingers between these two ropey parts and your spine—it is a small area and there are surface muscles that you need to work past so gently roll your fingers into your neck either side of your spine. Keeping your fingers still and pressing gently, slowly move your eyes as far as you can to the left and then to the right, then upwards and downwards, without moving your head. Only your eyes should be moving but you will feel movement in these suboccipital muscles as your eyes move. This is the area you are working on with your client.

With your client lying facing upward, cradle their head in your hands so that your fingers are curving into these muscles just below the base of the skull; warm the muscles up by gently stretching the neck, pulling the head towards yourself—this should be a pleasurable not a painful stretch. Do not use this stretch if your client has had spinal fusion surgery in their neck or if they have Down Syndrome. Release the stretch a little but still support the head and slowly tilt the head so that the chin moves

toward the chest by no more than half an inch. Keeping your fingers still, press gently onto the suboccipital muscles. Ask the client to look directly at the ceiling above them and to relax; now ask them, without moving their head, to look at their toes and then to relax their gaze back to the ceiling, then again without moving their head, to look up to you, then back to the ceiling. Ask them to look to the left and back to the ceiling and then to the right and back to the ceiling, all only with eye movements and keeping the head still.

Securely lift the head by another half an inch, keeping a firm contact with the suboccipital muscles and repeat the looking down, up, left and right movements, always returning to look at the ceiling between eye movements. This will help relax the muscles at the top of the back of the neck. Gently replace the client's head on the couch. This may cause some short-term eye-strain and you can help to relieve this by gently cupping your hands over the client's eyes for 20–30 seconds—without making contact with the eyes. The eyes should return to normal within a few moments and reassure your client that this is normal.

You can now repeat the circling of your fingers on the skull and the press and release moves along the centreline.

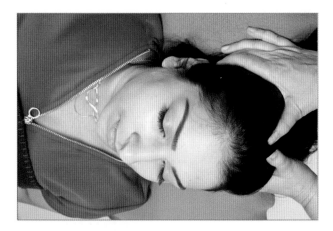

If your client has long hair then you can also pull the hair to help release the scalp—done well this feels like your scalp can breathe, but done badly it will take your client back to the school yard. It is important to grasp a good amount of hair, about an inch's worth between your fingers, and pull straight out. Make sure that you are not pulling one area more than another or this will hurt, and do make sure that you pull with equal pressure on both sides of the head at the same time. Get feedback from your client—if you don't hear something along the lines of it being "wonderful," stop and practice on yourself first. If this is good for your client, work all the way around the head with this technique.

Finally for this part of the head and face massage, ask the client to relax the jaw and let it fall open a little. Place your three middle fingers at the jaw joint (you can find this by asking the client to open and close the mouth) and, without moving your fingers from the contact point they have with the skin (so that you are moving the skin and not just moving around on top of it), make small circles with your fingers to help to release the jaw tension.

These are all techniques that can be self-administered as headache "first aid" in a work settling. The following massage processes are for prevention between headaches or for a fuller treatment during headaches. As long as the headache is not accompanied by other symptoms, these can be carried out while the client has a headache to give a deeper level of relief.

Tension headaches can also be made worse by tension in the neck and back, so for a more complete treatment you should also follow the back and neck massage protocol given in Chapter 5, and this can give you longer-lasting results. If you are restricted for time you can always add in the back and shoulder massage every second or third treatment, but do try not to neglect this area as it will help address the problem in the longer term.

Finish the treatment by returning to the eyebrows and forehead for a soothing conclusion to the massage session. Allow your client to relax for a few minutes and ensure that he or she has plenty of water to drink for the rest of the day.

Trigeminal Neuralgia

Background to the Condition

Trigeminal neuralgia (TN) causes sudden, severe facial nerve pain. The pain can last from just a few seconds to two minutes each time[180] and attacks can follow in quick succession. An episode of multiple attacks could last for several hours. Symptoms usually gradually increase and worsen over time. In most cases it only affects one side of the face (unilateral), more commonly the right side. Rarely, people with trigeminal neuralgia have pain on both sides of their face (bilateral).[181] The pain is often described as an electric shock, or a stabbing or piercing pain. Historically TN was commonly known as the "suicide disease" because of the numbers taking their own lives because of the pain in the days before there were any effective treatments. Trigeminal neuralgia is considered to be among "the most excruciatingly painful conditions known to medical practice."[182] Attacks are often described by patients as being severe enough to rivet them to the spot or bring them to their knees.[183]

The trigeminal nerve is one of 12 pairs of nerves known as the cranial nerves. The trigeminal nerve is the fifth and largest of these. While damage to or pressure on this nerve does not change the appearance of the face, this is the nerve whose job it is to allow us to feel touch, temperature, and pain in the face. There are three branches to this nerve: the

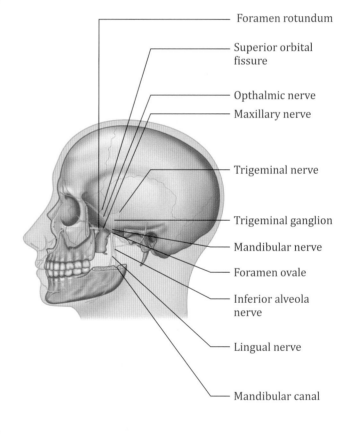

- Foramen rotundum
- Superior orbital fissure
- Opthalmic nerve
- Maxillary nerve
- Trigeminal nerve
- Trigeminal ganglion
- Mandibular nerve
- Foramen ovale
- Inferior alveola nerve
- Lingual nerve
- Mandibular canal

180 http://www.nhs.uk/conditions/trigeminal-neuralgia/pages/symptoms.aspx

181 http://www.nhsdirect.wales.nhs.uk/encyclopaedia/t/article/trigeminalneuralgia/

182 http://uspainfoundation.org/eNewsletters/Understanding-TN.pdf

183 http://www.tna.org.uk/pages/trigeminal_neuralgia.html

ophthalmic branch, which carries sensation to the forehead, scalp, and front of the head; the maxillary branch, which serves the ear, eye, cheek, and nose; and lastly the mandibular branch, whose job it is to carry sensation to the jawline, chin, and lips.

TN occurs when the trigeminal nerve "misfires." It is thought that this misfiring occurs owing to damage in the nerve's protective myelin sheath. The myelin sheath can be damaged by pressure from blood vessels (veins or arteries), multiple sclerosis (MS), injury to the nerve, or simply as part of the ageing process. In a small number of cases, the cause may be a tumor or a benign growth pressing on the nerve.[184] The medical world divides TN into three categories: type one with the standard symptoms as described above, where there is no known cause; type two, where the pain is more consistent but is more of an aching, throbbing, or burning (atypical trigeminal neuralgia); and symptomatic trigeminal neuralgia, where the problems occur as a result of an underlying cause, such as MS.

An episode of trigeminal neuralgia can be triggered by a very small event, including simple skin contact such as shaving, washing, or brushing teeth. Being outside on a windy day can be enough to trigger an attack in some people, as can eating, drinking, or even talking.

There is no one test to diagnose trigeminal neuralgia—diagnosis is instead based on symptoms and it is commonly diagnosed by family doctors or dentists. There is no set cure, and because of the intensity of the pain standard painkillers, even morphine, may not be effective. For some sufferers anticonvulsant drugs (used to treat epilepsy) or antidepressants can be effective under close medical monitoring. Surgery can be an option for some people.

Specific Contraindications

Some sufferers can get temporary relief through massage; at the very least you should do no harm with massage, so long as you avoid the trigger points of the condition by not touching the face you may be able to help with massage. Facial massage should be avoided, it is contraindicated as it will be far too painful for the client. Throughout any massage treatment you need to be sure that you get feedback, that your client tells you immediately if pain has been triggered, and that you take great care in positioning your client so that you avoid any pressure or touch on the face. Your client will need to be faceup or seated, as being facedown is likely to be far too painful. Unfortunately you are not going to cure the trigeminal neuralgia but some clients will experience temporary relief from the symptoms.

Massage Treatments

Begin the massage by warming up the head, shoulders, and neck. With the client faceup, begin by stroking down the neck and across the top of the shoulders to allow the client to relax while being touched in massage. With your hands at the top of the shoulders glide upward, stroking up the back of neck in slow, rhythmic, and gentle movements, with constant feedback from the client.

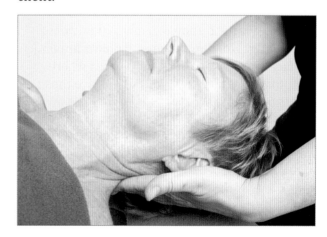

[184] http://www.tna.org.uk/data/files/Pamphlets/trigeminal_neuralgia__an_overview__february_20111.pdf

Ask the client to turn the head to one side and work with slow, gentle circles with two or three fingers down the side of the neck, working down and backward and out across the top of the shoulders. Hold the trapezius muscles at the top of the shoulder in a gentle squeeze. Repeat on the other side and always get feedback from your client. The final stage of the warm-up is to stretch the back of the neck and begin to work on the muscles at the base of the skull. Curl your fingers underneath the skull and pull gently upward—this will work on both the semispinalis and trapezius muscles as they attach into the head, and will stretch the neck, helping to release tension in these muscles.

A number of patients with trigeminal neuralgia have experienced relief with acupuncture,[185/186] and provided the massage practitioner works in close conjunction with the client, gaining constant feedback to check that symptoms are not triggered, then trying an acupressure treatment to assist will do no harm and may be beneficial to individual clients.

These are shown on the chart as triple heater 17 and 21; gall bladder 2 (be careful not to brush the face while treating with this point); small intestine 18; stomach 2, 3, and 7 (avoid 2 and 3 if they trigger symptoms); governing vessel 26 (avoid if this triggers symptoms); and large intestine 20 (again avoid if this triggers symptoms).

The last three of these groups of points are on the face—if any of them are in an area where symptoms could be triggered, then leave those points out. Some clients can tolerate their own touch as that gives some sense of control over and above being touched by someone else, but this will only be likely for milder or early-onset cases. In classic acupuncture there are two complementary (not opposing) techniques, known as reducing and reinforcing;[187] the

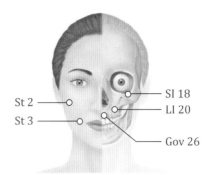

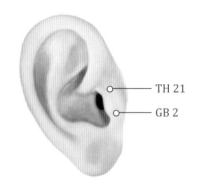

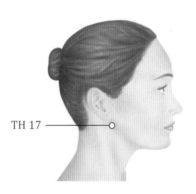

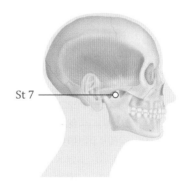

---

[185] http://www.ncbi.nlm.nih.gov/pmc/articles/PMC2797593/#!po=16.6667

[186] http://www.naturalnews.com/026126_acupuncture_Chi_treatment.html

[187] http://www.geocities.ws/altmedd/acupuncture/acupuncture_technique/ReinforcingandReducingMethods.html

finer points of this take some detailed training and mastery and referring the client to a fully qualified acupuncturist is worth considering, but you can also try treating these points at home on a friend or family member with acupressure. In acupressure, the same points are used but pressure is applied with fingers or a blunt instrument, not a needle. As the points we are using in this treatment are on the head and, if tolerated, the face, finger pressure would be more suitable.

There are two techniques to consider using and it is worth experimenting with both to see what works for individual clients. The first is firm (but easily tolerated) constant fingertip pressure directly onto the acupressure point. The pressure needs to be maintained for one to two minutes and either the client or the person administering the treatment should feel a change in the area being pressed—it might become softer or warmer, or may tingle. If you do not get any of these results it can be one of two things: either you have not yet developed the sensitivity in your fingers to be able to detect it, or you are in the wrong place—acupressure points are around just two hundredths of an inch in width, so move around close to the area on the diagram and try again. You will not do any damage with this and may also be releasing muscular tension as you work.

The second technique is to find the acupressure point again and, instead of a consistent pressure, you circle your finger—without moving it around on the skin—so that the pressure is constantly moving. Circle clockwise for one to two minutes and, again, you should feel a change to that area.

The final point to remember in treating someone with trigeminal neuralgia is that pain in the face or head tends to make us pull our shoulders upward and this tenses the neck and shoulders, causing knock-on problems here. Working these areas can be a problem for people who cannot stand the pressure of the massage table face hole if they are lying facedown. You can work around this either by working with them seated or in side position. If seated, ask them to straddle a chair so that the back of the chair is in front of them—this will allow you to work more deeply

into their shoulders and give them something to lean on to counter your pressure. Be careful with your draping—using a sheet or blanket will allow the person still to feel covered as it can be wrapped around the front of the body and draped over the back and sides.

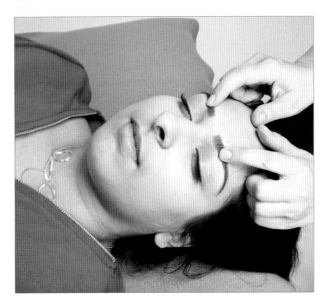

You may also be treating someone with TN for a different complaint and need to be able to massage the lower body or back—you can adapt your massage to use the side position to do this. If you are working with someone lying down in the side position, provide pillows to be positioned under the head so that it is supported, but ensuring the person is not lying on his or her face. Provide two pillows for the body: one needs to go between the knees so that the person doesn't get pushed forward into a rotation that will then bring the face into contact with the table, and the other is to tuck into the chest/belly to give added support, again, to stop the person rolling forward while you work on the shoulders.

These precautions, along with constant and open feedback, may allow you to treat the person with trigeminal neuralgia with a full massage treatment but geared toward his or her specific needs.

For further reading, I recommend: George Weigal, *Striking Back: The Trigeminal Neuralgia and Face Pain Handbook*, 2004, published by the Trigeminal Neuralgia Association.

Whiplash

Background to the Condition

Whiplash, more correctly known as whiplash-associated disorders (WAD) is a term used, fairly loosely, to describe a neck injury where the head is either suddenly jolted backward and then forward, or forward and then backward, in a whip-like movement, or it may be suddenly and forcibly rotated depending on the angle of the neck when the incident occurs. This sudden force can stretch and/or tear the muscles and tendons in the neck. Most commonly this is as a result of a road traffic accident, but it can also be from a sports injury, a fall, or being struck on the head by a heavy object.

As the term whiplash covers a multiple of both symptoms and severities of injury, and with the rise in litigation following motor vehicle accidents, it was thought within the insurance industry that some standardization was needed to define the type and severity of injury. The Canadian car industry led the way, and established a task force of experts to investigate whiplash injuries. Although it was originally devised to assist the insurance industry, the Quebec Task Force (QTF) criteria are often used as a standard format to define and describe whiplash injuries. There have been updates, and various other groups have modified the criteria to develop their own standards, but the baseline descriptions are as follows:

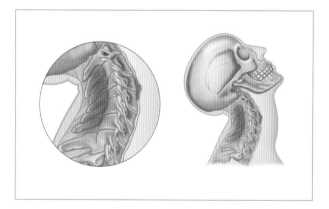 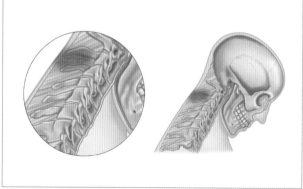

- *Grade 0*—No complaint about the neck, no physical sign(s)

- *Grade 1*—Neck complaint of pain, stiffness, or tenderness only, no physical sign(s)

- *Grade 2*—Neck complaint AND musculoskeletal sign(s); musculoskeletal signs include decreased range of motion and point tenderness

- *Grade 3*—Neck complaint AND neurological sign(s); neurological signs include decreased or absent tendon reflexes, weakness, and sensory deficits

- *Grade 4*—Neck complaint AND fracture or dislocation,[188] or damage to the spinal cord.

Prior to QTF there was controversy within the massage world, with some advocating treatment for whiplash and others identifying whiplash as a contraindication. The QTF allowed differentiation between the different levels of whiplash and therefore new treatment guidelines.

For a client with grade 4 whiplash massage is strictly contraindicated: to massage a dislocated or fractured neck would be dangerous at all levels and the person with whiplash needs referring to urgent medical care. Grade 3 whiplash should also be referred to a medical practitioner to rule out any grade 4 injuries, as some of the symptoms may be similar.

The South Australian Centre for Trauma and Injury Recovery produced guidelines for the management of WAD,[189] and this recommended massage for whiplash once the level of whiplash has been established for all but level 4.

In medical terms, whiplash is divided into four stages:[190] the acute stage is the first one to two weeks following the accident, this is followed by the early subacute (weeks three to four), and the late subacute (weeks five to six). At six weeks plus, the whiplash is considered chronic. While most people will recover fully from whiplash injuries the speed of recovery can vary from person to person. One study reports that up to 50% of patients will still have some symptoms after 12 months,[191] others put this at 65%,[192] whilst the UK NHS suggests just 12%.[193]

Specific Contraindications

For a grade 4 whiplash, massage is strictly contraindicated. If the client presents with any of the following symptoms referral to emergency medical services is necessary for a full checkup: blurring of vision, numbness in shoulders and arms, pins and needles or tingling and/or weakness in the arms and legs, swelling in the back of the throat or a difficulty in swallowing, or any disturbance to bowel or bladder function.

A client presenting with grade 3 whiplash symptoms should be referred urgently to a medical practitioner to rule out any grade 4 injuries, as some of the symptoms will be similar and massage should wait until they have been given the all clear of severe injury.

---

[188] http://www.nhmrc.gov.au/_files_nhmrc/publications/attachments/cp112.pdf

[189] Ibid.

[190] http://www.massagetherapyreference.com/whiplash-massage/

[191] Prognosis of patients with whiplash-associated disorders consulting physiotherapy: development of a predictive model for recovery, T Bohman et al., http://www.biomedcentral.com/1471-2474/13/264

[192] http://www.nhmrc.gov.au/_files_nhmrc/publications/attachments/cp112.pdf

[193] http://www.nhs.uk/Conditions/Whiplash/Pages/Complications.aspx

Massage Treatments

The neck is a complex and multidirectional part of the body. It is made up of seven cervical vertebrae (C1–C7) connected with muscles and ligaments, intervertebral discs that act as shock absorbers, and within this a complex system of nerves. The complexity of the neck's anatomy makes it incredibly versatile in how it can move, but it also leaves it susceptible to whiplash injury.

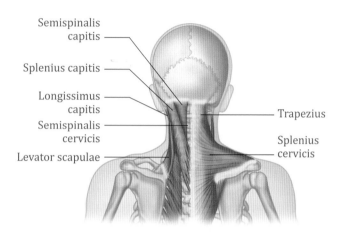

Semispinalis capitis
Splenius capitis
Longissimus capitis
Semispinalis cervicis
Levator scapulae
Trapezius
Splenius cervicis

There are a number of ways that massage can help with the recovery from whiplash, but it is important to work gently and progressively with clients and only at a depth that they can readily tolerate. Provided that a more serious injury has been ruled out medically, then treatment can begin as soon as the client can bear touch. You can use the diagram above to direct your work; where someone feels the pain and which muscles are affected most will depend on the nature and direction of the injury, so listen carefully to where your client is saying it hurts the most and use the diagram to ensure that you are working with the direction of the muscle, stroking up and down the muscle rather than across it.

In the initial stages the area of the neck, shoulders, and even arms may be tender and swollen. Gentle lymphatic drainage massage, along with ice treatment, can be helpful; full details for lymphatic drainage massage are given on page 68. Use long and gentle stroking movements to stimulate the muscles, and at this early stage focus just on the main belly of the muscle, avoiding the insertion points where the

muscle becomes tendon and meets the bone, as these areas may have small tears that need time to heal before they are treated. Use massage oil to lubricate the skin and ensure that the neck is fully supported at all times. When the client needs to move position allow time and let the client move his or her own head rather than you moving it. It is important to work very, very lightly in the early stages, using just finger-light touch so that you do not irritate inflamed muscles, and the client is likely to feel more comfortable and more confident if facing upward.

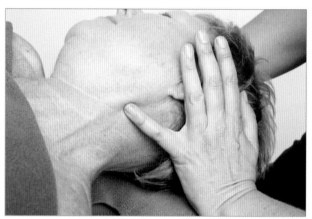

As the injury starts to heal and the client moves into the early subacute stage it is possible to work a little more deeply, particularly into the shoulders, but still always within easy tolerance for the client. Begin by gently massaging the head in small circular movements (see Chapter 4 for more details), then moving to warm up the muscles running from the back of the neck down across the top of the shoulders and from the top of the neck down to the middle of the neck.

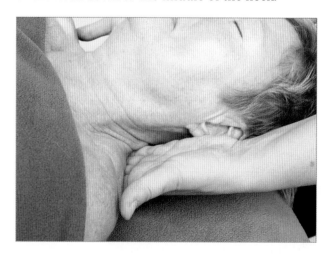

Use slow sweeping movements downward and begin by simply warming up the muscle and releasing any surface tension that may have become "stuck." As the client is likely to have been holding the head more stiffly than usual and restricting its movement, the connective tissue around the neck may have stiffened.

These next instructions are in common with the general neck and back massage but are adapted to be gentler for treating whiplash. Cradle the client's head in your hands so that your fingers are curving into the muscles just below the base of the skull. Do not stretch the neck, but ask your client to slowly tilt the head so that the chin moves toward the chest by no more than half an inch. Keep your fingers still; you will be very gently pressing onto the suboccipital muscles.

These muscles not only control some important aspects of eye movement but they also play an important role in the stabilization and fine movement control of the head—you can work these muscles with eye movement rather than needing to press into the muscles themselves.

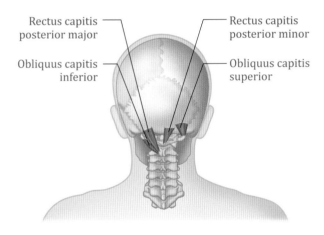

Rectus capitis posterior major
Rectus capitis posterior minor
Obliquus capitis inferior
Obliquus capitis superior

Ask the client to look directly at the ceiling above and to relax, and then ask them to look at their toes, without moving their head, and then to relax their gaze back to the ceiling. Then, again without moving their head, to look up to you, then back to the ceiling. Ask them to look to the left and back to the ceiling and then to the right and back to the ceiling, all only with eye movements and keeping the head still.

Securely and very gently lift the head by another half an inch—let your client know that you are going to do this before you move so he or she does not tighten up to protect against the unexpected movement. Keeping firm but gentle contact with the suboccipital muscles, repeat the looking down, up, left, and right movements, always returning to look at the ceiling between eye movements. This will help relax the suboccipital muscles.

Gently and securely replace the client's head on the massage table. The eye movements may cause some short-term eye strain and you can help to relieve this by gently cupping your hands over the client's eyes for 20–30 seconds, without making contact with the eyes. The eyes should return to normal within a few moments—reassure your client that this is nothing to be alarmed about.

Repeat the neck warm-up massage, stroking upward from the top of the shoulders to the base of the skull or hairline, without losing contact with the skin, then stroking back down from the base of the skull to the top of the shoulders and being very gentle as you get to the area you have just worked in more depth as this still may be a little tender to the touch.

Next, ask your client to carefully turn the head; it does not matter which direction this is in to start with as you will eventually work both sides. If your client is nervous about this neck movement, you can place a small folded towel just to the side they are turning into so the face can rest against this and he or she does not need to self-support the head with already-tender neck muscles. You will be able to feel a group of strong, ropey muscles that come down from behind the ear and go down toward the shoulder and collar bone. This is where we are now going to work, being careful not to slip forward to touch the throat.

Using a little massage oil so that you do not drag the skin, place the flat of your index finger so that you are gently pressing with the finger pad on the top of the sternocleidomastoid (SCM) muscle, and slowly follow the muscle down to where it inserts toward the center of the collar bone.

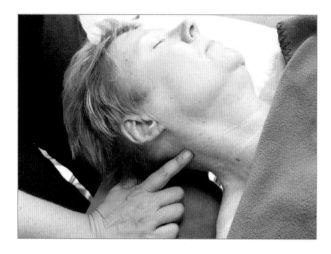

Now you are coming to work on the levator scapulae (below). The levator scapulae muscle has the nickname "shrug muscle" because when it contracts you lift your shoulders up and shrug. If you are very tense then your shoulders may feel like they are in a permanent upward shrug, and this shortens the levator scapulae. One of the things that someone with whiplash is likely to do is to pull the shoulders up and forward in a "protective hug," but longer term this does not help solve the problem. The levator scapulae originates on the first four cervical vertebrae and inserts into the shoulder blade.

Repeat this move slowly, three or four times. Always work downward from head to collar bone, never upward. If there are particular spots that are resistant to your touch and that the client reports are tender, simply hold your finger still on each point, maintaining (never deepening) your pressure, and you will feel the muscle relax under your touch.

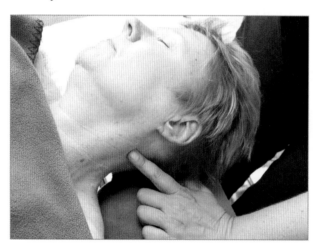

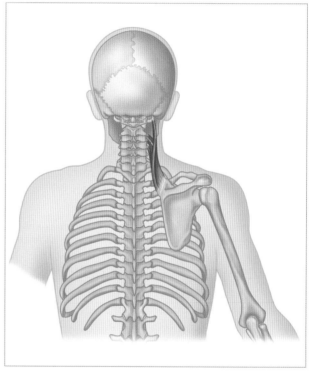

When the muscle gets shortened it pulls the four vertebrae down and to the side.

Ask your client to return the head to center and then to turn it to the other side, and repeat the work to the SCM on the other side. Having completed that, again repeat the warm-up massage sequence—although you are no longer warming up the muscles you are applying massage over a wider area, and this is good practice having worked specific muscles within that overall muscle group.

You can do this work with your client faceup, or if you have a massage table with a face hole and your client is comfortable lying facedown, then you may find it easier to work that way. Work all the way down the levator scapulae muscle using very small circles with two fingertips placed together.

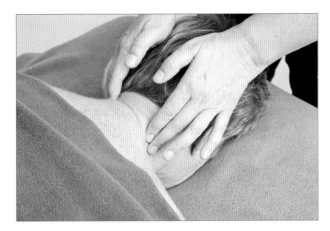

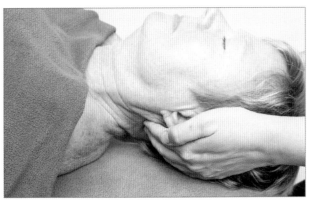

You now need to extend your working to the back of the neck and the trapezius muscle below, and those that underlie it. This is a large, powerful diamond-shaped muscle that links from the back of the neck, across the back of the shoulder to the tip of the shoulder, and down to the center of the back.

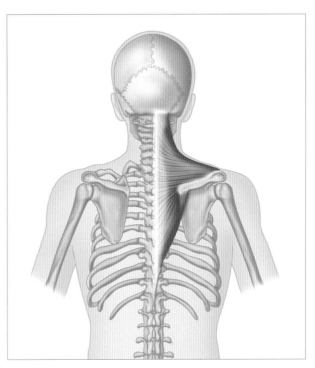

If your client is faceup, ask him or her to turn the head very slightly to reveal the muscle; once you have worked down the muscle three or four times you can then work a little more deeply but always within the client's easy tolerance. The area being massaged may feel tender but you should not be causing pain; if you feel your client tighten up against your touch, reduce your pressure. As you repeat the massage you will begin to feel the muscle soften to your touch. Remember that the muscles will be very tender because of the whiplash and you do not want to aggravate them with your massage—err on the side of gentleness.

If the client is experiencing back pain as a result of the whiplash you can now follow the instructions for the rest of the back massage in Chapter 5.

You main aim at this stage is to stretch out the muscle to encourage its full range of movement. You can do this by gently restricting the muscle at the top of the neck and stroking downward with the other thumb; be very careful with your pressure levels so that you are not aggravating the injury and setting back the healing process.

This stretch should give the recipient a sense of relief. Work across the whole trapezius with this stretch. If as you work you find particular areas of the muscle that are more tender or are resistant to touch, then apply static compression by pressing gently and holding this area. You may need to hold the pressure for 30–40 seconds before you feel the muscle start to relax; once you feel this relaxation you can move on. If the muscle doesn't relax, release the pressure and move very slightly up or down the muscle—you should find the point at which the muscle relaxation is triggered.

If after six weeks the whiplash is not resolving, then a more thorough and far-ranging treatment is called for. Tension in the upper body can be held by tightness in the hands; gripping a steering wheel, especially for people who could see the impact of a crash coming, can tighten the muscles all the way up the arm and into the shoulder. There is a detailed description of how to massage hands in Chapter 2. This will need much more time than previous treatments and you could easily spend one and a half to two hours working to release the whole area. Begin with the hands and work up the arms until you reach the shoulders. Then work on the head and move down to the neck, following the descriptions above and in Chapter 4 on head massage, and only then move on to the shoulder and rotator cuff treatments. After such a long and detailed treatment your client will need some recovery time, so you should allow 10–15 minutes for the client to "come round" from what should be a deeply relaxing, but in places challenging, treatment.

Whiplash can be a complex injury that needs time and care to heal. It is important to encourage your client to maintain as normal a life as possible. The pain of whiplash is normal but restricting movement will slow recovery and increase the chance of long-term complications. Massage, applied sensitively and progressively, should help recovery.

Winged Scapula

Background to the Condition

The scapula, or shoulder blade, is the largest bone of the shoulder and has 17 different muscles attached to it. These muscles both stabilize the arm and allow it to move. The muscles move together like a well-oiled machine but when things go wrong it can be difficult to address and can lead to the scapula "winging," so that the shoulder blade sticks out on the back, rather than lying flat against the back of the chest wall. This gives the scapula a wing-like appearance, hence its name.

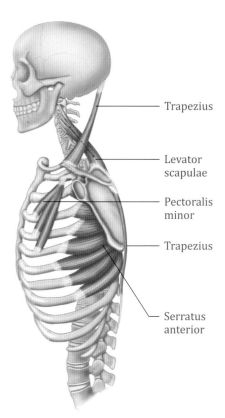

Trapezius

Levator scapulae

Pectoralis minor

Trapezius

Serratus anterior

Some mild cases may produce no symptoms—there will be no loss of power or control and no pain. More severe cases may be very painful and there can be significant loss of movement and control over the shoulder. The winging can be caused by poor control or imbalance in the muscles, or by injury or dysfunction of the muscles or the nerves that supply the muscles. It can also be symptomatic of muscle wasting, for example in people with muscular dystrophy. Poor posture can contribute to or trigger the problem, and overuse of specific muscles can be to blame, for example with weightlifters. It is a problem that affects a small, but wide-ranging, part of the population.

Ultimately it can lead to an inability to lift, pull, or push heavy objects or to perform daily activities such as brushing teeth, combing hair, or carrying things around. While some people will experience little or no pain, for others the pain will be excruciating.

There are a number of causes of the condition, so treatment will vary depending on the underlying cause. The most common cause is weakness in the serratus anterior muscle or damage to the long thoracic nerve that supplies the serratus anterior muscle. The serratus anterior is the muscle underneath the shoulder blade, lying over the top of and between the ribcage at the outside of the body and attaching to the ribs, from the second to the ninth.

While severe cases of winged scapula may need surgery, a lot of cases will respond well to strengthening exercises and to massage. If the problem arises suddenly after a trauma or injury then the individual needs to be seen by a medical practitioner prior to any massage treatment being administered.

Less common causes of a winged scapula include loss of trapezius muscle function, this is extremely rare and usually only occurs following radical surgery, for example in removal of a tumor. If this is the cause of a winged scapula then treatment should only be given by a professional trained therapist under the supervision of the patient's medical practitioner or surgeon.

When the underlying cause of the winged scapular is overall muscle degeneration with a condition such as muscular dystrophy, then there will be a weakness in all the scapula stabilizers. In this instance it is important to treat the arms, shoulders, and back on both sides and not just one. The muscles are likely to be tight and smaller owing to the muscle degeneration.

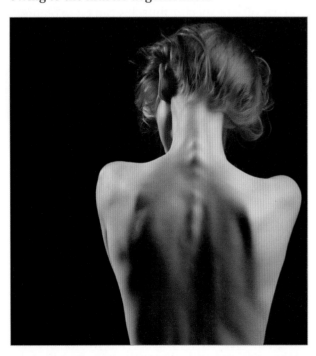

Be careful not to slip off the muscles onto bone as this would be painful, and you may need to alter the area of your own body used to massage to suit the needs of the recipient—so a thumb may be

needed in place of an elbow, depending on the size of individual's muscles. It is important to work all areas of the scapula so that tension in one area isn't released at the expense of another.

Another cause of a winged scapular is dislocation of the acromioclavicular joint or a fracture of the outer third of the clavicle. This would normally follow a specific trauma or injury; it isn't painful and mainly affects athletes or people whose work requires them to have their hands stretched above their head for a prolonged period of time. If you are treating an individual with this background it is important to liaise with his or her medical practitioner or physiotherapist before beginning treatment as this would normally involve severe ligament damage.

If there has been a repeated dislocation of the shoulder, for example with a football player, then the winged scapula is secondary to the shoulder dislocation and strengthening exercises under the supervision of a physiotherapist would normally be the treatment of choice; if this is not successful then surgery may be required. There are other, more rare, conditions that can result in a winged scapula, but all would follow trauma or injury so clients would be under the supervision of a medical practitioner.

Specific Contraindications

- If there has been a recent trauma to the area that has resulted in the winged scapula, this should be checked by a doctor prior to treatment. If the area is swollen or inflamed, wait until that has fully settled before treatment.

- If there is significant muscle degeneration around the shoulder due to a long-term condition, take extra care not to slip onto the bones when massaging.

- If there is a history of shoulder dislocation with a client, work with his or her physiotherapist.

Massage Treatments

Massage can assist in the recovery of a winged scapula, apart from the minor exceptions above. Massage should be carried out in conjunction with strengthening work, and your client's physiotherapist or doctor will be able to provide strengthening exercises aimed at his or her specific problem. This chapter deals with only the major muscular cause of a winged scapula; other causes may respond well to specialized treatment but would be best treated by a specialist practitioner.

The aim of the massage is to relax the musculature of the shoulder joint to allow the scapula to return to a normal position. As the muscles are able to relax, the scapula will retract against the back and normal function can return. As with any massage to the elbow or shoulder, it is important to release the tension from where it might be held—in this case that requires detailed work on the hands so begin your treatment by following the treatment for hand massage in Chapter 2. Having massaged the hands, work your way up the arms to the shoulder, using massage oil to lubricate the skin as you work. Start by warming up the muscles on the inner forearm and then use your thumb to knead the muscles working up from the hand to the elbow.

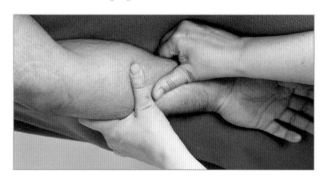

After you have worked the inner forearm you can gently massage the outer forearm; you will feel the radius and ulna bones and you are now slowly working up between these, warming up and softening the muscles running between and across the two bones.

Avoid massaging over or behind the elbow, and you may find that as you move to the upper arm

it becomes very tender to the touch. Follow the direction of the muscles, upward from just above the elbow to just below the shoulder, without working close to either joint and avoiding the armpit. You can work the upper arm by first warming up the muscles with long strokes, by slowly kneading the muscles with your hand, or by gently pressing into the muscle with your thumb, holding that pressure for a 30–60 seconds and then releasing, and repeating this until you have covered the entire upper arm.

The hand and arm work should be completed before treating the shoulders directly.

If the serratus anterior is tight then working on it may be very tender for your client, so be sure to work within his or her tolerance. Ask clients to lie on their side with the arm on the affected side raised above the head—support this with a pillow if necessary so that clients can maintain their position for a period of time.

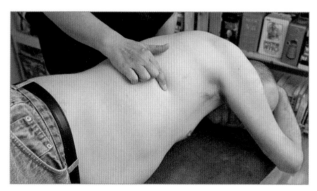

In women you will only be able to access the muscle as it emerges from underneath the breast tissue, so unless you are working on a very close friend or family member you may want to ask women to wear a soft nonwired bra to allow you to access this muscle without compromising on your draping. The rest of the body can be covered, and a towel or blanket can cover the breasts. With male clients you will be able to work a little further in; if you use the nipple as the guideline, you are starting the work about an inch to the outside of the nipple.

To begin with work *gently* to warm up this area. Starting from the ribs, as discussed above, work backward toward the scapula—as you move away from the breast area you can work backward and forward with the aim of warming up the muscle and releasing the surface fascia. Once you have done this, with your thumb, and using massage oil, work in quick movements against the run of the muscle, in this case up and down the body as the muscle is sitting front to back. Your movements should be fairly small and gentle, with your thumb moving just around an inch each time. You can also use both thumbs and work in a quick cross-friction movement.

Once you have warmed up the area for at least three or four minutes you can begin very specific treatment. Be careful to differentiate between muscle and rib, and slowly pull back toward the scapula. This may be tender but should not be excruciating for your client; work from bottom to top, starting at the ninth rib.

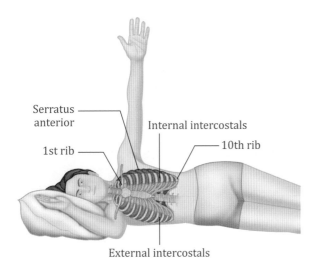

Serratus anterior

1st rib

Internal intercostals

10th rib

External intercostals

It is important that, to begin with, until you get to the seventh rib, you do not go too far forward into the rib cage. You will see on the diagram the area colored red for the muscle—you are not going in front of this into the front of the rib cage or you may cause further damage and pain. Work slowly and methodically up, rib by rib; if you look to where the line of the arm follows on into the trunk you will have the line to work to in terms of where to start the treatment.

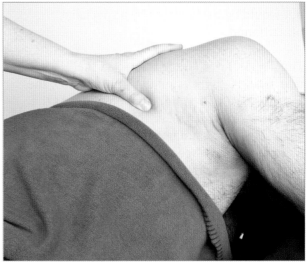

As you move upward toward the armpit, be careful to move toward the back so that you avoid the armpit as you do not want to be putting pressure on glands.

Treatment for a winged scapula is a long-term commitment—it can take several months of work to see any significant improvement, but it is worth persevering with massage twice a week and even more frequent exercises to build strength.

Wrist-Drop

Background to the Condition

A dropped wrist, wrist-drop, radial nerve palsy, and radial neuropathy all refer to the same thing, and are almost always caused by damage to the radial nerve that leaves the client unable to use the hand. A person with wrist-drop will not be able to extend the hand or to raise the hand using the wrist. The hand or wrist may be weak, and the fingers may also be affected.

The radial nerve runs down the underside of the arm and controls movement in the triceps (the muscle located at the back of the upper arm).

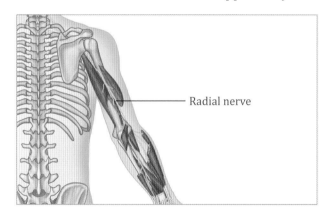

Radial nerve

The radial nerve is also responsible for extending the wrist and fingers, and controls sensation in a portion of the hand. It is one of three nerves that carry signals from the brain to the hand.[194]

An injury to this nerve can block normal nerve function. The person may experience widespread numbness and or tingling throughout the wrist, hand, and fingers. Other symptoms include wrist pain, tenderness, and swelling or pain in the forearm close to the elbow. Someone with a dropped wrist will find it almost impossible to turn the hand over and there will be a loss of strength and mobility in the affected hand, making it impossible to grasp or hold anything or to control the movement of the hand. The client will also be unable to raise the thumb as though they are asking for a lift.

The cause of wrist-drop is usually physical trauma, infection, or exposure to toxins. In the past, when lead was used in paint, it was a common symptom of lead poisoning. It can also be caused by drinking too much illicitly brewed strong alcohol where the chemicals are not controlled or monitored properly. It may also be caused by a specific trauma to the nerve such as a cut or puncture wound, a fracture of the upper arm, and even handcuffs.

Two common slang terms for wrist-drop are used: "Saturday night palsy" and "lover's palsy." Saturday night palsy is usually related to alcohol or recreational drug use, where the person falls asleep with the arm draped over the back of a chair while intoxicated, and sleeps in that

[194] http://www.healthline.com/health/radial-nerve-dysfunction#Overview

position all night. This results in damage to the radial nerve, which can then lead to radial neuropathy, or wrist-drop. The other cause, in lover's palsy, or "honeymoon palsy," is falling asleep with a partner asleep on your arm and not wanting to move.

These cases usually recover fully but can take anything from days to a year to resolve. In the meantime the hand is unable to be used or controlled. There is usually pain and swelling before the point of damage is reached but there have been cases of this being ignored, or even not noticed, depending on the level of intoxication involved. Carpal tunnel syndrome can produce some similar symptoms and even if a late binge-filled night is the suspected cause, the symptoms can be frightening and full medical checks should still be carried out to make sure that there is no other underlying cause.

Specific Contraindications

If any of the following symptoms occur alongside the wrist-drop then immediate emergency medical attention should be sought: increasing swelling or increasing pain in the arm; numbness or weakness of the face or leg or slurred speech; confusion; trouble speaking, walking, or seeing.

While the symptoms of wrist-drop can be very frightening, unless the nerve has been completely severed because of a significant trauma full recovery should be expected—it just takes time.

Massage Treatments

The radial nerve supplies the extensor muscles, which allow the wrist and fingers to extend, and the triceps, which allows the elbow to be extended. In some cases the injury will be such that both the wrist and the elbow will be affected.

Treatments are usually conservative; the wrist may be splinted for support and to prevent further injury from the hand "getting in the way," and physiotherapy will usually be recommended. Massage can be an integral part of this as it is vital to maintain muscle strength while the nerve repairs and to prevent muscle contracture, which could cause much longer-term problems. Surgery may an option where the injury has been caused by a fracture or where the nerve does not repair itself over time. Gentle stretches can be included in massage treatments unless they have been advised against by the client's doctor.

Massage work needs to focus on the whole arm, starting at the fingers. As the hand is not used the muscles can contract and pull the fingers inward toward the palm, and it is vital to work this area to prevent this. Focus your attention initially on the palm of the hand, turning the client's hand so that you are supporting it in your own hands, palm up. Begin by gently stretching the fingers backward, to within their normal limits, and supporting the last knuckle joint as the fingers join the hand.

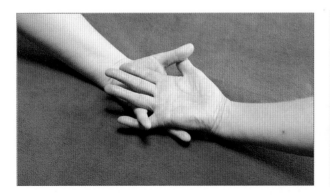
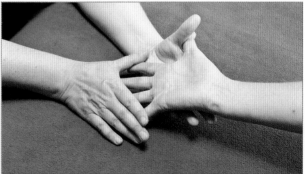

Next you need to work the soft tissue around each finger in detail. Use your own thumb to make small circles around each section of each finger, avoiding working directly over the knuckles. Do not worry what kind of tissue you are working on—everything interconnects so it does not matter too much at this stage if you are palpating fascia, tendon, ligament or, as you work down the finger into the palm, muscle. Make sure you cover every part of the fingers (with the exception of the knuckle joints), kneading the fingers with your own thumb. This will take time to do properly; expect to spend around 10 minutes just on this part of the massage.

Next bring your attention to the palm of the hand. You may notice that the fingers are drawn upward, not through any control of the muscles, but tension and contracture within the hand. Supporting the client's hand in your own hand and using your thumb to make deep strokes from the base of the fingers, across the palm, and to the wrist, and then back from the wrist to where the palm meets the fingers. Work your way across the whole palm in this movement and repeat so that you have worked the entire palm three or four times.

A gentle wrist stretch is helpful and doing this now and again after you have massaged the arm should show you how much more movement there is post massage. Supporting the client's arm, first gently and slowly flex the wrist upward toward the ceiling and then downward toward the floor; repeat this four or five times. Do not force the hand, as you risk further damage to the wrist; stretch only within the natural movement of the wrist.

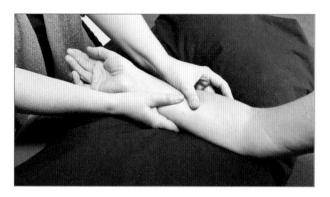

Having worked the hand fully, you can now move up to work the extensor muscles in the forearm. It is important to work the whole muscle group as all will be affected by an injury. Using a little massage oil, rest the client's arm on a folded-up towel on your own knees or on a desk top for support. Although the main muscles affected are in the back of the forearm, it is best to release the inner forearm first as this will usually allow tension in the back of the forearm to free more easily. Place your hands so that your thumbs are on the inner forearm and then use your thumbs to work upward toward the elbow.

Work in small sweeping motions starting with your thumbs at the wrist and working upward and outward until you are just below the elbow; do not massage into the elbow joint. Then turn the client's arm so that it is palm down and repeat the same motions as for the inner forearm, being careful not to press onto bones.

Finally, you can work the upper arm. For some people this will be incredibly tender so work gently here, repeating the movements that you have just completed for the forearm. When you are working on the inner arm, stop short of the armpit by a couple of inches. While you can complete the hand and forearm work with both you and your client seated, it may be easier to work the upper arm with your client seated and you kneeling or standing, but be careful not to put strain on your back while you work. Try to avoid having the client lying facedown on a massage couch as this can put pressure on the underside of the arm, which is the area already damaged.

You do not need to work the other arm when treating a case of wrist-drop but, of course, your client may appreciate it if you do. Aim to carry out this treatment as often as possible; daily will do no harm and twice weekly should be the minimum where possible but, as with most massage treatments, some treatment is better than none.

INDEX

Achilles tendon, 167, 168, 229
Acupressure, 145
Acupuncture, 145
Adhesive capsulitis. *See* Frozen shoulder
Amenorrhea, 131. *See also* Gynecological issues
Ankylosing spondylitis (AS), 42
    advantages of massage, 48
    background, 42
    contraindications, 43
    erector spinae muscles, 46
    foot massage, 43
    massage and tension, 43
    massage treatments, 43
    muscles surrounding spine, 45
    sacroiliitis, 46
    sacrum, 46
    stretching, 44
Anterior tibial tenosynovitis, 211–212, 213–215. *See also* Shin splint syndrome
Anxiety disorders, 49
    adrenalin, 49–50
    background, 49
    complaints associated with, 52
    contraindications, 53
    cortisol release, 50
    drugs, 52
    levels and subcategories, 49
    massage treatments, 53–55
    stomach-churning feeling, 52
AS. *See* Ankylosing spondylitis (AS)
Asthma, 56
    background, 56–57
    cause of, 56
    contraindications, 57
    massage treatments, 57–61
    symptoms of, 57
Atypical anorexia nervosa, 104. *See also* Eating disorders
Ayurveda, 9. *See* also Massage

Back massage, 31. *See also* Massage
    back of the shoulder blade, 37
    levator scapulae muscle, 34–35
    massage treatments, 32
    neck warm-up massage, 33–34
    sacrum, 38–39
    specific contraindications, 31
    suboccipitals, 33
    teres major and infraspinatus, 38

Baihui, 88
BCE (before the Common Era), 9
Brain, 110

Cancer, 62
    background, 62–64
    case study, 67
    chemotherapy, 66
    contraindications, 64–66
    lymphedema, 65
    massage treatments, 66–67
    metastasis, 64
    MLD massage, 68–74
    nadir period, 65
    specialist oncology massage training, 66
Cerebral palsy, 75
    background, 75–76
    classifications of, 75
    contraindication, 76
    massage treatments, 76–79
Cervical myelopathy, 81
Cervical spondylosis, 80
    background, 80–81
    contraindications, 81
    massage treatment, 82–84
    symptoms of, 80
CFS. *See* Chronic fatigue syndrome (CFS)
Chemotherapy, 66. *See also* Cancer
Chronic fatigue syndrome (CFS), 86
    background, 86–87
    contraindications, 87
    Du 20, 88
    massage treatments, 87–88
    PC 6, 88
    ST 36, 88
Chronic low back pain, 137. *See also* Lumbar spondylosis
Client, 9
Compartment syndrome, 210. *See also* Shin splint syndrome
Constipation, 89
    background, 89
    contraindications, 89
    massage treatments, 90–91
Contracture, 156
Cramp, 92
    background, 92
    contraindications, 92
    massage treatments, 92–96

Dead tissue, 178
Diaphragm, 158
DNA, 63
Dorsiflexion, 120
Down syndrome, 97
    background, 97–98
    contraindications, 98
    massage treatments, 99–100
    mosaicism, 97
    nondisjunction, 97
    physical characteristics of, 98
Drop foot. *See* Foot drop
Dropped foot. *See* Foot drop
Dual relationship, 107
Dupuytren's contracture, 101
    background, 101
    contraindications, 101
    massage treatments, 102–103
Dysmenorrhea, 131–132. *See* also Gynecological issues

EARLS. *See* European Alliance for Restless Legs Syndrome (EARLS)
Eating disorders, 104
    background, 104–105
    contraindications, 106
    dual relationship, 107
    massage treatments, 107
    types of, 104
Elimination points, 172
Encephalopathy, 86
Endometriosis, 133. *See also* Gynecological issues
Epinephrine, 49
Erector spinae muscles, 46
Essential oils, 147
European Alliance for Restless Legs Syndrome (EARLS), 184

Fascia, 118. *See also* Fibromyalgia
Fibromyalgia, 116
    background, 116–117
    contraindications, 117
    fascia, 118
    massage treatments, 118–119
    symptoms of, 116
Fingers, 15. *See also* Hand massage
Foot drop, 120
    background, 120
    contraindications, 120
    massage treatment, 120–123

Foot massage, 21, 43
    detailed, 21–26
    toes, 21–22
Frozen shoulder, 124
    background, 124–125
    contraindications, 125
    massage treatments, 125–129

Golfer's elbow, 231
Great eliminator, 18. *See also* Hand massage
Gynecological issues, 130
    amenorrhea, 131
    backgrounds, 130
    contraindications, 130
    dysmenorrhea, 131–132
    endometriosis, 133
    massage treatments, 130
    menorrhagia, 132–133
    polycystic ovary syndrome, 134
    unexplained infertility, 134

Hamstring muscles, 187
Hand massage, 14
    detailed, 14–20
    fingers, 15
    great eliminator, 18
    hands, 14
    soft tissue work, 15–16
Hands, 14
Head massage, 27, 112
    centerline, 28
    clients' vision, 27
    jaw, 30
    temple area, 28
Healing crisis, 88
Hippocampus, 111
Hippocrates, 10
Hypertrophy, 156

IBS. *See* Irritable bowel syndrome (IBS)
Irritable bowel syndrome (IBS), 135
    background, 135
    contraindications, 135–136
    massage treatments, 136

Lateral epicondylitis. See Tennis elbow
Levator scapulae muscle, 34–35, 246
Lumbar spondylosis, 137
    background, 137–139
    contraindications, 139

massage treatments, 139–143
sacrum, 142
spine, 137
Lumbar spondylosis, 80. *See also* Cervical
spondylosis
Lymph, 68
Lymphatic massage, 69
Lymphatic system, 68–69
Lymphatic vessels, 68
Lymphedema, 65, 69

Manual lymphatic drainage massage (MLD
massage), 68–74. *See* also Cancer
Massage, 8
    breathing, 12
    conditions benefitting from, 8
    contraindication to, 9, 11
    Eastern approaches, 9–10
    history, 9
    hygiene, 13
    oil, 10
    rest, 13
    tables,12
    water, 13
    Western traditions, 10
Mastoid process, 225
MD. *See* Muscular dystrophy (MD)
ME. *See* Myalgic encephalopathy (ME)
Medial epicondylitis. See Golfer's elbow
Menopause, 144
    background, 144–145
    contraindications, 145
    essential oils, 147
    massage treatments, 145–148
Menorrhagia, 132–133. *See also* Gynecological
issues
Metastasis, 64. *See also* Cancer
MLD massage. *See* Manual lymphatic drainage
massage (MLD massage)
Mosaicism, 97. *See also* Down syndrome
MS. *See* Multiple sclerosis (MS)
Multiple sclerosis (MS), 149
    background, 149–150
    contraindications, 150–151
    massage treatments, 151–153
    symptoms of, 149
    types, 150
Muscular dystrophy (MD), 154
    background, 154–155
    contraindications, 155–156

massage treatments, 156–158
    varieties of, 155
Myalgia, 86
Myalgic encephalomyelitis. *See* Myalgic
encephalopathy (ME)
Myalgic encephalopathy (ME), 86. *See also*
Chronic fatigue syndrome (CFS)
Myofascial system, 118. *See also* Fibromyalgia

Nadir period, 65
Night eating syndrome, 104. *See also* Eating
disorders
Nondisjunction, 97

Obliquus capitis inferior (OCI), 32
Obliquus capitis superior (OCS), 32
OCI. *See* Obliquus capitis inferior (OCI)
OCS. *See* Obliquus capitis superior (OCS)

Parkinson's disease, 159
    background, 159
    contraindications, 159–160
    massage treatments, 160–162
PCOS. *See* Polycystic ovary syndrome (PCOS)
Peripheral neuropathy, 163
    background, 163
    contraindications, 163–164
    massage treatments, 164–165
Peristalsis, 90
PF. *See* Plantar fasciitis (PF)
Plantar fasciitis (PF), 166
    background, 166
    causes, 166
    contraindications, 167
    massage treatments, 167–170
Polycystic ovary syndrome (PCOS), 134. *See also*
Gynecological issues
Posterior tibial muscle, 212. *See also* Shin splint
syndrome
Posterior tibial tendonitis, 215–217. *See also* Shin
splint syndrome
Posterior tibial tendonitis of ankle, 212. *See also*
Shin splint syndrome
Post-traumatic stress disorder (PTSD), 108, 109
    background, 108–111
    brain, 110
    contraindications, 111
    head massage, 112
    massage treatments, 112–115
    types of symptoms, 110

western vs. traditional massage, 108–109
PPMS. See Primary progressive MS (PPMS)
Pregnancy, 171
    background, 171
    contraindications, 172–174
    elimination points, 172–173
    massage treatments, 174–176
Primary progressive MS (PPMS), 150
Psoriasis, 42
PTSD. See Post-traumatic stress disorder (PTSD)
Purging disorder, 104. See also Eating disorders

Qi, 145
QTF. See Quebec Task Force (QTF)
Quebec Task Force (QTF), 242

Raynaud's syndrome, 177
    background, 177–178
    contraindications, 178
    forms of, 177
    massage treatments, 178–179
RCP. See Royal College of Psychiatrists (RCP)
RCPM. See Rectus capitis posterior minor (RCPM)
RCPMaj. See Rectus capitis posterior major
(RCPMaj)
Rectus capitis posterior major (RCPMaj), 32
Rectus capitis posterior minor (RCPM), 32
Relapsing remitting MS (RRMS), 150
Repetitive strain injuries (RSI), 180
    background, 180–181
    cause of, 181
    contraindications, 182
    groups, 181
    massage treatments, 182–183
Restless legs syndrome (RLS), 184
    background, 184–185
    contraindications, 185
    forms of, 184
    massage treatments, 185–190
RLS. See Restless legs syndrome (RLS)
Rotator cuff, 191
    impingement syndrome, 192
Rotator cuff injury, 191
    background, 191–193
    contraindications, 193
    massage treatments, 193–194
    subacromial space, 192
Royal College of Psychiatrists (RCP), 109
RRMS. See Relapsing remitting MS (RRMS)
RSI. See Repetitive strain injuries (RSI)

Sacroiliac joints (SI joints), 46
Sacroiliitis, 46. See also Ankylosing
spondylitis (AS)
Sacrum, 38–39, 46, 142
Sangha, 10
Scar tissue, 195
    background, 195–196
    contraindications, 196
    deep transverse friction massage, 197
    massage treatments, 196–197
    stretching, 197
Sciatica, 198
    background, 198–199
    causes of, 198
    contraindications, 199
    massage for appendicular sciatica, 201–202
    massage for axial sciatica, 202
    massage treatments, 199–202
Scleroderma, 177
SCM. See Sternocleidomastoid (SCM)
Scoliosis, 203
    aims of massage for, 205
    background, 203–204
    contraindications, 204
    massage treatments, 204–209
    Secondary progressive MS (SPMS), 150
Shiatsu, 9
Shin splint syndrome, 210
    anterior tibial tenosynovitis, 211–212, 213–215
    background, 210
    compartment syndrome, 210
    contraindications, 212
    massage treatments, 213–217
    posterior tibial tendonitis, 212, 215–217
    stress fractures of tibia and/or fibula, 211
Shivago, 10
Shoulder, 124. See also Frozen shoulder
Shrug muscle. See Levator scapulae muscle
SI joints. See Sacroiliac joints (SI joints)
Sinusitis, 218
    background, 218–219
    chronic, 218
    contraindications, 219
    massage treatments, 219–221
Sjögren's syndrome, 178
Soleus muscles, 95
Specialist oncology massage training, 66. See also
Cancer
Spine, 137. See also Lumbar spondylosis
Spleen, 69

Splenius capitis muscles, 84
SPMS. *See* Secondary progressive MS (SPMS)
Spondylosis, 80. *See also* Cervical spondylosis; Lumbar spondylosis
Sternocleidomastoid (SCM), 34, 71, 221
Stress fractures, 211. *See also* Shin splint syndrome
Subacromial space, 192
Suboccipitals, 33, 236
Suicide disease. *See* Trigeminal Neuralgia (TN)
Supraspinatus tendonitis, 228. *See also* Tendonitis
Swimmer's shoulders. *See* Supraspinatus tendonitis
Synergy, 148

TCM. *See* Traditional Chinese Medicine (TCM)
Temporomandibular joint disorders (TJDs), 222
    contraindications, 223
    massage treatments, 223–226
    types of, 222
Temporomandibular joints (TMJs), 222. *See also* Temporomandibular joint disorders (TJDs)
Tendinopathy, 227. *See also* Tendonitis
Tendinosis, 227. *See also* Tendonitis
Tendonitis, 227
    background, 227
    contraindications, 227
    heel, 229–230
    knee, 229
    massage treatments, 228
    shoulder, 228
    wrist, 228
Tendons, 227. *See also* Tendonitis
Tennis elbow, 231
    background, 231–232
    contraindication, 232
    massage treatments, 232–233
Tenosynovitis, 227. *See also* Tendonitis
Tension headaches, 234
    background, 234–235
    contraindications, 235
    massage treatments, 235–237
    suboccipitals, 236
Thai yoga therapy, 10. *See also* Massage
Thoracic spondylosis, 80
    background, 81
    contraindications, 81
    massage treatment, 85
Tibialis anterior, 121

muscle, 211. *See also* Shin splint syndrome
TJDs. *See* Temporomandibular joint disorders (TJDs)
TMJs. *See* Temporomandibular joints (TMJs)
TN. *See* Trigeminal neuralgia (TN)
Traditional Chinese Medicine (TCM), 9
Traumatic event, 109. *See also* Post-traumatic stress disorder (PTSD)
Trigeminal nerve, 238
Trigeminal neuralgia (TN), 238
    background, 238–239
    categories, 239
    contraindications, 239
    massage treatments, 239–241
Ulna bones, 20

WAD. *See* Whiplash associated disorders (WAD)
Whiplash, 242
    background, 242–243
    contraindications, 243
    massage treatments, 244–248
    stages, 243
Whiplash associated disorders (WAD), 242
WHO. *See* World Health Organization (WHO)
Willis–Ekbom disease. *See* Restless legs syndrome (RLS)
Winged scapula, 249
    background, 249–250
    causes of, 250
    contraindications, 250
    massage treatments, 251–252
World Health Organization (WHO), 56
Wrist-drop, 253
    background, 253–254
    contraindications, 254
    massage treatments, 254–255

Yang, 145
Yin, 145